GESTATIONAL DIABETES

Origins, Complications, and Treatment

Edited by
CLIVE J. PETRY

GESTATIONAL DIABETES
Origins, Complications, and Treatment

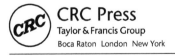

CRC Press is an imprint of the
Taylor & Francis Group, an **informa** business

CRC Press
Taylor & Francis Group
6000 Broken Sound Parkway NW, Suite 300
Boca Raton, FL 33487-2742

First issued in paperback 2019

ISBN-13: 978-1-4398-7996-2 (hbk)
ISBN-13: 978-0-367-37890-5 (pbk)

Library of Congress Cataloging-in-Publication Data

Gestational diabetes (Petry)
   Gestational diabetes : origins, complications, and treatment / editor, Clive J. Petry.
   p. ; cm.
   Includes bibliographical references and index.
   ISBN 978-1-4398-7996-2 (hardcover)
   I. Petry, Clive J., editor of compilation. II. Title.
   [DNLM: 1. Diabetes, Gestational. 2. Evidence-Based Medicine. WQ 248]

   RG580.D5
   618.3'646--dc23   2013047331

Visit the Taylor & Francis Web site at
http://www.taylorandfrancis.com

and the CRC Press Web site at
http://www.crcpress.com

Contents

SECTION I   Gestational Diabetes

SECTION II   Origins

SECTION III   Complications

SECTION IV   Treatments

SECTION V   *Future Prospects*

Preface

Gestational diabetes, defined as diabetes that first develops in a pregnant woman, is coming of age. Although this has been recognised as a distinct form of diabetes since the 1960s, recent large studies such as the Hyperglycemia and Adverse Pregnancy Outcome Study and the Australian Carbohydrate Intolerance Study in Pregnant Women are only now helping to precisely define the risks associated with having raised glucose concentrations in pregnancy, as well as the benefits that may be gained by reducing such glucose intolerance. As such, they may end up making the contribution to gestational diabetes that the Diabetes Control and Complications Trial and the UK Prospective Diabetes Study have made to type 1 and 2 diabetes, respectively. The need for this is great given that the worldwide incidence of gestational diabetes is increasing rapidly in line with the increased prevalence of obesity, and the risks associated with a gestational diabetes pregnancy stretch beyond those to the mother (such as a massively increased risk of developing type 2 diabetes) and the newborn (e.g., macrosomia) to long-term, transgenerational risks in the offspring (such as for obesity and type 2 diabetes, and in females for gestational diabetes). The complications of these transmitted conditions could lead to potentially catastrophic effects, such as the offspring's generation being the first in modern times to die at younger ages than their parents (Zimmet et al., 2007).[*]

This book therefore sets out to provide timely reviews relating to what may be considered some of the most important aspects of gestational diabetes, in particular its causes, consequences, and ways of treating it. The book is split into five main sections to encompass this. The initial section is based around metabolism in pregnancy and gestational diabetes. The first chapter, by Dr. Chen and Professor Scholl, deals with the important area of maternal and foetal glucose metabolism in pregnancy, particularly in relation to insulin resistance. The second chapter, by Dr. Lindsay, deals with the controversial topic of what actually constitutes gestational diabetes, an area that is currently receiving much attention in the literature.

Section II contains chapters about risk factors and causes of gestational diabetes. The most obvious risk factors for gestational diabetes, almost by definition but often overlooked, are the subject being female and pregnant! However, whilst these factors are sensitive for the development of gestational diabetes, they carry no specificity, as only a fraction of pregnant women develop gestational diabetes. Environmental risk factors with greater specificity for gestational diabetes are outlined in Chapter 3 by Dr. Hadar and Professor Hod. In Chapter 4 I then outline the rapidly expanding field of genetic risk factors for gestational diabetes and how these are closely linked to genetic risk factors for other forms of diabetes.

Having outlined the causes of gestational diabetes, the succeeding section then deals with the consequences of having this condition, namely, the potential

---

[*] Zimmet, P. et al. 2007. The International Diabetes Federation Consensus Definition of the Metabolic Syndrome in Children and Adolescents. Brussels, Belgium: IDF Communications. Available at http://www.idf.org/webdata/docs/Mets_definition_children.pdf.

complications for both the mother and her offspring. In Chapter 5 Dr. Salzer and Professor Yogev outline the potential short- and long-term effects of gestational diabetes for both the mother and her offspring, a vital consideration given the rising prevalence of this condition and the potential risk of transmitting this condition and type 2 diabetes on to the next generation.

The largest section in the book then deals with treating gestational diabetes in an effort to improve the outcome for both the mother and baby. In Chapter 6 Dr. Walsh and Professor McAuliffe deal with the nutritional approach to treating gestational diabetes, which has been described as the cornerstone of its treatment. Then in Chapter 7 Dr. Boulvain examines the evidence for the role of exercise in treating this condition, including what benefits it brings and its potential risks. In Chapter 8 Professor Simmons presents a highly useful strategy for treating gestational diabetes pharmacologically, including recent advances in the use of insulin analogues and the use of alternatives to insulin.

The final section contains a chapter in which I speculate on the future prospects for the condition of gestational diabetes, including areas not covered by other chapters in the book, such as how the need for screening correlates with maternal obesity. Clearly in a volume of this size it is impossible to write about every clinical and scientific aspect of gestational diabetes, but in this chapter I briefly try to fill in some of the gaps and suggest likely areas of progress in the forthcoming years.

Each chapter of this book is therefore designed to provide a summary of the current state of practice and knowledge in its particular subject area, with an emphasis on highlighting key recent research. Key points are condensed into a single summary diagram for each chapter to provide an *aide mémoire* for those trying to hold many aspects of gestational diabetes in their mind at one time. Hopefully these may also prove useful for those wanting to revise current knowledge about gestational diabetes in preparation for exams. In addition, for those wanting greater detail than can be provided in a book of this size, recent key references are bold (with an explanation as to why) to help direct areas of further research. We hope that you will find it useful.

Clive J. Petry, PhD
Department of Paediatrics, University of Cambridge,
Addenbrooke's Hospital, Cambridge, UK

About the Editor

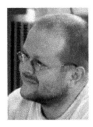 **Clive J. Petry, PhD,** earned a BSc in biochemistry (medical) from the University of Surrey, Guildford, UK, in 1991 and then an MSc in clinical biochemistry in 1993 from the same institution. In 1998, he earned a PhD in clinical biochemistry from the University of Cambridge, Cambridge, UK. Since then, he has worked at the University of Cambridge as a postdoctoral research associate, first in the Department of Clinical Biochemistry (from 1997 to 2000) and then in the Department of Paediatrics (from 2001). In 2006, he was promoted to senior research associate. Dr. Petry has authored over 50 scientific publications and currently serves on the editorial board of the *British Journal of Nutrition, Journal of Nutritional Science, Human Reproduction,* and *ISRN Obstetrics and Gynecology.* He is a member of the Association for Clinical Biochemistry, the Biochemical Society, the Nutrition Society, and the European Association for the Study of Diabetes. His research involves trying to understand the mechanisms and consequences of the link between altered foetal growth and the short- and long-term risk of the development of diseases such as gestational and type 2 diabetes and hypertension.

Contributors

Michel Boulvain
Department of Gynecology and
  Obstetrics
Geneva University Hospitals
Faculty of Medicine
University of Geneva
Geneva, Switzerland

Xinhua Chen
Department of Obstetrics and
  Gynecology
School of Osteopathic Medicine
Rowan University
Stratford, New Jersey

Eran Hadar
Helen Schneider Hospital for Women
Rabin Medical Center
Petah Tikva, Israel
and
The Sackler Faculty of Medicine
Tel Aviv University
Tel Aviv, Israel

Moshe Hod
Helen Schneider Hospital for Women
Rabin Medical Center
Petah Tikva, Israel
and
The Sackler Faculty of Medicine
Tel Aviv University
Tel Aviv, Israel

Robert Lindsay
BHF Glasgow Cardiovascular Research
  Centre
University of Glasgow
Glasgow, United Kingdom

Fionnuala M. McAuliffe
Department of Maternal–Fetal
  Medicine
National Maternity Hospital
Dublin, Ireland
and
UCD Obstetrics and Gynaecology
University College Dublin
National Maternity Hospital
Dublin, Ireland

Clive J. Petry
Department of Paediatrics
University of Cambridge
Addenbrooke's Hospital
Cambridge, United Kingdom

Liat Salzer
Helen Schneider Hospital for Women
Rabin Medical Center
Petah Tikva, Israel
and
The Sackler Faculty of Medicine
Tel Aviv University
Tel Aviv, Israel

Theresa O. Scholl
Department of Obstetrics and
  Gynecology
School of Osteopathic Medicine
Rowan University
Stratford, New Jersey

David Simmons
Wolfson Diabetes and Endocrinology
    Clinic
Institute of Metabolic Science
Cambridge University Hospitals NHS
    Foundation Trust
Addenbrooke's Hospital
Cambridge, United Kingdom

and

Department of Rural Health
University of Melbourne, Shepparton
Victoria, Australia

Colin A. Walsh
Department of Maternal–Fetal
    Medicine
Royal North Shore Hospital
Sydney, Australia

Yariv Yogev
Helen Schneider Hospital for Women
Rabin Medical Center
Petah Tikva, Israel

and

The Sackler Faculty of Medicine
Tel Aviv University
Tel Aviv, Israel

Section I

Gestational Diabetes

1 Glucose, Foetal Growth, and Pregnancy

Xinhua Chen and Theresa O. Scholl
School of Osteopathic Medicine, Rowan
University, Stratford, New Jersey

CONTENTS

1.1   INTRODUCTION

Normal pregnancy is marked by significant changes in maternal insulin resistance and hyperinsulinaemia from progressively increasing insulin secretion during gestation. The regulation of glucose metabolism during pregnancy is complex. After a successful implantation of a genetically normal foetus, the placenta plays a critical role in the delivery of nutrients and in the tissue-specific regulation of normal foetal growth. In addition to its metabolic and endocrine function, the placenta secretes cytokines that significantly impact foetal growth. Pregnancies complicated by gestational diabetes mellitus (GDM) have an increased risk of foetal overgrowth (macrosomia or large for gestational age birth), higher perinatal morbidity and mortality, and presage a long-term risk of developing type 2 diabetes for the mother.

This chapter outlines the current knowledge in maternal and foetal glucose metabolism, and the pathophysiologic and molecular mechanisms of insulin resistance in both normal pregnancy and pregnancies complicated by GDM. We first focus on foetal growth and placental function and the role of growth factors, including hormones, cytokines, and adipocytokines. Next, we discuss other factors, including maternal obesity and pregnancy weight gain and the epigenetic modification of the foetal phenotype. Finally, we review the significance of gestational hyperglycaemia, including hyperglycaemia less severe than GDM, from the Hyperglycemia and Adverse Pregnancy Outcome (HAPO) study and elsewhere.

1.2   MATERNAL GLUCOSE METABOLISM IN NORMAL PREGNANCY AND GESTATIONAL DIABETES MELLITUS

1.2.1   INSULIN RESISTANCE AND ITS PHYSIOLOGICAL ROLE DURING PREGNANCY

Pregnancy is characterised by increased insulin resistance (i.e., decreased insulin sensitivity) defined as the diminished biological response of a nutrient (glucose, free fatty acid) to a given concentration of insulin at the target tissue, e.g., liver, skeletal muscle, or adipose tissue.[1,2] During early gestation (<20 weeks) insulin sensitivity is either normal or slightly increased, and progressively decreases during mid to late pregnancy, with compensatory increases in insulin secretion.[3,4] Resistance to the action of insulin on glucose is supported by data from the euglycaemic-hyperinsulinaemic clamp, which show that insulin-stimulated glucose disposal declined by 40–50% in nondiabetic pregnant women (lean and obese) at the end of the third trimester compared to earlier in gestation.[3] In addition, resistance to the action of insulin on lipolysis (in response to the hyperinsulinaemic clamp, the rate of lipolysis declined by 51% and 30% in the second and third trimesters, respectively) and fat oxidation (decreases of 51% and 38% in the second and third trimesters, respectively) developed during late gestation in nondiabetic overweight/obese women.[4–6]

Increased maternal insulin resistance is physiologically important during pregnancy. Late gestation is characterised by foetal growth and a maternal response to the increasing foetal need for nutrients. Carbohydrate is of particular importance, since it is the major fuel for the foetal and maternal central nervous system.[7–9] Maternal resistance to the action of insulin on glucose uptake and oxidation preserves glucose by reducing its use in insulin-sensitive tissues (muscles and adipose), while resistance to the action of insulin on lipolysis and fat oxidation preserves fatty acids as an alternate fuel for foetal oxidation.[4–6]

1.2.2   GLUCOSE METABOLISM IN WOMEN WITH GDM

Between 1989 and 2004 the prevalence of GDM in the United States increased from 1.9% to 4.2% in parallel with the well-documented obesity epidemic.[10,11] Metabolic features of GDM (hyperglycaemia, insulin resistance, and hyperlipidaemia) are components of type 2 diabetes mellitus (T2DM) and the metabolic syndrome.[12,13] Women with GDM have both increased peripheral insulin resistance (mainly in skeletal muscle) and impaired insulin secretion.[14,15] Insulin sensitivity is reduced 30–40% in women with GDM compared to controls, and insulin secretion is significantly impaired in response to hyperglycaemia.[15] This suggests a major β-cell defect that makes compensation for increased insulin resistance difficult to achieve and implies multiple defects in insulin action along with impaired compensatory insulin secretion in the aetiology of GDM.[6,14,15]

1.2.3   MECHANISMS FOR INSULIN RESISTANCE IN NORMAL PREGNANCY AND GDM

Insulin resistance during pregnancy is multifactorial. In this section we review recent data on the placental hormones, cytokines, adipocytokines, increased lipids, and oxidative stress in relation to pregnancy-induced insulin resistance and GDM.

1.2.3.1   Placental Hormones

The placental hormones reprogramme maternal physiology to achieve an insulin-resistant state.[16] Placental lactogen (hPL) is significantly increased during pregnancy and induces insulin secretion.[17] Experimental studies outside of human pregnancy suggested that hPL also increases peripheral insulin resistance[18] and may be a potent insulin antagonist. Placental growth hormone (hPGH), structurally similar to pituitary growth hormone, causes severe peripheral insulin resistance by the third trimester.[19] Hormones important for placental and foetal development and growth are discussed in Section 1.4.

1.2.3.2   Cytokines/Adipocytokines

Normal pregnancy is now considered to be a state of mild systemic inflammation.[20] Circulating maternal levels of pro-inflammatory and anti-inflammatory cytokines, including tumour necrosis factor-alpha (TNF-α), interleukin-6 (IL-6), and C-reactive protein (CRP), are raised compared to the nonpregnant state similar to sepsis.[20,21] Pregnancies complicated by obesity and GDM stimulate the dysregulation of metabolic vascular and inflammatory pathways by increasing circulating concentrations of inflammatory molecules.[21,22] It has also been observed that the increased cytokine levels parallel increasing insulin resistance.[20]

Several cytokines synthesised within the placenta itself are preferentially released into the maternal rather than the foetal circulation.[22,23] Most maternal cytokines are not readily transferred across the placenta in humans.[21] Like the placenta, maternal adipose tissue, a key player on the endocrine-inflammatory axis, secretes common molecules (adipocytokines like TNF-α, IL-6, CRP, and leptin).[22] Adiponectin is an adipocytokine that is specially secreted by adipocytes. Whether expression of adiponectin and its receptors is present in placental tissue remains controversial.[22,24] In vitro experiments demonstrated high levels of expression for inflammation-related genes in both white adipose tissue and term placenta. They suggested that the placenta promotes a molecular interplay between maternal immune function and metabolism, which subsequently influences foetal growth (Table 1.1).[22]

1.2.3.3   Cytokines and Gestational Hyperglycaemia

TNF-α induces inflammation by inhibiting production of adiponectin. TNF-α-induced insulin resistance is mediated by placental hormones; thus, TNF-α may be the preferable predictor of insulin resistance in pregnancy.[21,25] TNF-α and IL-6 are key regulators of acute phase protein CRP. Insulin inhibits IL-6-mediated CRP stimulation.[26-28] Elevated CRP levels predict insulin resistance and other features of the metabolic syndrome.[26-28] An elevated CRP level is consistently associated with an increased risk of GDM.[29,30] The relationship is often but not always found to be dependent on maternal adiposity.[31]

1.2.3.4   Cytokines and Hyperglycaemia in Camden

We examined the relation of two adipocytokines (CRP and adiponectin) to GDM and mild maternal hyperglycaemia in women from Camden, New Jersey. The Camden Study is a prospective cohort study of pregnancy outcome and complications in young, generally healthy women residing in one of the poorest cities in the continental United States.[32] Women with a serious nonobstetric problem (e.g., lupus, type 1 or 2 diabetes, seizure disorders, malignancies, acute or chronic liver disease, drug or alcohol abuse, and psychiatric problems) were excluded from participation. Gestational hyperglycaemia was classified as either GDM or as a glucose impairment that did not meet the diagnostic criteria for GDM (>140 mg/dl [7.8 mmol/L],

TABLE 1.1

Expression of Inflammation-Related Genes in White Adipose Tissue and Term Placenta and Their Regulation in Obesity and Gestational Diabetes

	Adipocyte	SVF	Placenta	Obesity	GDM
TNF-α	+	+++	+	+	+
IL-6	+	+	+	+	+
IL-1b		++		+	+
IL-8	+	++	+	+	+
IL-1Ra	+	++	+		
IL-10	+	++	+	+	+
Leptin	++	0	+	+	+
Adiponectin	++	0	–	0	
Resistin	0	++	+	+	+
MCP-1	+	++	+	+	+
MIF	++	+	+	+	–
VEGF	+	++	+	+	
PAI-1	+	++	+	+	+
Cathepsin S	+	++	+	+	+

Source: Adapted from Hauguel-de Mouzon, S., and Guerre-Millo, M., *Placenta,* 27, 794–98, 2006. With permission from Elsevier.

Note: SVF, stroma vascular fraction of white adipose tissue; GDM, gestational diabetes mellitus; MCP-1, monocyte chemoattractant protein 1; MIF, migration inhibiting factor; PAI-1, plasminogen activator inhibitor-1; VEGF, vascular endothelial growth factor; IL-1b, interleukin 1 beta; IL-1Ra: interleukin 1 receptor beta.

1 h after a 50 g oral glucose load). Both of these groups were compared to normal controls (as described previously).[33]

Elevated serum CRP was associated with a twofold increased risk for GDM during early as well as late gestation compared to controls ($p < 0.05$; Table 1.2),[34] but did not differ significantly between women with an impaired glucose challenge test non-GDM and normal controls ($p > 0.05$; Table 1.2). The association of high CRP with risk of GDM was attenuated and became nonsignificant after additional adjustment for pregravid body mass indices (BMIs). Thus, our data suggest that elevated maternal CRP levels during pregnancy reflect chronic inflammation that depends upon maternal pregravid BMI.

Adiponectin is a novel protein highly specific to adipose tissue and acts in an opposite manner to other cytokines.[35,36] Adiponectin exhibits potent anti-inflammatory and atheroprotective responses in vascular tissue and is a regulator of insulin sensitivity and glucose homeostasis.[35-37] It is also found in cord blood, but its role in the foetal growth is not confirmed. Low concentrations of circulating adiponectin in

TABLE 1.2
Association of Elevated Serum CRP with GDM and Impaired GCT but Non-GDM

	GDM	Impaired GCT but Non-GDM	Controls
Entry			
CRP (≥8.2 mg/L)[a] N (%)	41 (51.3)	47 (36.7)	166 (29.9)
Model 1 AOR (95% CI)[c]	1.98 (1.19, 3.20)	1.19 (0.78, 1.81)	1.00
Model 2 AOR (95% CI)[d]	1.26 (0.73, 2.19)	1.09 (0.70, 1.71)	1.00
Third Trimester			
CRP (≥8.4 mg/L)[b] N (%)	36 (45.0)	44 (34.4)	166 (29.8)
Model 1 AOR (95% CI)[c]	1.67 (1.02, 2.76)	0.93 (0.61, 1.41)	1.00
Model 2 AOR (95% CI)[d]	1.15 (0.67, 1.97)	0.90 (0.58, 1.41)	1.00

Source: Adapted from Scholl, T.O., and Chen, X., Increased Inflammatory Response in Women with Gestational Hyperglycemia, paper presented at the 69th American Diabetes Association Scientific Sessions, New Orleans, LA, 2009.

Note: AOR, adjusted odds ratio; CI, confidence interval; GDM, gestational diabetes mellitus; impaired GCT non-GDM, glucose > 140 mg/dl during a glucose challenge test (GCT) at 28 week's gestation and a normal diagnostic oral glucose tolerance test; normal controls, glucose ≤ 140 mg/dl during a glucose challenge test (same in Tables 1.3–1.5).

[a] The highest tertile of serum CRP concentration at entry.
[b] The highest tertile of serum CRP concentration at the third trimester.
[c] Model 1, models were adjusted for age, parity, ethnicity, and cigarette smoking.
[d] Model 2, additional adjustment for prepregnant BMI.

mid to late pregnancy are consistently associated with an increased risk of GDM.[38,39] Whether the association of hypoadiponectinaemia with risk of GDM is independent of maternal adiposity is uncertain.[38–40]

In a nested case-control study using data from Camden, we demonstrated that hypoadiponectinaemia (the lowest tertile) during early and late pregnancy was strongly associated with risk of gestational hyperglycaemia, including GDM (2.5-fold increased risk) and less severe hyperglycaemia non-GDM (1.5-fold increased risk). This association did not differ significantly between lean and obese women (Table 1.3).[41] Thus, our data suggest that, unlike CRP, the association of hypoadiponectinaemia and gestational hyperglycaemia is independent of prepregnant BMI.

1.2.3.5 Cellular Mechanisms of Insulin Resistance

Insulin resistance in GDM is best characterised as a post-receptor defect resulting in the decreased ability of insulin to bring about glucose transporter-4 (GLUT-4) mobilisation from the interior of the cell to the cell surface.[13,16] The cellular mechanisms

TABLE 1.3

Association of Hypoadiponectinaemia with GDM and Impaired GCT but Non-GDM

	GDM	Impaired GCT but Non-GDM	Controls
Entry Adiponectin Tertile (μg/ml)[a]			
Lowest (<10.7), N (%)	40 (50.0)	49 (38.3)	165 (29.6)
Middle (10.7–16.3), N (%)	23 (28.8)	41 (32.0)	192 (34.5)
Highest (>16.3), N (%)	17 (21.3)	38 (29.7)	200 (35.9)
Model 1 AOR (95% CI)[b]	2.68 (1.62, 4.41)	1.58 (1.05, 2.38)	1.00
Model 2 AOR (95% CI)[c]	1.92 (1.14, 3.24)	1.53 (1.02, 2.33)	1.00
Third Trimester Adiponectin Tertile (μg/ml)[d]			
Lowest (<9.0), N (%)	39 (50.7)	53 (41.4)	149 (28.4)
Middle (9.0–13.5), N (%)	20 (25.9)	40 (31.6)	185 (35.2)
Highest (>13.5), N (%)	18 (23.4)	35 (27.1)	191 (36.4)
Model 1 AOR (95% CI)[b]	2.53 (1.53, 4.19)	1.59 (1.06, 2.40)	1.00
Model 2 AOR (95% CI)[c]	2.03 (1.21, 3.42)	1.58 (1.04, 2.40)	1.00

Source: Adapted from Chen, X. et al., *J. Diabetes Mellitus*, 2, 196–202, 2012. With permission.

Note: AOR, adjusted odds ratio; CI, confidence interval.

[a] The lowest tertile of serum adiponectin concentration at entry was compared to other tertiles pooled.

[b] Model 1, models were adjusted for age, parity, ethnicity, and cigarette smoking; p for trend < 0.0001.

[c] Model 2, additional adjustment for prepregnant BMI; p for trend < 0.01.

[d] The lowest tertile of serum adiponectin concentration at the third trimester was compared to other tertiles pooled.

that give rise to insulin resistance in normal pregnancy as well as in pregnancies complicated by GDM are not completely understood.

The insulin receptor is a protein tyrosine kinase that results in the phosphorylation of intracellular substrates after binding insulin. Upon phosphorylation, these substrates interact and activate other molecules that modulate intracellular metabolism.[12,42] Thus, normal insulin receptor tyrosine kinase (IRTK) activity is a key step in the insulin signalling pathway. Cytokines are implicated in insulin resistance in type 2 diabetes because they interfere with intracellular insulin receptor signalling.[12,42,43]

In GDM, defective insulin receptor signalling, as indicated by less than maximal tyrosine phosphorylation of the insulin receptor, occurs without changes in receptor binding capacity or receptor number.[44,45] Increased expression of the inhibitors of the IRTK also could lead to impaired insulin action. Tomazic et al.[46] found that in GDM impaired adipocyte glucose transport was characterised by a defect in insulin receptor substrate-1 (IRS-1) tyrosine phosphorylation, from reduced expression of the IRS-1 protein. An increase in plasma cell membrane glycoprotein (PC-1) contents, one of the inhibitors of IRTK, could underlie the mechanism for impaired glucose uptake in adipocytes from these women.[46] While changes in the number of insulin signalling proteins may play a role in the induction of insulin resistance, there is undoubtedly much to be learned about the cellular mechanisms of insulin resistance during pregnancy.

1.2.3.6   Free Fatty Acids and Insulin Resistance

Maternal circulation free (nonesterified) fatty acids (FFAs) are elevated in late pregnancy[4,14,33] and are a direct source of energy for foetal growth. All of the omega 3 and omega 6 FFA structures are acquired by the foetus from the mother, and cross the placenta, in the form of either essential FFAs (linoleic acid, α-linolenic acid) or their derivatives, of which arachidonic acid and docosahexaenoic acid are metabolically the most important.[47,48] Physiologically elevated FFAs induce insulin resistance and inhibit insulin-stimulated glucose uptake by ~30% in healthy pregnant women but have no effect on hepatic glucose production.[4,6] Reducing FFA levels improved insulin action in nondiabetic males.[4,12] In Camden the concentration of total fatty acids, individual fatty acids, and grouped FAs (saturated FA, monounsaturated FA, polyunsaturated FA) was elevated not only in women with GDM, but also in women with impaired glucose challenge test non-GDM when compared with controls. Maternal pregravid overweight or obesity (BMI ≥ 25 kg/m²) appears to contribute to increased level of serum FFAs.[33]

In 1963, Randle et al. proposed a connection between muscle insulin resistance and elevated FFAs.[49] FFAs compete with glucose as an energy substrate in muscle and adipose tissue, a relationship described as the glucose–fatty acid cycle. In vitro experiments suggested that elevated FFAs inhibited insulin-stimulated glucose uptake at the level of glucose transport/phosphorylation[12,49] by inhibiting insulin signalling pathways, decreasing IRS-1 tyrosine phosphorylation, suppressing phosphatidylinositol 3-kinase (PI-3 kinase) activity, increasing protein kinase C theta (PCKθ) activity, and decreasing GLUT-4 transport, culminating in reduced glucose transport and causing insulin resistance in muscle (Figure 1.1).[12,42] Other mechanisms may involve peroxisome proliferator-activated receptor gamma (PPARγ) and insulin receptor substrate-2 (IRS-2).[12,42] These findings seemingly support the notion of a causal relationship between elevated FFAs and peripheral insulin resistance. During pregnancy, a rise in FFA concentration has important physiological consequences, inducing insulin resistance so that glucose is reserved for the developing foetus.[1–3] Additionally, FFAs impact insulin secretion: elevated levels reduce insulin secretion in GDM women.[50]

1.2.3.7   Oxidative Stress and Insulin Resistance
during Normal Pregnancy and GDM

Oxidative stress is an imbalance between the production of free radicals and the synthesis of antioxidant defences. Human pregnancy is susceptible to oxidative stress.[51,52] The human placenta is haemomonochorial, rich in mitochondria, and significantly vascularised with a high metabolic rate. There is increased generation of reactive oxygen species (ROS) in normal pregnancy with increased leakage of electrons from the mitochondrial respiratory chain.[52] In addition, the increase in insulin

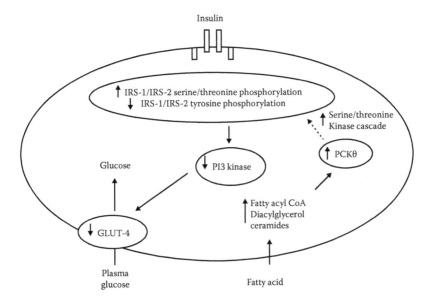

FIGURE 1.1 Proposed alternative mechanism for fatty acid-induced insulin resistance in human skeletal muscle. IRS-1, insulin receptor substrate-1; IRS-2, insulin receptor substrate-2; PI-3 kinase, phosphatidylinositol 3-kinase; PCKθ, protein kinase C theta. (From Shulman, G.I., *J. Clin. Invest.*, 106, 171–76, 2000. Permission granted by the American Society for Clinical Investigation.)

resistance during late gestation results in higher circulating lipid levels, including total cholesterol and low-density lipoprotein (LDL), which contribute to an increased lipid hydroperoxation.[25,53]

A family of antioxidant/detoxification enzymes that enhance cellular ROS-scavenging capacity is key to the maintenance of cellular redox homeostasis and to reducing oxidative damage.[54] There is an increase in oxidative stress accompanied by an altered antioxidant defence during normal pregnancy and with GDM.[52] In our prospective study, normal pregnant women from Camden showed that erythrocyte glutathione peroxidase (GPx) activity at weeks ~16 and ~30 was positively associated with markers of insulin resistance—an increased fasting insulin concentration and increased homoeostasis model for insulin resistance (HOMA-IR)—which suggested a link between insulin resistance and antioxidant defences in nondiabetic pregnancy.[52,54] However, while a correlation is present, it is unclear whether the relationship between diabetes and oxidative stress is causal.

Hyperglycaemia in T2DM is known to enhance free radical production and induce oxidative stress; glucose oxidation is a powerful source of hydrogen peroxide. β-cells have a low expression of and activity for many of the enzymes involved in antioxidant defence, which makes them susceptible to oxidative damage.[51,55] ROS are a natural by-product of metabolism, and even modest ROS production has an important role in cell signalling. Glucose levels that stimulate basal insulin secretion also generate ROS. However, high amounts of ROS cause damage to cells. ROS are essential and sufficient signals for the hypersecretion of insulin.[51,55] Whether or not oxidative stress and excess ROS contribute to induction of insulin secretion and increased insulin resistance with gestational hyperglycaemia has not been confirmed.

1.2.3.8 Other Factors That Alter Insulin Resistance in Pregnancy

Other factors that influence the insulin resistance of pregnancy include body composition, the prevalence of metabolic syndrome, and other obesity-related chronic diseases.[56,57] There are also ethnic differences in insulin secretion and resistance in healthy nondiabetic adults, children, and adolescents.[58] We observed such differences in the concentration of C-peptide and the C-peptide/insulin ratio in women from Camden. Both were consistently lower in African Americans and significantly different during the second and third trimesters from Hispanics and Caucasians. African Americans and Hispanics had comparable insulin and insulin/glucose ratios (an index of insulin resistance) that exceeded the ratios in Caucasians; fasting glucose did not differ among the three groups. Our data thus suggested that pregnant nondiabetic African Americans had lower insulin production and a delayed hepatic insulin extraction or clearance.[59] Furthermore, African Americans of every glycaemic status had third trimester adiponectin concentrations that were consistently and significantly lower than those in Hispanics or Caucasians of the same group, i.e., GDM, less severe hyperglycaemia, and controls.[41] We propose that the ethnic difference in serum adiponectin may be a response to a different degree of insulin resistance in African Americans where the greater the insulin resistance, the greater the suppression of adiponectin production.

In summary, many factors and mechanisms have a causal relation to insulin resistance during pregnancy (inflammatory cytokines/adipocytokines, FFAs, hyperglycaemia-induced oxidative stress). The cellular mechanisms underlying these factors that lead to increased insulin resistance require further study.

1.3 GLUCOSE AND FOETAL GROWTH

The human foetus is dependent on maternal metabolic substrates, including glucose, lactate, amino acids, and free fatty acids, for energy, protein synthesis, and the growth of new tissues.[60] Glucose is the most important substrate passing through the placenta to the foetus. Approximately 80% of foetal energy comes from glucose oxidation; the foetus has minimal ability to produce glucose on its own.[61] The enzymes related to glycogen synthesis and gluconeogenesis are found in sheep or rat foetal liver in early gestation and significantly increase closer to term, suggesting that the foetus can synthesise glycogen from pyruvate, acetate, alanine, glycerol, and glucose.[62,63]

1.3.1 MECHANISMS OF GLUCOSE TRANSFER

Maternal glucose is transferred to the foetus across the placenta by carrier-mediated diffusion.[60,61] A glucose molecule must use glucose transporters to cross from the maternal to the foetal circulation.[60] The glucose transporter-1 (GLUT-1) is the major placental glucose transporter isoform. During the second half of gestation, placental glucose transfer increases to meet the rising metabolic requirement of the larger growing foetus. Increased glucose transport occurs by increasing transplacental glucose concentration gradient (as foetal glucose decreases relative to maternal glucose concentration), by increasing placental GLUT-1 capability, as well as by hormonal (insulin and IGF-1) regulation.[61]

1.3.2 Foetal Glucose Metabolism

The foetal pancreas develops in the late first to early second trimester, producing measureable insulin by mid-gestation.[61,64] Basal insulin and glucose-stimulated insulin secretion gradually increase toward term.[61] Foetal glucose metabolism (utilisation and oxidation) is dependent on the simultaneous interaction of foetal plasma glucose and foetal insulin.[60,61] High glucose downregulates and low glucose upregulates foetal insulin secretion. Foetal insulin increases the permeability of insulin-sensitive cells to glucose, enhancing foetal glucose uptake and utilisation.[64] However, the mechanism and time course of insulin action in the foetus have been difficult to determine. In foetal sheep, increases in the principal insulin signal transduction proteins (insulin receptor, IRS-1, PI-3 kinase) with acute insulin stimulation of skeletal muscle suggest that insulin-regulated pathways for glucose uptake and metabolism, the initiation of mRNA translation, protein synthesis, and growth are well developed by late gestation.[64]

1.4 PLACENTAL FUNCTION AND FOETAL GROWTH

The placenta is the interface between the mother and foetus that transfers nutrients and waste products for normal foetal growth and development.[65] It is the source of hormonal regulators and the network of cytokine and insulin receptors that act as growth factors.[66] Foetal growth is conditioned by normal placental development. Patterns of placental transfer vary for different types of nutrients. For example, simple diffusion is limited by placental blood flow and the exchange area for oxygen and urea transfer; active transport for amino acids involves carrier proteins on the cell surface and requires additional energy.[66] Glucose is transported by facilitated diffusion and is carrier mediated, as described (Section 1.3.1).

1.4.1 Placental Hormones

The placenta is an active endocrine organ that produces steroid and protein hormones and growth factors, including human placental lactogen (hPL), placental growth hormone (hPGH), insulin-like growth factor-1 (IGF-1), and a range of unique cytokines and bioactive molecules and their corresponding receptors.[65,66] Placental transport is influenced by hormones of the somatotrophic axis (GH/IGF-1 axis). Foetal nutritional status also influences the foetal somatotrophin axis and insulin regulation.[67–69]

1.4.1.1 Human Placental Lactogen and Growth Hormone

The hPGH and hPL family consists of growth hormone and placental lactogen genes; the hormones are structurally related and share several biological features.[70] hPL, also called human chorionic somatomammotropic hormone, is a product of hPLa and hPLb genes secreted by the syncytiotrophoblast.[49,71] hPL is found in maternal blood from the sixth week of gestation and increases continuously until 35 weeks.[70,71] Although radiolabelled, hPL does not cross the placenta; it is detectable in the foetal circulation and stimulates IGF production in foetal tissues.[49,70] It is also possible that hPL is directly secreted into both the maternal and the foetal circulation.[71]

hPGH is a GH variant (hPGH-V) expressed by placenta. Its structure and function are similar to those of human pituitary growth hormone, differing by 13 amino acid residues.[68–70,72] hPGH gradually replaces pituitary growth hormone during pregnancy. Unlike pituitary GH, hPGH secretion is nonpulsatile and not regulated by growth hormone-releasing hormone (GHRH). Instead, hPGH secretion is regulated (inhibited) by glucose.[69,70] hPGH is not detectable in the foetal circulation and appears not to have a direct effect on foetal growth.[68,69] hPGH modifies the metabolic state of the mother during pregnancy by exerting a strong effect on gluconeogenesis and lipolysis in maternal liver and other organs, thereby increasing the energy supply for the foetal-placental unit.[69,73] Additionally, hPGH is the key regulator of maternal IGF-1.[74]

1.4.1.2 Insulin-Like Growth Factor (IGF) System

The IGF family includes IGF-1, IGF-2, six binding proteins, and several IGF binding protein proteases with major effects on foetal growth and development.[69] IGF-1 is produced by cells of mesenchymal origin and is protein bound.[68] Only free IGF-1 is biologically active.[75] IGF-1 and IGF-2 are single-chain peptides related to proinsulin, which interact with GH, insulin, and other hormones to regulate somatic and tissue growth.[74]

IGF-1 acts at endocrine, paracrine, and autocrine levels via specific receptors.[76] The IGF-1 receptor is similar in structure to the classic insulin receptor. Both the IGF-1 receptor and the insulin receptor bind to IGF-1; both the IGF-1 receptor and the IGF-2 receptor bind to IGF-2.[68,74] IGF-1 secretion is primarily regulated by nutrient intake. hPGH is the key regulator of IGF-1 concentration.[76] In addition, IGF-1 action is modulated by binding proteins, which themselves are modified by several mechanisms.[77,78] IGF-1 shares structural and functional similarities with insulin and has mitogenetic (cell growth and multiplication, inhibition of cell death) and anabolic (glucose uptake and utilisation and protein anabolism) actions.[69,75] In contrast, the action of IGF-2, which depends upon insulin, is primarily on foetal growth.[60,68]

1.4.1.3 Foetal Glucose–Insulin–IGF Axis and Maternal Nutritional Supply to Foetal Growth

Data on the relationship between the maternal IGF system and foetal IGF system are inconclusive. It was suggested that maternal and foetal IGFs are independent since maternal IGF-1 and binding protein 3 correlate with gestational age, whereas foetal IGF-1, IGF-2, and their binding proteins do not.[67] In contrast, other investigators reported that maternal IGF-1 levels rise progressively through pregnancy, and are positively associated with foetal size and infant birth weight.[66,67] These data support the idea that maternal IGF-1 influences foetal growth by enhancing placental function, especially substrate transfer.[68,74] Foetal insulin and IGF-1 control foetal growth by responding to nutritional and metabolic signals.[60,66,67]

1.4.2 Cytokines/Adipocytokines and Foetal Growth

The association of inflammatory cytokines/adipocytokines with maternal insulin resistance in normal pregnancy and in pregnancy complicated with GDM was described in Sections 1.2.3.2 and 1.2.3.3. Like the placental hormones, most maternal cytokines do not cross the trophoblastic barrier and thus do not reach the foetal circulation.[21,24] How maternal cytokines regulate foetal growth is unclear. Placental TNF-α, derived from macrophages and likely modulated by TNF-α and its receptor signalling, facilitates trophoblast differentiation and has a role in developmental differentiation.[21] Growth of foetal adipose tissue is regulated by the complex interaction of transcription factors, nutrients, and adipocytokines.[23,24] Radaelli et al.[23] found an association between maternal systemic IL-6 and the foetal fat mass, a correlation not found with cytokines in cord blood. They hypothesised that inflammatory reactions taking place in the placenta modified placental structure and indirectly influenced the availability of substrates for foetal growth.[23,24]

Leptin is a product of the obesity gene that is synthesised by white adipose tissue and produced within the intrauterine environment.[24,79] Leptin expression and its receptors are widespread in foetal adipose tissue and placental tissue.[24] In adults leptin acts as an endocrine signal of energy reserves, to coordinate appetite and metabolism with nutrient availability, and regulate body weight and the metabolic response to fasting.[70,79]

There is a substantial body of data linking foetal leptin to foetal growth. Umbilical leptin concentration at term is positively correlated to placental weight and indices of foetal growth, such as birth weight, infant length, and bone mineral content, as well as IGF-1 level.[24] Foetal leptin is positively related to foetal fat mass.[23,60] It was also reported that infants from obese mothers had higher cord blood leptin as well as increased HOMA-IR, like their mothers.[69,80] Thus, foetal leptin is an endocrine marker for foetal adiposity that participates in the control of metabolism and maturation of foetal tissue and foetal energy reserves. In addition, lower levels of maternal and placental leptin were found in infants with an intrauterine growth-restricted infant (IUGR), and higher leptin levels were found in macrosomic offspring of diabetic mothers.[24]

1.5 MATERNAL HYPERGLYCAEMIA AND OTHER FACTORS CONTRIBUTING TO FOETAL OVERGROWTH

1.5.1 Foetal Overgrowth

Two important consequences are associated with foetal growth that is either restricted or excessive. Foetal overgrowth, defined as macrosomia (birth weight > 4000 g independent of gestational age or sex) or a large for gestational age (LGA) birth (birth weight > 90th percentile for a given gestational age), increases maternal morbidity from operative delivery and also causes serious consequences to the offspring, including birth trauma, obesity during childhood, and type 2 diabetes and metabolic syndrome in adult life.[81-85] The prevalence of foetal overgrowth was reported as 8–16% from women without GDM and 15–40% from women with gestational hyperglycaemia.[83–86] Despite different diagnostic criteria, many studies confirmed that GDM increases the risk of macrosomia or LGA birth.[87–89] However, under certain circumstances, because of the interaction of genetics and environment, GDM can give rise to an IUGR infant.[90] For example, a glucokinase gene mutation in mother or foetus, or both, causes defects in foetal insulin secretion and results in decreased foetal growth and possible IUGR.[90,91] Because foetal growth and development are determined by multiple factors, we will focus on several topics that are related to maternal hyperglycaemia and the epidemic of obesity.

1.5.2 MATERNAL GLYCAEMIC STATUS AND FOETAL OVERGROWTH

Maternal glucose concentrations originate from both dietary sources and endogenous production.[2,8] The foetus obtains its glucose almost entirely from circulating levels in the mother because the foetus has a minimal capability for glucose production.[2,8,43] More than 50 years ago, Pedersen suggested that in maternal diabetes foetal overgrowth was related to increased transplacental transfer of glucose, stimulating the release of insulin by the foetal β-cell and subsequent macrosomia.[92] This hypothesis was supported by observations that GDM women undergoing intensive diabetic care had neonatal birth weights and rates of macrosomia similar to those of non-GDM women.[93] A clinical trial of continuous glucose monitoring in GDM resulted in a significant improvement in infant birth weight with a reduced risk of macrosomia.[94] Pedersen's hypothesis also applies to foetal growth when the mother is not diabetic.[95] In Camden, higher plasma glucose (>99 mg/dl (5.5 mmol/L) after a 1 h 50 g oral glucose load) was associated with increased infant birth weight ($p < 0.005$), decreased duration of gestation ($p < 0.05$), increased risk for an LGA infant, and reduced risk for small for gestational age (SGA) birth.[95] Higher plasma glucose was also associated with other pregnancy complications (such as chorioamnionitis and caesarean delivery).

The maternal glycaemic response is dependent on the type of carbohydrate eaten.[96] The dietary glycaemic index (GI) is a qualitative measure that classifies the type of carbohydrate according to the metabolic response that it elicits. A high dietary GI was associated with increased infant birth weight, whereas low GI is associated with lower birth weight and higher risk of SGA birth (adjusted odds ratio 1.75, 95% CI 1.10–2.77).[96] These data showed that foetal growth and development are exquisitely sensitive to fluctuations in maternal fuel levels. Even a minor degree of elevation in maternal glucose in nondiabetic women is associated with adverse pregnancy outcomes.

1.5.3 MATERNAL OBESITY, GDM, AND LGA BIRTH

There has been a significant increase in obesity worldwide in the last 20 years, and a subsequent increase in the prevalence of GDM and T2DM. Exposure of the developing foetus to the maternal environment of GDM or T2DM is different from exposure to maternal T1DM, the type of diabetic patient that was in Pedersen's care.[5,92] Maternal obesity is a common problem during pregnancy and is a risk factor for LGA birth.[97] Data on whether obesity-associated LGA is independent of hyperglycaemia are inconsistent.[97] We examined the influence of maternal hyperglycaemia and obesity on risk of LGA in Camden women comparing three groups (GDM, impaired glucose challenge test (GCT) non-GDM, and normal GCT) (Table 1.4).[98] Infant birth weight was significantly higher in obese women with GDM, impaired GCT non-GDM, or normal GCT compared to nonobese women with normal GCT ($p < 0.001$). A stratified analysis was performed to explore the independent and combined effects of hyperglycaemia and maternal obesity on risk of LGA. Using nonobese women (prepregnant BMI ≤ 30 kg/m²) with normal GCT as a reference group, we found that obese women, regardless of whether they were diagnosed with GDM or impaired GCT non-GDM, had a three- to sixfold increased risk for delivering an LGA infant (Table 1.4, model 1). Additionally, obese women with a normal GCT had a twofold increased risk for delivering an LGA infant. We tested the contribution of hyperglycaemia alone by using obese and nonobese women with a normal GCT as separate reference groups (Table 1.4, model 2). Impaired GCT non-GDM was associated with a 2.7-fold increased risk of LGA in obese and nonobese women, whereas risk for LGA among GDM women, all of whom were treated with insulin or diet, was

TABLE 1.4

Maternal Hyperglycaemia and Delivery of an LGA Infant Stratified by Maternal Obesity

	N	Birth Weight (g)[a]	LGA Unadjusted %	Model 1[b] AOR (95% CI)	Model 2[c] AOR (95% CI)
			Obese		
GDM	40	3496 ± 6	15.0	3.73 (1.50, 9.31)	1.69 (0.65, 4.38)
Impaired GCT non-GDM	45	3537 ± 68	23.3	6.12 (2.89, 12.99)	2.79 (1.26, 6.18)
Normal GCT	398	3269 ± 21	9.6	2.26 (1.50, 3.41)	Reference
			Nonobese		
GDM	60	3223 ± 54	6.7	1.42 (0.49, 4.07)	1.45 (0.50, 4.21)
Impaired GCT non-GDM	140	3189 ± 39	10.8	2.17 (1.16, 4.05)	2.19 (1.17, 4.10)
Normal GCT	1716	3169 ± 10[d,e]	4.3	Reference	Reference

Source: Adapted from Chen, X., and Scholl, T.O., Mild Maternal Hyperglycemia Increases Risk of Fetal Overgrowth in Minority Pregnant Women: Camden Study, paper presented at the 68th American Diabetes Association Scientific Sessions, San Francisco, CA, 2008.

[a] Data are mean (SE) and adjusted for age, parity, ethnicity, gestational age at delivery, and cigarette smoking.

[b] Model 1 was adjusted for age, parity, ethnicity, cigarette smoking, and infant gender and with nonobese normal GCT as a reference.

[c] Model 2 was adjusted for age, parity, ethnicity, cigarette smoking, and infant gender and with obese or nonobese normal GCT as a reference.

[d] p for linear trend < 0.0001.

[e] $p < 0.001$ vs. obese women with any glycaemic status.

not significant when compared to the appropriate obese or nonobese control. These observations suggest that maternal obesity and untreated gestational hyperglycaemia are independently associated with LGA birth. This is supported by recent data from the HAPO study where high maternal BMI was independently associated with pregnancy complications, especially foetal overgrowth and foetal adiposity.[99,100]

1.5.4   INCREASED FOETAL ADIPOSITY OF GDM MOTHER

Although risk of foetal overgrowth has been improved by glycaemic control in pregnancies complicated by GDM, it was unclear if foetal growth from a diabetic mother is normal and if birth weight is the best indicator. Catalano et al. examined changes in infant body weight and infant body fat mass between women with normal glucose tolerance and GDM.[5,62] A significantly increased infant fat mass and percent body fat remained in the infants of GDM mothers whose hyperglycaemia was well controlled compared to mothers with normal glucose tolerance, suggesting infant birth weight alone may be insensitive to subtle differences in foetal growth during GDM pregnancies.[22,62] Mechanisms likely to increase foetal adiposity with maternal diabetes include exposure to higher maternal levels of lipids and cytokines. Overweight or obesity in the mother increases lipids supplied to the foetus; high maternal lipids are in turn related to elevated maternal and foetal cytokines.[22,23] Cytokines increase placental transport of lipid (FFAs) and foetal lipogenic activity, thus increasing foetal lipogenesis.[22,23] This hypothesis is supported by a study in mice where mothers fed high-fat diets had elevated inflammatory cytokines and lipids levels, as well as marked upregulation of placental nutrient transport and foetal overgrowth.[101] Thus, the foetus exposed to a high-fat diet receives more nutrients to stimulate foetal insulin secretion and promote foetal lipogenesis and growth.

1.5.5   PREGNANCY WEIGHT GAIN AND FOETAL OVERGROWTH

GDM and excessive pregnancy weight gain, especially in obese women, are known risk factors for foetal overgrowth.[88] Optimising gestational weight gain for both mother and foetus is critical but remains controversial. A large number of studies have found that excess gestational weight gain is associated with decreased risk of small for gestational age birth and with increased risk for LGA birth,[102] regardless of the definition or the scales used for excess pregnancy weight gain.[103] Even in women with a normal prepregnant BMI, a higher pregnancy weight gain was associated with an increased risk of LGA, while a normal weight gain by the 1990 Institute of Medicine (IOM) guidelines was associated with a decreased risk of LGA.[104] We explored the associations between gestational weight gain assessed throughout pregnancy with LGA using the 2009 IOM guidelines for weight gain during pregnancy. Inadequate, adequate, and excessive pregnancy weight gains at weeks 24, 28, 32, and at delivery were categorised according to IOM recommendations.[105] Compared to women with adequate weight gain, excessive weight gain was associated with a 1.56- to 2.66-fold increased risk of LGA birth (p for trend < 0.0001 for each model). In addition, women with inadequate weight gain had a reduced risk of LGA birth at weeks 28 and 32 ($p < 0.05$).[97]

TABLE 1.5

Maternal Hyperglycaemia and LGA Infant Stratified by Excess Weight Gain[a]

	Weight Gain at Week 24		Weight Gain at Week 28		Weight Gain at Week 32		Weight Gain at Delivery	
	LGA (%)	AOR (95% CI)[c]	LGA (%)	AOR (95% CI)[c]	LGA (%)	AOR (95% CI)[c]	LGA (%)	AOR (95% CI)[c]
Excess Weight Gain								
GDM	11.5	4.03 (1.67, 9.73)	10.5	3.31 (1.39, 7.90)	11.3	3.20 (1.34, 7.63)	14.3	6.07 (2.58, 14.70)
Impaired GCT non-GDM	16.0	6.14 (3.16, 11.90)	14.6	4.97 (2.53, 9.71)	14.1	4.62 (2.18, 8.31)	14.9	6.42 (3.20, 12.88)
Normal GCT	7.8	2.91 (1.88, 4.48)	7.2	2.43 (1.58, 3.73)	6.8	2.02 (1.33, 3.10)	8.2	3.58 (2.29, 5.60)
Nonexcess Weight Gain[b]								
GDM	5.6	1.64 (0.37, 7.21)	6.7	1.69 (0.38, 7.50)	5.9	1.31 (0.30, 5.71)	4.7	1.62 (0.37, 7.11)
Impaired GCT non-GDM	8.1	2.78 (1.17, 6.59)	9.5	2.98 (1.31, 6.77)	9.9	2.69 (1.19, 6.08)	9.1	3.79 (1.65, 8.68)
Normal GCT	2.8	Reference	3.1	Reference	3.6	Reference	2.5	Reference

Source: Adapted from Chen, X. et al., in *Gestational Diabetes*, ed. M. Radenkovic, InTech open-access publisher, 2011. With permission.

[a] Model was adjusted for age, prepregnant BMI, and cigarette smoking, in addition to using a standard that adjusted LGA for maternal ethnicity, parity, and foetal gender.

[b] Adequate and inadequate weight gains are combined.

[c] p for trend < 0.0001.

We also examined the independent and combined contributions of hyperglycaemia and excess weight gain on risk of LGA. Our results showed that excess weight gain by mid-gestation at weeks 24, 28, or 32 or by delivery was positively associated with a two- to sixfold increased risk for delivering an LGA infant regardless of whether the women were diagnosed with GDM, impaired GCT but non-GDM, or normal GCT. Furthermore, women with nonexcess weight gain and (untreated) mild hyperglycaemia (impaired GCT but non-GDM) also had a two- to threefold increased risk of LGA birth at all of four time points; risk of LGA was not increased in the GDM group with nonexcess weight gain (Table 1.5).[97] These data showed that excess pregnancy weight gain and untreated gestational hyperglycaemia (even mild hyperglycaemia) are independent risk factors for LGA.

1.5.6 Epigenetic Modifications in Phenotype of Foetal Growth

It is now widely accepted that the processes of growth and development are mediated directly or indirectly by epigenetic processes. Epigenetics is the study of stable genetic modifications that result in changes in gene expression and function without a corresponding alteration in the gDNA sequence.[106,107] The epigenetic modification is largely impacted by environmental and developmental factors. The best-known epigenetic marker is DNA methylation in which the addition of a methyl group to DNA is at the 5-carbon of the cytosine pyrimidine ring that precedes guanine. DNA methylation occurs in a complex chromatin network and is influenced by a number of modifications in the histone structure.[107]

1.5.6.1 Maternal Nutritional Status and Epigenetic Modification in Offspring

Maternal nutritional status may influence epigenetic mechanisms that could affect chromosomal stability and gene expression. Early maternal metabolism, nutritional status (dietary intake of methyl donors and cofactors), and chronic inflammation affect foetal growth, potentially via persistent alteration in DNA methylation.[108]

Data from animal models showed that intrauterine exposure to maternal nutrition affected DNA methylation, offspring phenotype, and had a long-term effect on offspring health.[109,110] The supplementation of the maternal diet with nutrients that provide methyl groups increased the extent of genomic DNA (gDNA) methylation, whereas restricting folate intake decreased gDNA methylation.[109,110]

Data from humans are limited. During the Second World War, well-nourished Dutch women experienced a serious food shortage in the course of pregnancy. A first trimester exposure at the peak of the famine, in combination with infection or another unknown factor, was linked to an excess of preterm birth, and to an increase in infants with low birth weight (<2000 g).[111] There was also a rise in the frequency of malformations of the central nervous system, including spina bifida, which is consistent with a deficiency in dietary folate.[109–111] Six decades later the lower methylation status of *IGF2* differentially methylated region (DMR) was noted among adults exposed to famine while in utero.[111] Thus, certain transient maternal environmental conditions may produce persistent changes in epigenetic marks that have lifelong phenotypic consequences.

1.5.6.2 Foetal Programming in GDM Pregnancies

Epidemiological observations have demonstrated that adaptive responses to the foetal environment can result in adverse effects later in life.[112] The effects of hypernutrition are best identified in offspring of mothers with T2DM or GDM.[113] At 22 years of age the offspring of diabetic mothers had an increased risk of T2DM compared to their background population.[90,114] Foetal macrosomia and a high-fat mass are linked to greater risk of childhood obesity and insulin resistance. Infants from obese mothers showed metabolic compromise, including higher body fat and insulin resistance at birth.[115] Small infants display catch-up growth in the first few years of life and have higher insulin resistance and body fat in childhood and adolescence.[112] It was hypothesised that the mother, in effect, gives the foetus a "forecast" of the nutrition it can expect at birth. The foetus is then "programmed" largely due to epigenetic changes to match that environment.[112,114] When the mother develops GDM, the developing foetus is exposed to high glucose levels that may trigger epigenetic changes in offspring

DNA, increasing the likelihood that exposed females will develop GDM. The epigenetic system is environmentally sensitive. Alternations in the epigenome may be a mechanism for deregulating gene expression during foetal development.[114,115]

1.6 GESTATIONAL HYPERGLYCAEMIA AND FOETAL OUTCOME—WHAT DID WE LEARN FROM HAPO STUDY?

1.6.1 WHY IT IS IMPORTANT TO STUDY GESTATIONAL HYPERGLYCAEMIA LESS SEVERE THAN OVERT GDM?

GDM increases the risk of perinatal morbidity and mortality in the mother and in the foetus.[116] Treatment to improve glycaemic control significantly reduces infant macrosomia.[7] An assessment of neonatal and perinatal outcomes in relation to varying degrees of maternal blood glucose levels less severe than GDM or overt diabetes was needed. It was also of interest to determine if maternal metabolic abnormalities were present; approximately 9–19% of pregnant women who have hyperglycaemia during fasting or after an oral glucose load do not meet the diagnostic criteria for GDM.[85,117] These patients generally are not provided the usual diabetes care. Like GDM, there is no consensus on the glucose threshold values.[84,85,118] This causes difficulty in the interpretation of the results.

Recent studies have reported that maternal glucose intolerance less severe than overt GDM is associated with an increased risk of adverse maternal/foetal outcomes.[117–119] Retnakaran et al. suggested that the metabolic implications of impaired glucose tolerance (non-GDM) in pregnancy vary in relation to the timing of the glucose abnormality during the oral glucose tolerance test (OGTT).[117] Italian women with a positive glucose challenge test followed by a normal OGTT ($n = 350$) had more LGA births (19%) than those with a negative glucose challenge test (8%), but were no different from the group with GDM (20.7%).[85] Swedish women not treated for impaired glucose tolerance (IGT) ($n = 213$, defined as 2 h plasma glucose in 160–199 mg/dl (8.9–11.1 mmol/L) by a 75 g OGTT) showed increases in rates of LGA, macrosomia, caesarean section, and admission to a neonatal intensive care unit (NICU) compared with women with normal glucose tolerance.[84] The proportions of LGA and macrosomia were similar in IGT and GDM in this report. Data from the Toronto Tri-Hospital Project, which involved a large cohort of Canadian women without GDM, demonstrated that increased glucose intolerance was associated with a graded increase in the incidence of caesarean section, preeclampsia, and macrosomia.[118] A study in the UK was an exception and showed no significant differences in infant birth weight and macrosomia (≥4000 g) when comparing women with IGT (diagnosed by WHO criteria) and women with a normal OGTT.[119]

1.6.2 HAPO STUDY AND ITS SIGNIFICANCE

One consequence of the secular increase in overweight and obesity has been a rise in the prevalence of gestational diabetes, i.e., glucose intolerance that is first recognised during pregnancy, a definition that includes women whose diabetes is pregestational as well as those with diabetes that is gestational in origin.[120]

An increasing frequency of GDM was detected among Northern California gravidae who were universally screened for gestational diabetes and diagnosed by National Diabetes Data Group criteria. Age-adjusted data showed a rise from 3.7% to 6.6% over a decade in every ethnic group. GDM was especially prevalent among minorities where type 2 diabetes is highest: Asians (~8.5%) and Hispanics (~7%) and African Americans (~6%), followed by non-Hispanic whites (~5%).[11] Likewise, hospital discharge data also showed substantial increases in GDM (122% increase) over a 15-year period[10] and among universally screened Colorado women (195% increase) between 1994 and 2002.[121] Worldwide, GDM is currently estimated to occur in 0.6 to 15% of pregnant women,[122] depending on presence or absence of risk factors (older maternal age, obesity, increased parity, positive family history of diabetes), whether or not the population is universally screened, the gestation when testing is done, and the type of test (a 75 g 2 h oral glucose tolerance test or 100 g 3 h OGTT). Diagnostic criteria also are not uniform; GDM prevalence is increased by 50% when results of the same 100 g oral glucose tolerance test are interpreted by different standards (Carpenter and Coustan vs. National Diabetes Data Group).[11] Recent recommendations derived from a global study that enrolled women from diverse ethnic groups, universally screened them, and diagnosed GDM using a common protocol with a sensitive cutoff point suggest a prevalence ranging from 9.3 to 25.5% among women from participating centres.[123]

Like type 1 and type 2 diabetes, gestational diabetes carries well-known risks for serious complications of pregnancy, such as preeclampsia, operative delivery, foetal macrosomia, birth defects, foetal demise, and other adverse pregnancy outcomes.[47] Following the index pregnancy, up to half of the women diagnosed with GDM will develop type 2 diabetes within the decade.[124] There are also long-term risks for children exposed to GDM while in utero: a threefold risk of developing obesity and a sevenfold risk of type 2 diabetes by young adulthood.[125,126] Maternal hyperglycaemia that does not meet the criteria for GDM also increases risk for adverse pregnancy outcomes.[127] Thus, it is likely that risks to the maternal–foetal unit during gestation, as well as afterward, will increase as the frequency of GDM continues to rise in reproductive age women. It is to be expected that mild maternal hyperglycaemia will increase in concert with GDM.

1.6.3   Findings from HAPO Study

The Hyperglycaemia and Adverse Pregnancy Outcomes (HAPO) study[128] was designed to study the influence of mild maternal hyperglycaemia on the outcome of pregnancy. The cohort was composed of more than 25,000 women from nine countries (UK, United States, Australia, Singapore, Thailand, Canada, Barbados, Israel, and China (Hong Kong)). Participants underwent a 75 g 2 h OGTT at 24–32 weeks gestation; providers were blinded to results except when plasma glucose was diagnostic of diabetes or met other predetermined criteria.[128] Primary outcomes of interest (high birth weight for gestation (>90th percentile), primary caesarean section, clinical neonatal hypoglycaemia, foetal hyperinsulinaemia (cord C-peptide > 90th percentile), and secondary outcomes (preterm delivery (<37 completed weeks), preeclampsia, shoulder dystocia/birth injury, and high bilirubin)) reflected an emphasis on foetal overgrowth and correlated risks to the maternal foetal unit from maternal hyperglycaemia.

The likelihood of high birth weight for gestation (37% increase), primary caesarean section (19% increase), and foetal hyperinsulinaemia (41% increase) increased monotonically as maternal plasma glucose rose and was first evidenced at very low levels of fasting (>75 mg/dl (4.2 mmol/L)), 1 and 2 h post-load glucose (>106 mg/dl (5.9 mmol/L) and >109 mg/dl (6.1 mmol/L)). At the highest categories of fasting (≥100 mg/dl (5.6 mmol/L)) and post-load glucose (≥212 mg/dl (11.8 mmol/L), ≥178 mg/dl (9.9 mmol/L) at 1 and 2 h, respectively), the adjusted odds ratio for high birth weight was increased ~5-fold; the likelihood of foetal hyperinsulinaemia (3.5- to 7.7-fold) and primary caesarean section (1.3- to 1.9-fold) was also raised. When examined as a continuous variable risk, clinical neonatal hypoglycaemia was weakly associated with maternal glycaemia (~10–13% increase). Of the secondary outcomes of interest, preeclampsia (20–28% increase) and shoulder dystocia/birth injury (18–23% increase) showed the strongest association with continuous levels of maternal fasting and post-load glucose. Increased risks of preterm delivery (16–18% increase), neonatal intensive care (7–9% increase), and high bilirubin (8–11% increase) were associated with 1 and 2 h plasma glucose concentrations but not fasting glucose.[128]

It was therefore concluded that maternal glucose far below the levels diagnostic of GDM or overt diabetes was associated with foetal hyperinsulinaemia and increased infant birth weight for gestation. Likewise, there was a strong, continuous, and positive relation between maternal glucose and excess infant skinfolds (sum of flank, triceps, and subscapular skinfolds > 90th percentile) and a percent body fat (>90th percentile derived from infant birth weight, length, and the flank skinfold). The infant's cord C-peptide showed the same relation with infant birth weight and excess fatness as maternal glucose; risks were increased 26% at low levels of cord C-peptide and five- to sixfold when infants at the highest and lowest levels were compared.[129] Thus, supporting Pedersen's hypothesis, rising maternal glucose and the foetal insulin response to maternal glycaemia not only resulted in increased foetal growth (high birth weight for gestation), but also increased infant adipose tissue stores.

Since HAPO showed an essentially linear relationship between maternal glucose, excess foetal growth, and correlated risks to mother and foetus, the findings were reviewed by the International Association of Diabetes and Pregnancy Study Group and resulted in new guidelines for the diagnosis of GDM.[130] Two separate steps were recommended: (1) early screening (by fasting or random plasma glucose or haemoglobin A1C) for the detection of overt diabetes—unrecognised or untreated—in women, with universal testing for populations with a high prevalence of type 2 diabetes, and (2) screening women not previously found to have overt diabetes or GDM by 75 g OGTT at 24–28 weeks gestation. These recommendations, if adopted, would result in a common protocol to evaluate GDM and separate overt but undiagnosed diabetes from diabetes that is gestational in origin.

1.7 CONCLUSIONS

As summarised in Figure 1.2, recent data support the influence of maternal obesity, pregnancy weight gain, increased oxidative stress, and elevated lipids (particularly free fatty acids) on insulin resistance during pregnancy, including GDM, and on foetal growth. Inflammatory cytokines and adipokines from white adipose tissue

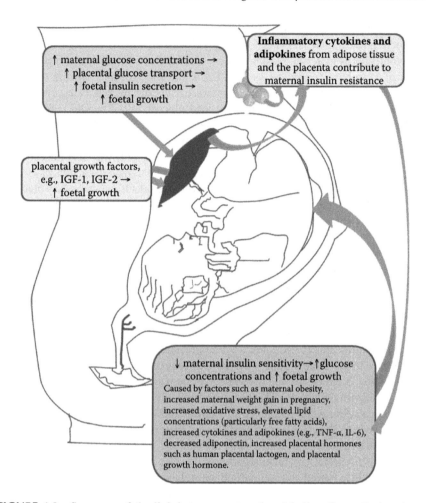

FIGURE 1.2 Summary of the link between maternal metabolism (in particular glucose levels and insulin sensitivity) and foetal growth.

also are derived from the placenta and, together with the placental hormones, give rise to increased insulin resistance and act as factors to promote foetal overgrowth and adiposity.

The cellular mechanisms underlying alterations in glucose metabolism during normal pregnancy, in complications like GDM as well as in the epigenetic regulation of foetal growth, require further investigation. However, there is mounting evidence that gestational hyperglycaemia less severe than overt GDM is associated with adverse foetal outcomes and abnormalities in maternal metabolism. Such data are important not only for GDM diagnosis but also for preventive interventions in the future.

REFERENCES

Key references are in bold.

1. Di Cianni, G., Miccoli, R., Volpe, L., Lencioni, C., and Del Prato, S. 2003. Intermediate Metabolism in Normal Pregnancy and in Gestational Diabetes. *Diabetes Metab Res Rev* 19:259–70.
2. Catalano, P.M., Huston, L., Amini, S.B., and Kalhan, S.C. 1999. Longitudinal Changes in Glucose Metabolism during Pregnancy in Obese Women with Normal Glucose Tolerance and Gestational Diabetes Mellitus. *Am J Obstet Gynecol* 180:903–16.
3. Catalano, P.M., Tyzbir, E.D., Wolfe, R.R., Calles, J., Roman, N.M., Amini, S.B., and Sims, E.A. 1993. Carbohydrate Metabolism during Pregnancy in Control Subjects and Women with Gestational Diabetes. *Am J Physiol* 264:E60–67.
4. Sivan, E., Homko, C.J., Whittaker, P.G., Reece, E.A., Chen, X., and Boden, G. 1998. Free Fatty Acids and Insulin Resistance during Pregnancy. *J Clin Endocrinol Metab* 83:2338–42.
5. Catalano, P.M., and Hauguel-De Mouzon, S. 2011. Is It Time to Revisit the Pedersen Hypothesis in the Face of the Obesity Epidemic? *Am J Obstet Gynecol* 204:479–87.
6. Sivan, E., Homko, C.J., Chen, X., Reece, E.A., and Boden, G. 1999. Effect of Insulin on Fat Metabolism during and after Normal Pregnancy. *Diabetes* 48:834–38.
7. Kalhan, S.C., D'Angelo, L.J., Savin, S.M., and Adam, P.A. 1979. Glucose Production in Pregnant Women at Term Gestation. Sources of Glucose for Human Fetus. *J Clin Invest* 63:388–94.
8. Kalhan, S., Rossi, K., Gruca, L., Burkett, E., and O'Brien, A. 1997. Glucose Turnover and Gluconeogenesis in Human Pregnancy. *J Clin Invest* 100:1775–81.
9. Catalano, P.M., Kirwan, J.P., Hauguel-de Mouzon, S., and King, J. 2003. Gestational Diabetes and Insulin Resistance: Role in Short- and Long-Term Implications for Mother and Fetus. *J Nutr* 133:1674S–83S.
10. Getahun, D., Nath, C., Ananth, C.V., Chavez, M.R., and Smulian, J.C. 2008. Gestational Diabetes in the United States: Temporal Trends 1989 through 2004. *Am J Obstet Gynecol* 198:525 e1–5.
11. Ferrara, A. 2007. Increasing Prevalence of Gestational Diabetes Mellitus: A Public Health Perspective. *Diabetes Care* 30(Suppl 2):S141–46.
12. Boden, G., and Shulman, G.I. 2002. Free Fatty Acids in Obesity and Type 2 Diabetes: Defining Their Role in the Development of Insulin Resistance and Beta-Cell Dysfunction. *Eur J Clin Invest* 32:14–23.
13. Catalano, P.M. 2010. Obesity, Insulin Resistance, and Pregnancy Outcome. *Reproduction* 140:365–71.
14. Xiang, A.H., Peters, R.K., Trigo, E., Kjos, S.L., Lee, W.P., and Buchanan, T.A. 1999. Multiple Metabolic Defects during Late Pregnancy in Women at High Risk for Type 2 Diabetes. *Diabetes* 48:848–54.
15. Homko, C., Sivan, E., Chen, X., Reece, E.A., and Boden, G. 2001. Insulin Secretion during and after Pregnancy in Patients with Gestational Diabetes Mellitus. *J Clin Endocrinol Metab* 86:568–73.
16. **Barbour, L.A., McCurdy, C.E., Hernandez, T.L., Kirwan, J.P., Catalano, P.M., and Friedman, J.E. 2007. Cellular Mechanisms for Insulin Resistance in Normal Pregnancy and Gestational Diabetes. *Diabetes Care* 30:S112–19.** *A comprehensive review on cellular mechanisms of insulin resistance in normal pregnancy and GDM.*
17. Brelje, T.C., Scharp, D.W., Lacy, P.E., Ogren, L., Talamantes, F., Robertson, M., Friesen, H.G., and Sorenson, R.L. 1993. Effect of Homologous Placental Lactogens, Prolactins, and Growth Hormones on Islet B-Cell Division and Insulin Secretion in Rat, Mouse, and Human Islets: Implication for Placental Lactogen Regulation of Islet Function during Pregnancy. *Endocrinology* 132:879–87.
18. Beck, P., and Daughaday, W.H. 1967. Human Placental Lactogen: Studies of Its Acute Metabolic Effects and Disposition in Normal Man. *J Clin Invest* 46:103–10.

19. Ryan, E.A., and Enns, L. 1988. Role of Gestational Hormones in the Induction of Insulin Resistance. *J Clin Endocrinol Metab* 67:341–47.
20. Richardson, A.C., and Carpenter, M.W. 2007. Inflammatory Mediators in Gestational Diabetes Mellitus. *Obstet Gynecol Clin North Am* 34:213–24.
21. Calleja-Agius, J., Muttukrishna, S., and Jauniaux, E. 2012. The Role of Tumor Necrosis Factor-Receptors in Pregnancy with Normal and Adverse Outcome. *Int J Interferon Cytokine Mediator Res* 4:1–15.
22. **Hauguel-de Mouzon, S., and Guerre-Millo, M. 2006. The Placenta Cytokine Network and Inflammatory Signals. *Placenta* 27:794–98.** *A review focused on the placental cytokine network and the cross talk between inflammation and metabolism pathways in pregnancy complicated by obesity or diabetes.*
23. **Radaelli, T., Uvena-Celebrezze, J., Minium, J., Huston-Presley, L., Catalano, P., and Hauguel-de Mouzon, S. 2006. Maternal Interleukin-6: Marker of Fetal Growth and Adiposity. *J Soc Gynecol Invest* 13:53–57.** *An original paper showing a strong association between increased foetal adiposity and maternal cytokine IL-6.*
24. Briana, D.D., and Malamitsi-Puchner, A. 2010. The Role of Adipocytokines in Fetal Growth. *Ann N Y Acad Sci* 1205:82–87.
25. Lappas, M., Permezel, M., and Rice, G.E. 2004. Release of Proinflammatory Cytokines and 8-Isoprostane from Placenta, Adipose Tissue, and Skeletal Muscle from Normal Pregnant Women and Women with Gestational Diabetes Mellitus. *J Clin Endocrinol Metab* 89:5627–33.
26. Kahn, S.E., Zinman, B., Haffner, S.M., O'Neill, M.C., Kravitz, B.G., Yu, D., Freed, M.I., Herman, W.H., Holman, R.R., Jones, N.P., Lachin, J.M., Viberti, G.C., and ADOPT Study Group. 2006. Obesity Is a Major Determinant of the Association of C-Reactive Protein Levels and the Metabolic Syndrome in Type 2 Diabetes. *Diabetes* 55:2357–64.
27. Kriketos, A.D., Greenfield, J.R., Peake, P.W., Furler, S.M., Denyer, G.S., Charlesworth, J.A., and Campbell, L.V. 2004. Inflammation, Insulin Resistance, and Adiposity: A Study of First-Degree Relatives of Type 2 Diabetic Subjects. *Diabetes Care* 27:2033–40.
28. Retnakaran, R., Hanley, A.J., Raif, N., Connelly, P.W., Sermer, M., and Zinman, B. 2003. C-Reactive Protein and Gestational Diabetes: The Central Role of Maternal Obesity. *J Clin Endocrinol Metab* 88:3507–12.
29. Wolf, M., Sandler, L., Hsu, K., Vossen-Smirnakis, K., Ecker, J.L., and Thadhani, R. 2003. First-Trimester C-Reactive Protein and Subsequent Gestational Diabetes. *Diabetes Care* 26:819–24.
30. Chen, X., Scholl, T.O., and Stein, T.P. 2006. Association of Elevated Serum Ferritin Levels and the Risk of Gestational Diabetes Mellitus in Pregnant Women: The Camden Study. *Diabetes Care* 29:1077–82.
31. Qiu, C., Sorensen, T.K., Luthy, D.A., and Williams, M.A. 2004. A Prospective Study of Maternal Serum C-Reactive Protein (CRP) Concentrations and Risk of Gestational Diabetes Mellitus. *Paediatr Perinat Epidemiol* 18:377–84.
32. Income, Earnings, and Poverty Data from the 2007 American Community Survey (online). 2008. Available from http:www.census.gov/prod/2008pubs/acs-09.pdf.
33. **Chen, X., Scholl, T.O., Leskiw, M., Savaille, J., and Stein, T.P. 2010. Differences in Maternal Circulating Fatty Acid Composition and Dietary Fat Intake in Women with Gestational Diabetes Mellitus or Mild Gestational Hyperglycemia. *Diabetes Care* 33:2049–54.** *Original paper that indicates the presence of elevated serum free fatty acid concentrations and composition in both GDM and gestational hyperglycaemia is less severe than overt GDM in multiethnic minority pregnant women.*
34. Scholl, T.O., and Chen, X. 2009. Increased Inflammatory Response in Women with Mild Gestational Hyperglycemia. Paper presented at the 69th American Diabetes Association Scientific Sessions, New Orleans, LA.

35. Krakoff, J., Funahashi, T., Stehouwer, C.D., Schalkwijk, C.G., Tanaka, S., Matsuzawa, Y., Kobes, S., Tataranni, P.A., Hanson, R.L., Knowler, W.C., and Lindsay, R.S. 2003. Inflammatory Markers, Adiponectin, and Risk of Type 2 Diabetes in the Pima Indian. *Diabetes Care* 26:1745–51.

36. Tan, K.C., Xu, A., Chow, W.S., Lam, M.C., Ai, V.H., Tam, S.C., and Lam, K.S. 2004. Hypoadiponectinemia Is Associated with Impaired Endothelium-Dependent Vasodilation. *J Clin Endocrinol Metab* 89:765–69.

37. Duncan, B.B., Schmidt, M.I., Pankow, J.S., Bang, H., Couper, D., Ballantyne, C.M., Hoogeveen, R.C., and Heiss, G. 2004. Adiponectin and the Development of Type 2 Diabetes: The Atherosclerosis Risk in Communities Study. *Diabetes* 53:2473–78.

38. Williams, M.A., Qiu, C., Muy-Rivera, M., Vadachkoria, S., Song, T., and Luthy, D.A. 2004. Plasma Adiponectin Concentrations in Early Pregnancy and Subsequent Risk of Gestational Diabetes Mellitus. *J Clin Endocrinol Metab* 89:2306–11.

39. Ranheim, T., Haugen, F., Staff, A.C., Braekke, K., Harsem, N.K., and Drevon, C.A. 2004. Adiponectin Is Reduced in Gestational Diabetes Mellitus in Normal Weight Women. *Acta Obstet Gynecol Scand* 83:341–47.

40. Tsai, P.J., Yu, C.H., Hsu, S.P., Lee, Y.H., Huang, I.T., Ho, S.C., and Chu, C.H. 2005. Maternal Plasma Adiponectin Concentrations at 24 to 31 Weeks of Gestation: Negative Association with Gestational Diabetes Mellitus. *Nutrition* 21:1095–99.

41. Chen, X., Scholl, T.O., and Stein, T.P. 2012. Hypoadiponectinemia during Pregnancy: Association with Risk of Varying Degrees of Gestational Hyperglycemia and with Maternal Ethnicity. *J Diabetes Mellitus* 2:196–202.

42. **Shulman, G.I. 2000. Cellular Mechanisms of Insulin Resistance.** *J Clin Invest* **106:171–76.** *A comprehensive review on recent advances in understanding of cellular mechanisms of human insulin resistance and the mechanisms of free fatty acid-induced insulin resistance.*

43. Yamashita, H., Shao, J. and Friedman, J.E. 2000. Physiologic and Molecular Alterations in Carbohydrate Metabolism during Pregnancy and Gestational Diabetes Mellitus. *Clin Obstet Gynecol* 43:87–98.

44. Buchanan, T.A., Xiang, A., Kjos, S.L., and Watanabe, R. 2007. What Is Gestational Diabetes? *Diabetes Care* 30:S105–11.

45. Shao, J., Catalano, P.M., Yamashita, H., Ishizuka, T., and Friedman, J.E. 2000. Vanadate Enhances but Does Not Normalize Glucose Transport and Insulin Receptor Phosphorylation in Skeletal Muscle from Obese Women with Gestational Diabetes Mellitus. *Am J Obstet Gynecol* 183:1263–70.

46. Tomazic, M., Janez, A., Sketelj, A., Kocijancic, A., Eckel, J., and Sharma, P.M. 2002. Comparison of Alterations in Insulin Signalling Pathway in Adipocytes from Type II Diabetic Pregnant Women and Women with Gestational Diabetes Mellitus. *Diabetologia* 45:502–8.

47. Shah, P., Vella, A., Basu, A., Basu, R., Adkins, A., Schwenk, W.F., Johnson, C.M., Nair, K.S., Jensen, M.D., and Rizza, R.A. 2003. Elevated Free Fatty Acids Impair Glucose Metabolism in Women: Decreased Stimulation of Muscle Glucose Uptake and Suppression of Splanchnic Glucose Production during Combined Hyperinsulinemia and Hyperglycemia. *Diabetes* 52:38–42.

48. King, J.C. 2006. Maternal Obesity, Metabolism, and Pregnancy Outcomes. *Annu Rev Nutr* 26:271–91.

49. Randle, P.J., Garland, P.B., Hales, C.N., and Newsholme, E.A. 1963. The Glucose Fatty-Acid Cycle. Its Role in Insulin Sensitivity and the Metabolic Disturbances of Diabetes Mellitus. *Lancet* 1:785–89.

50. McLachlan, K.A., Boston, R., and Alford, F.P. 2005. Impaired Non-Esterified Fatty Acid Suppression to Intravenous Glucose during Late Pregnancy Persists Postpartum in Gestational Diabetes: A Dominant Role for Decreased Insulin Secretion Rather Than Insulin Resistance. *Diabetologia* 48:1373–79.

51. Corkey, B.E. 2012. Banting Lecture 2011: Hyperinsulinemia: Cause or Consequence? *Diabetes* 61:4–13.
52. Chen, X., and Scholl, T.O. 2005. Oxidative Stress: Changes in Pregnancy and with Gestational Diabetes Mellitus. *Curr Diabetes Rep* 5:282–88.
53. Toescu, V., Nuttall, S.L., Martin, U., Nightingale, P., Kendall, M.J., Brydon, P., and Dunne, F. 2004. Changes in Plasma Lipids and Markers of Oxidative Stress in Normal Pregnancy and Pregnancies Complicated by Diabetes. *Clin Sci (London)* 106:93–98.
54. Chen, X., Scholl, T.O., Leskiw, M.J., Donaldson, M.R., and Stein, T.P. 2003. Association of Glutathione Peroxidase Activity with Insulin Resistance and Dietary Fat Intake during Normal Pregnancy. *J Clin Endocrinol Metab* 88:5963–68.
55. Pi, J., Bai, Y., Zhang, Q., Wong, V., Floering, L.M., Daniel, K., Reece, J.M., Deeney, J.T., Andersen, M.E., Corkey, B.E., and Collins, S. 2007. Reactive Oxygen Species as a Signal in Glucose-Stimulated Insulin Secretion. *Diabetes* 56:1783–91.
56. Ervin, R.B. 2009. Prevalence of Metabolic Syndrome among Adults 20 Years of Age and over, by Sex, Age, Race and Ethnicity, and Body Mass Index: United States, 2003–2006. *Natl Health Stat Report* 13:1–7.
57. Cossrow, N., and Falkner, B. 2004. Race/Ethnic Issues in Obesity and Obesity-Related Comorbidities. *J Clin Endocrinol Metab* 89:2590–94.
58. Ku, C.Y., Gower, B.A., Hunter, G.R., and Goran, M.I. 2000. Racial Differences in Insulin Secretion and Sensitivity in Prepubertal Children: Role of Physical Fitness and Physical Activity. *Obes Res* 8:506–15.
59. Chen, X., and Scholl, T.O. 2002. Ethnic Differences in C-Peptide/Insulin/Glucose Dynamics in Young Pregnant Women. *J Clin Endocrinol Metab* 87:4642–46.
60. Desoye, G., and Hauguel-de Mouzon, S. 2007. The Human Placenta in Gestational Diabetes Mellitus. The Insulin and Cytokine Network. *Diabetes Care* 30:S120–26.
61. Hay, W.W., Jr. 2006. Placental-Fetal Glucose Exchange and Fetal Glucose Metabolism. *Trans Am Clin Climatol Assoc* 117:321–39.
62. Beaudoin, A.R. 1983. The Effect of Aminothiadiazole on Glycogenesis and Glycogenolysis in Fetal and Neonatal Rat Liver. *Teratology* 28:369–74.
63. Ballard, F.J., and Oliver, I.T. 1965. Carbohydrate Metabolism in Liver from Foetal and Neonatal Sheep. *Biochem J* 95:191–200.
64. Hay, W.W., Jr. 2006. Recent Observations on the Regulation of Fetal Metabolism by Glucose. *J Physiol* 572:17–24.
65. Jansson, T., and Powell, T.L. 2000. Placental Nutrient Transfer and Fetal Growth. *Nutrition* 16:500–2.
66. Bauer, M.K., Harding, J.E., Bassett, N.S., Breier, B.H., Oliver, M.H., Gallaher, B.H., Evans, P.C., Woodall, S.M., and Gluckman, P.D. 1998. Fetal Growth and Placental Function. *Mol Cell Endocrinol* 140:115–20.
67. Holmes, R., Montemagno, R., Jones, J., Preece, M., Rodeck, C., and Soothill, P. 1997. Fetal and Maternal Plasma Insulin-Like Growth Factors and Binding Proteins in Pregnancies with Appropriate or Retarded Fetal Growth. *Early Hum Dev* 49:7–17.
68. Hill, D.J., Petrik, J., and Arany, E. 1998. Growth Factors and the Regulation of Fetal Growth. *Diabetes Care* 21(Suppl 2):B60–69.
69. Higgins, M., and McAuliffe, F. 2010. A Review of Maternal and Fetal Growth Factors in Diabetic Pregnancy. *Curr Diabetes Rev* 6:116–25.
70. Lacroix, M.C., Guibourdenche, J., Frendo, J.L., Muller, F., and Evain-Brion, D. 2002. Human Placental Growth Hormone—A Review. *Placenta* 23:S87–94.
71. Handwerger, S., and Freemark, M. 2000. The Roles of Placental Growth Hormone and Placental Lactogen in the Regulation of Human Fetal Growth and Development. *J Pediatr Endocrinol Metab* 13:343–56.

72. Barbour, L.A., Shao, J., Qiao, L., Pulawa, L.K., Jensen, D.R., Bartke, A., Garrity, M., Draznin, B., and Friedman, J.E. 2002. Human Placental Growth Hormone Causes Severe Insulin Resistance in Transgenic Mice. *Am J Obstet Gynecol* 186:512–17.
73. Haig, D. 2008. Placental Growth Hormone-Related Proteins and Prolactin-Related Proteins. *Placenta* 29:S36–41.
74. Boyne, M.S., Thame, M., Bennett, F.I., Osmond, C., Miell, J.P., and Forrester, T.E. 2003. The Relationship among Circulating Insulin-Like Growth Factor (IGF)-I, IGF-Binding Proteins-1 and -2, and Birth Anthropometry: A Prospective Study. *J Clin Endocrinol Metab* 88:1687–91.
75. Pratipanawatr, T., Pratipanawatr, W., Rosen, C., Berria, R., Bajaj, M., Cusi, K., Mandarino, L., Kashyap, S., Belfort, R., and DeFronzo, R.A. 2002. Effect of IGF-I on FFA and Glucose Metabolism in Control and Type 2 Diabetic Subjects. *Am J Physiol Endocrinol Metab* 282:E1360–68.
76. Clemmons, D.R. 2004. The Relative Roles of Growth Hormone and IGF-1 in Controlling Insulin Sensitivity. *J Clin Invest* 113:25–27.
77. Jensen, E.C., Harding, J.E., Bauer, M.K., and Gluckman, P.D. 1999. Metabolic Effects of Igf-I in the Growth Retarded Fetal Sheep. *J Endocrinol* 161:485–94.
78. Bauer, M.K., Breier, B.B., Bloomfield, F.H., Jensen, E.C., Gluckman, P.D., and Harding, J.E. 2003. Chronic Pulsatile Infusion of Growth Hormone to Growth-Restricted Fetal Sheep Increases Circulating Fetal Insulin-Like Growth Factor-I Levels but Not Fetal Growth. *J Endocrinol* 177:83–92.
79. Wauters, M., Considine, R.V., and Van Gaal, L.F. 2000. Human Leptin: From an Adipocyte Hormone to an Endocrine Mediator. *Eur J Endocrinol* 143:293–311.
80. Forhead, A.J., and Fowden, A.L. 2009. The Hungry Fetus? Role of Leptin as a Nutritional Signal before Birth. *J Physiol* 587:1145–52.
81. Zhang, J., and Bowes, W.A., Jr. 1995. Birth-Weight-for-Gestational-Age Patterns by Race, Sex, and Parity in the United States Population. *Obstet Gynecol* 86:200–8.
82. Brenner, W.E., Edelman, D.A., and Hendricks, C.H. 1976. A Standard of Fetal Growth for the United States of America. *Am J Obstet Gynecol* 126:555–64.
83. Mello, G., Parretti, E., Mecacci, F., Lucchetti, R., Lagazio, C., Pratesi, M., and Scarselli, G. 1997. Risk Factors for Fetal Macrosomia: The Importance of a Positive Oral Glucose Challenge Test. *Eur J Endocrinol* 137:27–33.
84. Ostlund, I., Hanson, U., Björklund, A., Hjertberg, R., Eva, N., Nordlander, E., Swahn, M.L., and Wager, J. 2003. Maternal and Fetal Outcomes if Gestational Impaired Glucose Tolerance Is Not Treated. *Diabetes Care* 26:2107–11.
85. Bo, S., Menato, G., Gallo, M.L., Bardelli, C., Lezo, A., Signorile, A., Gambino, R., Cassader, M., Massobrio, M., and Pagano, G. 2004. Mild Gestational Hyperglycemia, the Metabolic Syndrome and Adverse Neonatal Outcomes. *Acta Obstet Gynecol Scand* 83:335–40.
86. Gruendhammer, M., Brezinka, C., and Lechleitner, M. 2003. The Number of Abnormal Plasma Glucose Values in the Oral Glucose Tolerance Test and the Feto-Maternal Outcome of Pregnancy. *Eur J Obstet Gynecol Reprod Biol* 108:131–36.
87. Ricart, W., López, J., Mozas, J., Pericot, A., Sancho, M.A., González, N., Balsells, M., Luna, R., Cortázar, A., Navarro, P., Ramírez, O., Flández, B., Pallardo, L.F., Hernández, A., Ampudia, J., Fernández-Real, J.M., Corcoy, R., and Spanish Group for the Study of the Impact of Carpenter and Coustan GDM Thresholds. 2005. Potential Impact of American Diabetes Association (2000) Criteria for Diagnosis of Gestational Diabetes Mellitus in Spain. *Diabetologia* 48:1135–41.
88. Ray, J.G., Vermeulen, M.J., Shapiro, J.L., and Kenshole, A.B. 2001. Maternal and Neonatal Outcomes in Pregestational and Gestational Diabetes Mellitus, and the Influence of Maternal Obesity and Weight Gain: The Deposit Study. Diabetes Endocrine Pregnancy Outcome Study in Toronto. *QJM* 94:347–56.

89. Ehrenberg, H.M., Mercer, B.M., and Catalano, P.M. 2004. The Influence of Obesity and Diabetes on the Prevalence of Macrosomia. *Am J Obstet Gynecol* 191:964–68.

90. Catalano, P.M., Thomas, A., Huston-Presley, L., and Amini, S.B. 2007. Phenotype of Infants of Mothers with Gestational Diabetes. *Diabetes Care* 30:S156–60.

91. Hattersley, A.T. 2006. Beyond the Beta Cell in Diabetes. *Nat Genet* 38:12–13.

92. Pedersen, J. 1954. Weight and Length at Birth of Infants of Diabetic Mothers. *Acta Endocrinol (Copenh)* 16:330–42.

93. Ogonowski, J., Miazgowski, T., Czeszyńska, M.B., Jaskot, B., Kuczyńska, M., and Celewicz, Z. 2008. Factors Influencing Risk of Macrosomia in Women with Gestational Diabetes Mellitus Undergoing Intensive Diabetic Care. *Diabetes Res Clin Pract* 80:405–10.

94. Murphy, H.R., Rayman, G., Lewis, K., Kelly, S., Johal, B., Duffield, K., Fowler, D., Campbell, P.J., and Temple, R.C. 2008. Effectiveness of Continuous Glucose Monitoring in Pregnant Women with Diabetes: Randomised Clinical Trial. *BMJ* 337:a1680.

95. Scholl, T.O., Sowers, M., Chen, X., and Lenders, C. 2001. Maternal Glucose Concentration Influences Fetal Growth, Gestation, and Pregnancy Complications. *Am J Epidemiol* 154:514–20.

96. Scholl, T.O., Chen, X., Khoo, C.S., and Lenders, C. 2004. The Dietary Glycemic Index during Pregnancy: Influence on Infant Birth Weight, Fetal Growth, and Biomarkers of Carbohydrate Metabolism. *Am J Epidemiol* 159:467–74.

97. Chen, X., Scholl, T.O., Steer, R.A. and Stein, T.P. 2011. Gestational Hyperglycemia, Excessive Pregnancy Weight Gain and Risk of Fetal Overgrowth. In *Gestational Diabetes*, ed. M. Radenkovic, chap. 13. InTech open-access publisher.

98. Chen, X, and Scholl, T.O. 2008. Mild Maternal Hyperglycemia Increases Risk of Fetal Overgrowth in Minority Pregnant Women: Camden Study. Paper presented at the 68th American Diabetes Association Scientific Sessions, San Francisco, CA.

99. **Catalano, P.M., McIntyre, H.D., Cruickshank, J.K., McCance, D.R., Dyer, A.R., Metzger, B.E., Lowe, L.P., Trimble, E.R., Coustan, D.R., Hadden, D.R., Persson, B., Hod, M., and Oats, J.J.; for the HAPO Study Cooperative Research Group. 2012. The Hyperglycemia and Adverse Pregnancy Outcome Study: Associations of GDM and Obesity with Pregnancy Outcomes.** *Diabetes Care* 35:780–86. *An original paper demonstrating that both maternal GDM and obesity are independently associated with adverse pregnancy outcomes in the HAPO study.*

100. HAPO Study Cooperative Research Group. 2010. Hyperglycaemia and Adverse Pregnancy Outcome (HAPO) Study: Associations with Maternal Body Mass Index. *BJOG* 117:575–84.

101. Jones, H.N., Woollett, L.A., Barbour, N., Prasad, P.D., Powell, T.L., and Jansson, T. 2009. High-Fat Diet before and during Pregnancy Causes Marked Up-Regulation of Placental Nutrient Transport and Fetal Overgrowth in C57/BL6 Mice. *FASEB J* 23:271–78.

102. Oken, E., Kleinman, K.P., Belfort, M.B., Hammitt, J.K., and Gillman, M.W. 2009. Associations of Gestational Weight Gain with Short- and Longer-Term Maternal and Child Health Outcomes. *Am J Epidemiol* 170:173–80.

103. Kiel, D.W., Dodson, E.A., Artal, R., Boehmer, T.K., and Leet, T.L. 2007. Gestational Weight Gain and Pregnancy Outcomes in Obese Women: How Much Is Enough? *Obstet Gynecol* 110:752–58.

104. DeVader, S.R., Neeley, H.L., Myles, T.D., and Leet, T.L. 2007. Evaluation of Gestational Weight Gain Guidelines for Women with Normal Prepregnancy Body Mass Index. *Obstet Gynecol* 110:745–51.

105. Institute of Medicine. 2009. *Weight Gain during Pregnancy: Reexamining the Guidelines*. Washington, DC: National Academies Press. Available from http://www.nap.edu/catalog/12584.html.

106. Paoloni-Giacobino, A. 2007. Epigenetics in Reproductive Medicine. *Pediatr Res* 61:51R–57R.
107. Pinney, S.E., and Simmons, R.A. 2012. Metabolic Programming, Epigenetics, and Gestational Diabetes Mellitus. *Curr Diabetes Rep* 12:67–74.
108. Fernández-Morera, J.L., Rodríguez-Rodero, S., Menéndez-Torre, E., and Fraga, M.F. 2010. The Possible Role of Epigenetics in Gestational Diabetes: Cause, Consequence, or Both. *Obstet Gynecol Int*, article 605163.
109. Cooney, C.A., Dave, A.A. and Wolff, G.L. 2002. Maternal Methyl Supplements in Mice Affect Epigenetic Variation and DNA Methylation of Offspring. *J Nutr* 132:2393S–400S.
110. Lillycrop, K.A., Phillips, E.S., Jackson, A.A., Hanson, M.A., and Burdge, G.C. 2005. Dietary Protein Restriction of Pregnant Rats Induces and Folic Acid Supplementation Prevents Epigenetic Modification of Hepatic Gene Expression in the Offspring. *J Nutr* 135:1382–86.
111. Heijmans, B.T., Tobi, E.W., Stein, A.D., Putter, H., Blauw, G.J., Susser, E.S., Slagboom, P.E., and Lumey, L.H. 2008. Persistent Epigenetic Differences Associated with Prenatal Exposure to Famine in Humans. *Proc Natl Acad Sci U S A* 105:17046–49.
112. Gicquel, C., El-Osta, A., and Le Bouc, Y. 2008. Epigenetic Regulation and Fetal Programming. *Best Pract Res Clin Endocrinol Metab* 22:1–16.
113. Gluckman, P.D., and Hanson, M.A. 2008. Developmental and Epigenetic Pathways to Obesity: An Evolutionary-Developmental Perspective. *Int J Obes* 32:S62–71.
114. Yajnik, C.S. 2010. Fetal Programming of Diabetes: Still So Much to Learn! *Diabetes Care* 33:1146–48.
115. Catalano, P.M., Presley, L., Minium, J., and Hauguel-de Mouzon, S. 2009. Fetuses of Obese Mothers Develop Insulin Resistance In Utero. *Diabetes Care* 32:1076–80.
116. Langer, O., Yogev, Y., Most, O., and Xenakis, E.M. 2005. Gestational Diabetes: The Consequences of Not Treating. *Am J Obstet Gynecol* 192:989–97.
117. Retnakaran, R., Zinman, B., Connelly, P.W., Sermer, M., and Hanley, A.J. 2006. Impaired Glucose Tolerance of Pregnancy Is a Heterogeneous Metabolic Disorder as Defined by the Glycemic Response to the Oral Glucose Tolerance Test. *Diabetes Care* 29:57–62.
118. Sermer, M., Naylor, C.D., Gare, D.J., Kenshole, A.B., Ritchie, J.W.K., Farine, D., Cohen, H.R., McArthur, K., Holzapfel, S., Biringer, A., Chen, E., and Toronto Tri-Hospital Gestational Diabetes Investigators. 1995. Impact of Increasing Carbohydrate Intolerance on Maternal-Fetal Outcomes in 3637 Women without Gestational Diabetes. The Toronto Tri-Hospital Gestational Diabetes Project. *Am J Obstet Gynecol* 173:146–56.
119. Roberts, R.N., Moohan, J.M., Foo, R.L., Harley, J.M., Traub, A.I., and Hadden, D.R. 1993. Fetal Outcome in Mothers with Impaired Glucose Tolerance in Pregnancy. *Diabet Med* 10:438–43.
120. World Health Organisation. 1999. Definition, Diagnosis and Classification of Diabetes Mellitus and Its Complications. Available from http://whqlibdoc.who.int/hq/1999/who_ncd_ncs_99.2.pdf.
121. Dabelea, D., Snell-Bergeon, J.K., Hartsfield, C.L., Bischoff, K.J., Hamman, R.F., McDuffie, R.S., and Kaiser Permanente of Colorado GDM Screening Program. 2005. Increasing Prevalence of Gestational Diabetes Mellitus (GDM) over Time and by Birth Cohort: Kaiser Permanente of Colorado GDM Screening Program. *Diabetes Care* 28:579–84.
122. King, H. 1998. Epidemiology of Glucose Intolerance and Gestational Diabetes in Women of Childbearing Age. *Diabetes Care* 21:B9–13.
123. Sacks, D.A., Hadden, D.R., Maresh, M., Deerochanawong, C., Dyer, A.R., Metzger, B.E., Lowe, L.P., Coustan, D.R., Hod, M., Oats, J.J., Persson, B., Trimble, E.R., and HAPO Study Cooperative Research Group. 2012. Frequency of Gestational Diabetes

Mellitus at Collaborating Centers Based on IADPSG Consensus Panel-Recommended Criteria: The Hyperglycemia and Adverse Pregnancy Outcome (HAPO) Study. *Diabetes Care* 35:526–28.

124. England, L.J., Dietz, P.M., Njoroge, T., Callaghan, W.M., Bruce, C., Buus, R.M., and Williamson, D.F. 2009. Preventing Type 2 Diabetes: Public Health Implications for Women with a History of Gestational Diabetes Mellitus. *Am J Obstet Gynecol* 200:365 e1–e8.

125. Pettitt, D.J., Baird, H.R., Aleck, K.A., Bennett, P.H., and Knowler, W.C. 1983. Excessive Obesity in Offspring of Pima Indian Women with Diabetes during Pregnancy. *N Engl J Med* 308:242–45.

126. Clausen, T.D., Mathiesen, E.R., Hansen, T., Pedersen, O., Jensen, D.M., Lauenborg, J., and Damm, P. 2008. High Prevalence of Type 2 Diabetes and Pre-Diabetes in Adult Offspring of Women with Gestational Diabetes Mellitus or Type 1 Diabetes: The Role of Intrauterine Hyperglycemia. *Diabetes Care* 31:340–46.

127. Han, S., Crowther, C.A., and Middleton, P. 2012. Interventions for Pregnant Women with Hyperglycaemia Not Meeting Gestational Diabetes and Type 2 Diabetes Diagnostic Criteria. *Cochrane Database Syst Rev* 1:CD009037.

128. **HAPO Study Cooperative Research Group, Metzger, B.E., Lowe, L.P., Dyer, A.R., Trimble, E.R., Chaovarindr, U., Coustan, D.R., Hadden, D.R., McCance, D.R., Hod, M., McIntyre, H.D., Oats, J.J., Persson, B., Rogers, M.S., and Sacks, D.A. 2008. Hyperglycemia and Adverse Pregnancy Outcomes. *N Engl J Med* 358:1991–2002.** *An original paper demonstrating strong and continuous associations between adverse pregnancy outcomes and various degrees of maternal glucose intolerance less severe than that in overt GDM in the HAPO study.*

129. HAPO Study Cooperative Research Group. 2009. Hyperglycemia and Adverse Pregnancy Outcome (HAPO) Study: Associations with Neonatal Anthropometrics. *Diabetes* 58:453–59.

130. International Association of Diabetes and Pregnancy Study Groups Consensus Panel, Metzger, B.E., Gabbe, S.G., Persson, B., Buchanan, T.A., Catalano, P.A., Damm, P., Dyer, A.R., Leiva, A., Hod, M., Kitzmiler, J.L., Lowe, L.P., McIntyre, H.D., Oats, J.J., Omori, Y., and Schmidt, M.I. 2010. International Association of Diabetes and Pregnancy Study Groups Recommendations on the Diagnosis and Classification of Hyperglycemia in Pregnancy. *Diabetes Care* 33:676–82.

2 What Is Gestational Diabetes?

Robert Lindsay
BHF Glasgow Cardiovascular Research Centre,
University of Glasgow, Glasgow, United Kingdom

CONTENTS

ABBREVIATIONS

ACHOIS	Australian Carbohydrate Intolerance Study in Pregnant Women
HAPO	Hyperglycaemia and Pregnancy Outcomes
HbA1c	Haemoglobin A1c
IADPSG	International Association of Diabetes and Pregnancy Study Groups
MFMU	Maternal–Fetal Medicine Units Network
NICE	National Institute for Health and Care Excellence
OGCT	Oral glucose challenge test
OGTT	Oral glucose tolerance test
RDS	Respiratory distress syndrome
SIGN	Scottish Intercollegiate Guidelines Network
TTN	Transient tachypnoea of the newborn
WHO	World Health Organisation

2.1   INTRODUCTION

Over many years the literature in gestational diabetes has been made complex by different definitions and testing strategies between different countries and often within countries. A major division internationally existed between those countries, like the United States, who followed a pattern of screening and testing ultimately derived from the National Diabetes Data Group (NDDG), and those following a pattern derived from the World Health Organisation (WHO). Broadly, the NDDG suggested a pattern of universal screening with 50 g oral glucose challenge test (OGCT), followed by 100 g oral glucose tolerance test (OGTT) and diagnostic criteria ultimately derived from the work of O'Sullivan and Mahan. WHO promoted a pattern of risk factor screening, diagnostic testing with the 75 g OGTT, and criteria initially reflecting diagnostic levels for diabetes and impaired glucose tolerance in the nonpregnant population.[1] Within these two broad schools there was further variation between countries in screening and diagnostic levels. Inevitably, this resulted in publications and clinic populations with different degrees of glucose abnormality and differing rates of complications. Comparisons between and interpretation of research studies proved difficult.

Beyond this, and perhaps partly because of this, the validity of gestational diabetes as a diagnosis has been challenged, although this is now changing with new trials showing the benefit of diagnosis and treatment. In this chapter I will summarise briefly how the diagnosis of gestational diabetes developed historically, highlight some of the important differences between gestational diabetes and preexisting diabetes in pregnancy, and discuss current attempts to unify diagnosis under the International Association of Diabetes and Pregnancy Study Groups (IADPSG). Finally, I will discuss what general principles might underpin the diagnosis of gestational diabetes and argue that considering gestational diabetes mellitus (GDM) as a risk factor rather than disease might be the best way of allowing clinicians and patients to come to terms with this difficult diagnosis (Figure 2.1).

2.2 GESTATIONAL DIABETES: A BRIEF HISTORY

Earliest clinical recognition of the importance of diabetes and pregnancy was dominated by the very poor outcomes of pregnancy in women with preexisting diabetes. Until the discovery of insulin in the 1920s, isolated case reports and small case series noted dismal outcomes of diabetes complicating pregnancy, with very high maternal and foetal mortality and high rates of ketoacidosis. Even after onset of use of insulin it took some decades for the numbers of cases to increase and outcomes to improve markedly. The vast majority of these women likely had established or early type 1 diabetes. Hadden has elegantly recorded what is likely to be the first historical case of what would now be termed gestational diabetes.[2] He found a case report of a woman recorded in 1823 with new onset thirst and glycosuria during a pregnancy and subsequent delivery of a macrosomic baby.

Interestingly, two important concepts arrived relatively early in the 20th century. That foetal macrosomia and adverse pregnancy outcomes could reflect a "prediabetic" state—and therefore that outcomes such as macrosomia might predict later development of diabetes in mother. Second, glucose tolerance was influenced by the pregnant state itself. It was only in the 1950s that the first major prospective studies of carbohydrate metabolism in pregnancy were carried out.[3,4] In a seminal study in 1964 O'Sullivan and Mahan measured glucose tolerance in 752 women during pregnancy and assessed perinatal mortality and later maternal glucose tolerance.[5] O'Sullivan and Mahan first defined a normal range for glucose values fasting and at 1, 2, and 3 h after a 100 g glucose load. They published cutoffs based on values 2

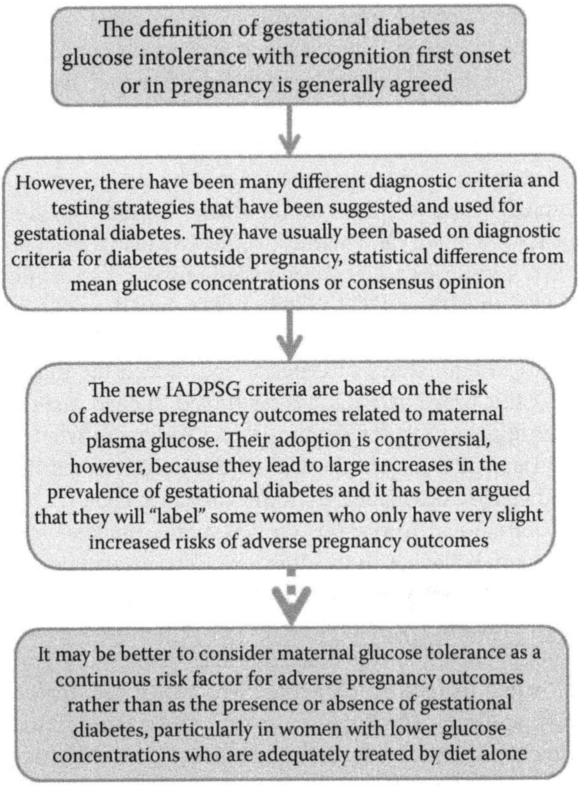

The definition of gestational diabetes as glucose intolerance with recognition first onset or in pregnancy is generally agreed

However, there have been many different diagnostic criteria and testing strategies that have been suggested and used for gestational diabetes. They have usually been based on diagnostic criteria for diabetes outside pregnancy, statistical difference from mean glucose concentrations or consensus opinion

The new IADPSG criteria are based on the risk of adverse pregnancy outcomes related to maternal plasma glucose. Their adoption is controversial, however, because they lead to large increases in the prevalence of gestational diabetes and it has been argued that they will "label" some women who only have very slight increased risks of adverse pregnancy outcomes

It may be better to consider maternal glucose tolerance as a continuous risk factor for adverse pregnancy outcomes rather than as the presence or absence of gestational diabetes, particularly in women with lower glucose concentrations who are adequately treated by diet alone

FIGURE 2.1   A summary of important factors relating to the question, "What is gestational diabetes?"

standard deviations above the mean at each of these times and defined women who had two or more raised values as having abnormal glucose tolerance.[5] This comprised around 3–4% of the pregnant population, and in later work, they showed that this group had a fourfold increase in perinatal mortality[6] and an increase in maternal diabetes up to 16 years later.[7] This work, with various later modifications for the assay techniques used, was to form the basis of diagnosis of gestational diabetes, at least in the United States, for over 40 years, and in some cases, to the present day.

At the end of the 1960s the term *gestational diabetes* was used by Pedersen and others,[2] but it was only toward the end of the 1970s that there was a move to formalise diagnostic criteria for gestational diabetes (along with diabetes more generally) by bodies both in the United States (the National Diabetes Data Group (NDDG)) and internationally under WHO. The work of the NDDG was also influenced by the International Workshop Conference on Gestational Diabetes held in 1979. This was the first of several consensus workshops. It was agreed that the definition of *gestational diabetes* was "glucose intolerance with recognition of onset during pregnancy." Agreement was reached that women should be universally screened in pregnancy, and that all women should have a measure of plasma glucose after the 24th week of pregnancy (if not already known to have diabetes). Notably, however, there was no agreement on the glucose load to be used or timing or type of blood sample for screening. Consensus was reached at the conference at least on use of a 100 g glucose load, 3 h oral glucose tolerance test interpreted by O'Sullivan criteria.

The reports of the NDDG in 1979 and WHO in 1980 led to largely concordant definitions of diabetes for those who were not pregnant. However, the WHO report suggested that diabetes and pregnancy be defined by the proposed criteria for diabetes and impaired glucose tolerance (at the time, ≥7.8 mmol/L (140 mg/dl) fasting and ≥11.1 mmol/L (200 mg/dl) at 2 h after the glucose load). By contrast, the NDDG (following the first consensus pattern) supported universal screening with 50 g glucose challenge test, the 100 g OGTT and criteria based on the O'Sullivan paper (Table 2.1). This is of more than simple historical interest because, while there have been modifications to both states of criteria (and indeed the diagnosis of diabetes out of pregnancy), this broad division has continued. Indeed, the two influential trials of "mild" gestational diabetes diagnosis and treatment from Crowther et al.[16] in Australia and Landon et al.[17] in the United States, published in 2005 and 2009, respectively, used criteria descended from this broad division (v.i.).

Subsequent international workshops on gestational diabetes in 1984, 1990, and 1998 made incremental changes to the diagnosis. The second conference consensus formalised use of the 50 g oral glucose challenge for diagnosis and use of a venous plasma cutoff of 140 mg/dl (7.8 mmol/L) for entry into the formal screening test.[18] In addition, formal recognition was made that the definition of gestational diabetes allowed for and would include those women who likely had unrecognised diabetes before the index pregnancy. The third conference noted other factors likely to influence outcome, including maternal obesity, ethnicity, past obstetric experience, and family history. In 1998 the WHO formalised its definition of gestational diabetes, stating that "gestational diabetes is carbohydrate intolerance resulting in hyperglycaemia of variable severity with onset or first recognition during pregnancy."[1] Again, this overtly included the important group of women with probable preexisting diabetes. Diagnostic criteria were revised for diabetes outwith pregnancy (to venous plasma glucose ≥ 7.0 mmol/L (126 mg/dl) fasting and ≥ 11.1 mmol/L (200 mg/dl) at 2 h after the glucose load).[1] The definition of gestational diabetes as a combination of the out-of-pregnancy groups of diabetes and impaired glucose tolerance was retained, albeit with this new fasting level. The WHO also effectively supported a risk factor-based approach rather than universal screening. It was recommended that a 75 g OGTT be used in women at "high risk for gestational diabetes," namely, those with a "history of large for gestational age babies, women from certain high-risk ethnic groups, and any pregnant woman who has elevated fasting, or casual, blood."

Finally, it can be noted that various other groups internationally have adopted their own modifications of these two broad approaches. For example, in Scotland the Scottish Intercollegiate Guidelines Network in 2001 supported a fasting glucose of >5.5 mmol/L (99 mg/dl) and >9 mmol/L (162 mg/dl) at 2 h. The Australian Diabetes in Pregnancy Society had a similar approach with ≥5.5 and ≥9 mmol/L at 2 h, although even here lower 2 h values were used in New Zealand (≥8 mmol/L (144 mg/dl)).

TABLE 2.1

Commonly Used Venous Plasma Glucose Concentration Cutoffs for Diagnosing Gestational Diabetes Using an Oral Glucose Tolerance Test[a]

Organisation	Glucose Load (g)	Fasting (mmol/L (mg/dl))	1 h Post-Glucose Load (mmol/L (mg/dl))	2 h Post-Glucose Load (mmol/L (mg/dl))	3 h Post-Glucose Load (mmol/L (mg/dl))	Reference
National Diabetes Data Group	100	5.8 (105)	10.6 (190)	9.2 (165)	8.1 (145)	8
American Diabetes Association (Carpenter and Coustan)	100	5.3 (95)	10.0 (180)	8.6 (155)	7.8 (140)	9, 10
World Health Organisation (1980 guidelines)	75	7.8 (140)	—	11.1 (200)	—	11
World Health Organisation (current (1999) guidelines)	75	7.0 (126)	—	7.8 (140)	—	12
European Association for the Study of Diabetes	75	6.0 (108)	—	9.0 (162)	—	13
Australasian Diabetes in Pregnancy Society	75	5.5 (99)	—	8.0 (144)	—	14
International Association of the Diabetes in Pregnancy Study Groups	75	5.1 (92)	10.0 (180)	8.5 (153)	—	15

Note: Gestational diabetes is generally diagnosed when one value is equal to or exceeds these values, except for the National Diabetes Data Group and American Diabetes Group criteria, where two or more values have to be met or exceeded.

[a] Some of these criteria are preceded by a 50 g glucose challenge with a cutoff of around 7.8 mmol/L (140 mg/dl).

Unsurprisingly, this web of different definitions and screening policies caused (and still causes) much confusion. In the early part of this century there was scepticism amongst several screening and obstetric groups about the diagnosis of gestational diabetes, notably in Canada and the UK,[19] and certainly no settled opinion over the best means of screening for and diagnosis of gestational diabetes. A number of factors have changed and led to revision of at least some of these earlier opinions.[20] Data from large-scale trials of diagnosis and treatment of gestational diabetes have defined the benefits of treatment.[16,17] The multinational Hyperglycaemia and Adverse Pregnancy Outcome (HAPO) study has explored the relationship of maternal glucose to pregnancy outcomes on an unprecedented scale, including over 23,000 women across nine countries.[21] This has led to a consensus effort led by the International Association of Diabetes and Pregnancy Study Groups (IADPSG) to achieve an agreed international pattern of screening and diagnosis published in 2010.[15] At present, it is not possible to define easily what current guidelines are, as these still differ between countries; however, several countries and the WHO in its most recent technical report on the subject[22] have adopted the IADPSG criteria, although these criteria have also been criticised.[23] Because of the influence of these guidelines, it is worth detailing them and the process by which they were developed, but first we will consider similarities and contrasts between diabetes first recognised in pregnancy and diabetes known and diagnosed before pregnancy.

2.3   GESTATIONAL AND PREGESTATIONAL DIABETES

Preexisting diabetes is associated with a broad range of complications for mother and child (Table 2.2). Similarities and contrasts between gestational and pregestational diabetes will depend on differences in the biochemical abnormality—with women with pregestational diabetes, at least potentially, having more abnormal blood glucose values on average—the effects of the stage of gestation at which these complications develop, and finally, the competing effects of long-term complications of diabetes. As detailed above, to some extent these divisions may be blurred due to the presence of women with existing but undiagnosed diabetes who are, by most definitions, included as gestational diabetes when the disease is first recognised in pregnancy.

One important contrast between gestational and pregestational diabetes comes in early pregnancy. Pregestational diabetes is associated with an increased risk of congenital anomalies. There is a three- to fivefold increased incidence in congenital anomalies relative to the general population that has shown little change over recent years,[24,25] with a similar increase in risk in mothers with type 1 and type 2 diabetes.[24] A linear relationship between haemoglobin A1c (HbA1c) concentrations and malformation rates has been reported, with poor glycaemic control in the pre- and early post-conception period being critical to subsequent malformation risk.[26] By contrast, the effect of gestational diabetes on congenital anomaly is controversial. A meta-analysis of available studies in 2009 concluded that there was a small but significant 20–40% increase in risk of major congenital anomalies—a much smaller effect than that seen in pregestational diabetes.[27] This will be influenced by the prevalence of undiagnosed diabetes in early pregnancy and effects of obesity and potentially other associated risk factors, including alcohol, smoking, and diet, leaving remaining

---

TABLE 2.2

Adverse Outcomes in Offspring of Mothers with Pregestational Diabetes

Biochemical

Hypocalcaemia

Polycythaemia and hyperviscosity

Hyperbilirubinaemia

Hypoglycaemia/hyperinsulinaemia

Diseases of Prematurity

Respiratory distress syndrome

Transient tachypnoea of the newborn

Growth and Development

Congenital anomalies

Foetal overgrowth

Increased adiposity

Growth restriction

Hypertrophic cardiomyopathy

Mortality

Increased perinatal mortality: Stillbirth and neonatal death

Late Effects

Offspring obesity

Impaired glucose tolerance, type 2 diabetes

---

influences of gestational diabetes per se uncertain, but probably very modest apart from effects of associated conditions and risk factors.

Babies born to mothers with pregestational diabetes are also prone to a range of changes in growth and biochemical abnormalities believed ultimately to be dependent on exposure to excess maternal glucose in later pregnancy and potentially mediated by foetal hyperinsulinaemia (Table 2.2). Numerous studies have delineated the association of gestational diabetes, variously defined, with foetal overgrowth.[28] The HAPO study, discussed below, has examined these relationships in detail, showing a clear relationship of maternal glucose across the reference range to foetal growth,[21] including foetal adiposity,[7,29] as well as cord blood C-peptide concentrations at birth.[21] Intervention studies have shown a reduction in foetal overgrowth with detection and treatment of gestational diabetes[16,17] (Table 2.3). Foetal overgrowth may cause obstetric concern in later pregnancy for a variety of reasons. There are increased risks of shoulder dystocia, obstructed labour, instrumented delivery, and caesarean section, with the potential for subsequent intrapartum compromise well described. Birth trauma, including brachial plexus injuries and similar nerve palsies, is also more frequent in macrosomic infants. An increase in shoulder dystocia is also described in gestational diabetes, and a reduction in the rate of shoulder dystocia is suggested in one of the two main studies of treatment of mild gestational diabetes.[16] It should be

TABLE 2.3

Relative Risk for Adverse Outcomes in ACHOIS and MFMU

	ACHOIS	MFMU
Primary outcome	↓ 0.33 (0.14–0.75) (p = 0.01)	↔ 0.87 (0.72–1.07) (p = NS)
Large for gestational age	↓ 0.62 (0.47–0.81) (p < 0.001)	↓ 0.49 (32–0.76) (p < 0.001)
Macrosomia birth weight > 4 kg	↓ 0.47 (0.34–0.64) (p < 0.001)	↓ 0.41 (0.26–0.66) (p < 0.001)
Neonatal fat mass	—	↓ (p = 0.003)
NICU admission	↑ 1.13 (1.03–1.23) (p = 0.04)	↔ 0.77 (0.51–1.18) (p = NS)
Shoulder dystocia	↔ 0.46 (0.19–1.10) (p = NS)	↓ 0.37 (0.14–0.97) (p = 0.02)
Induction	↑ 1.36 (1.15–1.62) (p < 0.001)	↔ 1.02 (0.81–1.29) (p = NS)
Preeclampsia	↓ 0.70 (0.51–0.95) (p = 0.02)	↓ 0.46 (0.22–0.97) (p = 0.02)
Caesarean section	↔ 0.97 (0.81–1.16) (p = NS)	↓ 0.79 (0.64–0.99) (p = 0.02)

Note: All figures are given as the relative risk (95% confidence intervals) in the intervention vs. control arms of the respective studies. ACHOIS, Australian Carbohydrate Intolerance Study; MFMU, Maternal–Fetal Medicine Units; NICU, neonatal intensive care unit; NS, not significant.

noted that the low rates of shoulder dystocia in this study and difficulty in clinically defining this make this a controversial result.[16] Caesarean section rates are increased by around 20–40% in women with gestational diabetes.[30] While reduction in foetal growth on treatment might be expected to reduce the need for caesarean section, there has been long-term concern that labelling a woman as having gestational diabetes might serve to paradoxically increase section rates.[30] Importantly then, the two large recent trials of treatment of gestational diabetes suggested either no change[16] or a decrease[17] in rates of caesarean section. This suggests at least the possibility that clinical effects of treatment to reduce foetal growth might result in reduced rates in certain clinical contexts.

Other abnormalities at birth include increases in respiratory distress in the form of either transient tachypnoea of the newborn (TTN) or relative surfactant deficiency of respiratory distress syndrome (RDS). This predominantly relates to earlier delivery in response to the recognised risk of late intrauterine death, but may also be increased as a function of maternal diabetes per se.[32] Similar effects would be expected in gestational diabetes, again relating to time of delivery. Offspring of mothers with pregestational diabetes also have increased risk of neonatal hypoglycaemia, neonatal hypocalcaemia, and polycythaemia[33] and jaundice[21] in the form of unconjugated hyperbilirubinaemia. Both bilirubin and neonatal hypoglycaemia relate to maternal glucose in the HAPO study,[21] but responses to treatment of neonatal jaundice, hypoglycaemia, and respiratory distress are less clear in intervention studies—although this may relate to relatively small numbers of cases.[16,17]

At the most severe end of the spectrum of complications, maternal type 1 and type 2 diabetes are associated with increased rates of perinatal mortality, with increases in both stillbirth and early neonatal death.[24] Meta-analyses have shown no significant increase in perinatal mortality in gestational diabetes.[28] It should be noted that some national surveys have shown an increase,[34] and this is one area where the underlying prevalence of undiagnosed pregestational diabetes may be having an important effect. In the studies of detection and treatment of mild gestational diabetes there was no significant effect on stillbirth or perinatal mortality, as there were no stillbirths in one of the studies[17] and very low rates of stillbirth or neonatal death in the other study, albeit concentrated in the nonintervention group.[16]

Offspring of mothers with pregestational diabetes have also been described from the 1940s as having cardiomegaly or cardiac hypertrophy. This hypertrophy appears to relate to maternal glycaemia control and foetal hyperinsulinaemia.[35] Generalised myocardial hypertrophy is the norm with disproportionate thickening of the ventricular septum. Severe hypertrophy with intermittent occlusion of the left ventricular outflow tract is required before clinical sequelae, which can result in intrauterine or neonatal death. The condition appears to be transient, with symptoms resolving by 4 weeks with complete regression of ventricular septal hypertrophy by 12 months or earlier without later-life sequelae[36]—equivalent rates in contemporary series in gestational diabetes are not known.

Maternal pregestational diabetes is also associated with worsening of complications, most notably retinopathy[37] and nephropathy. Apart from a very tiny number of women with previously undiagnosed diabetes long-standing enough to have caused complications, this should not be a major consideration in gestational diabetes. Maternal diabetes is also associated with increased risk of preeclampsia, particularly in the presence of nephropathy.[30] Gestational diabetes is also associated with an approximately 70% increase in risk of preeclampsia.[28] This is particularly important, as detection and treatment of gestational diabetes are also associated with a reduction in this risk[16,17] (Table 2.3).

Finally, maternal diabetes has also been suggested to increase the risk of obesity and type 2 diabetes in their offspring.[38,39] These late-life effects are usually suggested to reflect in utero "programming" by aspects of the intrauterine environment, most likely hyperglycaemia. This is an important area, as while effects are best described in mothers with pregestational diabetes, such an influence in gestational diabetes would, because of the greater numbers involved, have a much larger public health impact. As described in early studies in the Pima Indian population, it appears clear that offspring of mothers with type 2 diabetes have an increase in adiposity and altered glucose tolerance.[38,39] Studies of mothers with type 2 diabetes have the potential for confounding by shared propensity to diabetes and obesity between mother and child; however, the presence of similar effects in offspring of mothers with type 1 diabetes[40,41] suggests that programming effects are occurring. Data for offspring of mothers with gestational diabetes are less clear—in part as the glycaemic programming effect might be expected to be more modest, and the potential confounders of maternal risk of type 2 diabetes and obesity are present. Longer-term follow-up of children born to mothers in the HAPO study[42] and intervention studies may clarify this with time.[43]

2.4   IADPSG CRITERIA

The adverse consequences of gestational diabetes have been known for some time, but the relationship of maternal glycaemia to pregnancy outcomes has been most clearly delineated by the multinational, multicentre HAPO study. This study examined over 23,000 women with glucose tolerance short of frank diabetes in pregnancy. Thus, women were included if fasting glucose was less than 5.8 mmol/L (104 mg/dl) and 2 h glucose was less than 11.1 mmol/L (200 mg/dl). Notably around 1.7% of women were *not* included in the study because of a raised fasting or 2 h value at baseline. A further 1.2% of women were omitted from the study due to raised random glucose (above 8.9 mmol/L (160 mg/dl)) later in pregnancy. These mothers were excluded as the results of blood glucose in the HAPO study were otherwise blinded, and it was felt unethical to not transmit results at this level to clinicians to start treatment. Thus, the HAPO population excludes both women with known pregestational diabetes and potentially 2.9% of the normal population with the highest glucose levels during pregnancy.

The HAPO study has indicated a continuous relationship of fasting, and 1 and 2 h glucose after a 75 g OGTT with a variety of pregnancy outcomes. For the primary outcomes of the HAPO study there was a continuous graded relationship with likelihood of macrosomia, cord C-peptide > 90th percentile, clinical neonatal hypoglycaemia, and caesarean section.[21] Later publications from the HAPO study indicated a continuous relationship of maternal glucose with neonatal adiposity[29] and weaker relationships with neonatal glycaemia.[44]

The HAPO investigators also examined a range of other important outcomes. Of these secondary outcomes, shoulder dystocia and preeclampsia were positively associated with maternal fasting and post-challenge blood glucose, while preterm delivery, hyperbilirubinaemia, and intensive neonatal care were related to post-challenge but not fasting glucose concentrations.[21] The study was not powered for, and did not show, any significant relationship with perinatal mortality—perhaps reflecting the exclusion of mothers at the highest level of blood glucose.[21]

The findings from HAPO are largely in keeping with previous results in the literature. Most notably, there has not been a convincing relationship of gestational diabetes to stillbirth or perinatal mortality in the past, with only a few studies suggesting such a relationship.[28,34]

2.5   WHAT IS GESTATIONAL DIABETES
(OR WHAT SHOULD IT BE?)

As will be apparent from much of the above discussion, there is still not a settled definition of gestational diabetes. More optimistically, there does seem to be substantial progress toward this and important new data that will inform this diagnosis. As a background, gestational diabetes has now been included among those conditions whose advocates are accused of overdiagnosing and "medicalising" parts of normal life.[45] Given that the new IADPSG criteria may increase prevalence to up to 20% of women in pregnancy, these are important concerns, and it is incumbent upon us to ensure that the diagnosis is associated both with tangible risks, as discussed above, and with clear benefits if detected and treated. A central issue is whether gestational diabetes is considered a disease or a risk factor. In current clinical practice, patients with gestational diabetes are rarely, if ever, symptomatic at the time of diagnosis, and treatment of the condition is essentially preventive. The diagnosis is made on the understanding that by intervention we can reduce adverse outcomes. In that light, perhaps the way ahead is clearer.

First, there are a group of women with high blood glucose values who benefit from immediate control of blood glucose. This is a small but important group and would include the occasional woman who is developing type 1 diabetes in pregnancy and a larger group with likely preexisting type 2 diabetes or monogenic forms of diabetes. In some of these women blood glucose can be markedly raised and, especially if antenatal glucocorticoids are used, metabolic complications such as ketoacidosis can ensue. While incident type 1 diabetes is rare, women with type 2 diabetes will be more commonly found, depending on broad risk factors, including ethnicity, rates of obesity, and age in the pregnant population, and the rate of undiagnosed type 2 diabetes in the background population. This will in turn be influenced by the presence or absence of screening programs in these groups. These women need to be diagnosed, and with effective screening and early case detection it would be hoped that rates of worsened diabetic complications and stillbirth in this group can be kept to a minimum.

The second, much larger group is those for whom gestational diabetes will act purely as a risk factor. That risk factor could be for immediate pregnancy outcomes for mother or child (preeclampsia, macrosomia, shoulder dystocia, caesarean section), long-term outcome for mother (predominantly longer-term type 2 diabetes), and longer-term outcomes for child (obesity and type 2 diabetes). While the latter two outcomes may be of great importance, it is important to concentrate on the immediate pregnancy outcomes.

In this regard we begin to have a stronger ground in considering a framework for the diagnosis. The HAPO study gives a clear relationship of maternal glucose as a risk factor to a number of outcomes (macrosomia, caesarean section). It should be noted that there was not a significant relationship with perinatal mortality or stillbirth.[21] At the same time, it is not sufficient to simply identify a risk factor to justify screening, but for gestational diabetes we can now identify that detection and treatment broadly are associated with improved outcomes. There is an issue. In the diagnosis of diabetes outwith pregnancy, diagnostic levels are based on increased risk of microvascular screening.[1] While there may be debate over the precise levels, and these have been revised with time, epidemiologic data would support this and suggest the presence of thresholds above which the patient is at risk of development of diabetic retinopathy and nephropathy. By contrast, the HAPO study has demonstrated a continuous relationship of maternal glucose to risk.[21] In that light, any cutoff point will be subject to debate and will require close scrutiny as to its predictive power. The IADPSG criteria have been criticised on a number of grounds. One frequent criticism is that the numbers of women are simply too high. While this might be a very real immediate practical concern, it does not bear greater scrutiny—where there is evidence of cost-effective benefit to patients, this should generally be applied independent of the numbers involved.

A second concern is that the cutoff for diagnosis is too low when considered in terms of risks and benefits to the woman. The IADPSG criteria were set with an increased rate of complications of 1.75-fold.[15] This is not arbitrary but could clearly be set at different levels capturing, as is clear from the HAPO study, different levels of risk. These arguments have been highlighted by Ryan,[23] suggesting an alternative set of cutoff points based around a twofold increase in complications and concomitantly fewer women with the diagnosis. Advocates of this approach also point to the relatively low reproducibility of the oral glucose tolerance test.[23] As background to this, it should be noted that while in Europe prevalence of gestational diabetes is likely 2–6%,[46] even these more "conservative" criteria are projected to result in 10% of the population being classed as having gestational diabetes. Most of this debate should be determined by how great a risk women at lower levels of blood glucose are and how great the benefit they will have from treatment. It might be noted that the rates of large for gestational age babies born to women diagnosed using the IADPSG criteria (16.2%) are similar to those in the untreated arms of the two main intervention studies (Crowther 22%, Landon 14.5%), suggesting that similar patient groups are involved. Neither study maps exactly to patients selected by IADPSG criteria, allowing much debate on whether this is the right level of risk. At the same time, the presence of the largely positive results of these studies renders a blinded study involving a control group without intervention potentially unethical.

As part of this debate it is also often noted that other risk factors, notably obesity, may be as or more important. This is apparent within the HAPO data set,[47] but it is also the case that we now have evidence-based interventions for maternal glucose without equivalent interventions for maternal obesity.

Finally, there is concern that the diagnosis leads to harm—either by increasing medical interventions such as caesarean section[31] or admission of babies to special care or neonatal units, or by causing anxiety in mothers. As noted above, the most recent studies suggest no change or even a decrease in caesarean section rates with diagnosis,[16,17] although there is still an increase in admission to neonatal units in at least one of the studies.[16,17] What is notable about these issues is that they are as much about the clinical culture of how women and their risks are perceived after a diagnosis of gestational diabetes. Crowther et al. looked carefully at women's mood and quality of life after diagnosis with gestational diabetes and found an improvement overall in the intervention group.[16] It is also noticeable that the great majority (80–90%) of women in these studies of mild gestational diabetes could be managed by dietary intervention alone.[16,17] This then may be the crux of how gestational diabetes should be considered in the future. If both women and clinicians can approach gestational diabetes—particularly in those women with lower levels of glucose who are adequately treated with diet alone—as a risk factor that does not lead to unnecessary clinical intervention and with positive effects on the mother's outlook, as is at least possible in the available studies,[16] then extension of the diagnosis may be supported.

REFERENCES

Key references are in bold.

1. World Health Organisation. 1999. *Definition, diagnosis and classification of diabetes mellitus and its complications*. Geneva: World Health Organisation.
2. Hadden, D.R. 1998. A historical perspective on gestational diabetes. *Diabetes Care* 21(Suppl. 2):B3–4.
3. Wilkerson, H.L, and Remein, Q.R. 1957. Studies of abnormal carbohydrate metabolism in pregnancy; the significance of impaired glucose tolerance. *Diabetes* 6:324–29.
4. Hoet, J.P., and Lukens, F.D. 1954. Carbohydrate metabolism during pregnancy. *Diabetes* 3:1–12.
5. O'Sullivan, J.B., and Mahan, C.M. 1964. Criteria for the oral glucose tolerance test in pregnancy. *Diabetes* 13:278–85.
6. O'Sullivan, J.B., Charles, D., Mahan, C.M., and Dandrow, R.V. 1973. Gestational diabetes and perinatal mortality rate. *Am J Obstet Gynecol* 116:901–4.
7. O'Sullivan, J.B. 1975. Long term follow up of gestational diabetics. In *Early diabetes in early life*, ed. R.A. Camerini-Davalos and H.S. Cole, 503–19. New York: Academic Press.
8. National Diabetes Data Group. 1979. Classification and diagnosis of diabetes mellitus and other categories of glucose intolerance. *Diabetes* 28:1039–57.
9. American Diabetes Association. 2004. Clinical Practice Recommendations 2004. Diagnosis and classification of diabetes mellitus. *Diabetes Care* 27:S5–10.
10. Carpenter, M.W., and Coustan, D.R. 1982. Criteria for screening tests for gestational diabetes. *Am J Obstet Gynecol* 144:768–73.
11. WHO Expert Committee. 1980. *WHO Expert Committee on Diabetes Mellitus*. World Health Organisation Technical Report Series 646. Geneva: World Health Organisation.
12. Alberti, K.G., and Zimmet, P.Z. 1998. Definition, diagnosis and classification of diabetes mellitus and its complications. Part 1. Diagnosis and classification of diabetes mellitus provisional report of a WHO consultation. *Diabet Med* 15:539–53.
13. European Association for the Study of Diabetes. 1996. Report of the Pregnancy and Neonatal Care Group of the European Association for the Study of Diabetes. *Diabet Med* 13:S43–53.
14. Martin, F.I.R., for the Ad Hoc Working Party. 1991. The diagnosis of gestational diabetes. *Med J Aust* 155:112.
15. **Metzger, B.E., Gabbe, S.G., Persson, B., et al. 2010. International Association of Diabetes and Pregnancy Study Groups recommendations on the diagnosis and classification of hyperglycemia in pregnancy. *Diabetes Care* 33:676–82.** *Hotly debated criteria recommended for the diagnosis of gestational diabetes, based on consensus opinion following the finding from the HAPO study that there was not a glucose tolerance threshold below which there was a large reduction in glucose-associated adverse pregnancy outcomes.*
16. **Crowther, C.A., Hiller, J.E., Moss, J.R., McPhee, A.J., Jeffries, W.S., and Robinson, J.S. 2005. Effect of treatment of gestational diabetes mellitus on pregnancy outcomes. *N Engl J Med* 52:2477–86.** *A large randomised controlled trial that found that treatment of women with gestational diabetes was associated with a reduction in serious perinatal morbidity and possibly women's health-related quality of life.*
17. **Landon, M.B., Spong, C.Y., Thom, E., et al. 2009. A multicenter, randomized trial of treatment for mild gestational diabetes. *N Engl J Med* 361:1339–48.** *Another large randomised controlled trial testing the effect of treating women with mild gestational diabetes. It found that treatment reduced the risk of foetal overgrowth, shoulder dystocia, caesarean delivery, and hypertensive disorders.*

18. Gabbe, S.G. 1986. Definition, detection, and management of gestational diabetes. *Obstet. Gynecol* 67:121–25.
19. Scott, D.A., Loveman, E., McIntyre, L., and Waugh, N. 2002. Screening for gestational diabetes: a systematic review and economic evaluation. *Health Technol Assess* 6:1–161.
20. Waugh, N., Royle, P., Clar, C., et al. 2010. Screening for hyperglycaemia in pregnancy: a rapid update for the National Screening Committee. *Health Technol Assess* 14:1–183.
21. **Metzger, B.E., Lowe, L.P., Dyer, A.R., et al. 2008. Hyperglycemia and adverse pregnancy outcomes. N Engl J Med 358:1991–2002.** *Landmark multinational study detecting linear associations between glucose concentrations in pregnancy and adverse pregnancy outcomes even in the range not considered at the time to constitute gestational diabetes.*
22. **World Health Organization (WHO). (2013). Diagnostic criteria and classification of hyperglycaemia first detected in pregnancy. Available at http://apps.who. int/iris/bitstream/10665/85975/1/WHO_NMH_MND_13.2_eng.pdf. (Accessed 16 September 2013.)** *A WHO technical report assessing the usefulness of different diagnostic criteria for GDM. Whilst ultimately endorsing the IADPSG recommendations for the diagnosis of GDM, the report also separates GDM from a more hyperglycaemic category labelled "diabetes in pregnancy."*
23. **Ryan, E.A. 2011. Diagnosing gestational diabetes. Diabetologia 54:480–86.** *Thought-provoking analysis of the likely consequences of implementing the IADPSG criteria for diagnosing gestational diabetes.*
24. Macintosh, M.C., Fleming, K.M., Bailey, J.A., et al. 2006. Perinatal mortality and congenital anomalies in babies of women with type 1 or type 2 diabetes in England, Wales, and Northern Ireland: population based study. *Br Med J* 333:177.
25. Penney, G.C., Mair, G., and Pearson, D.W. 2003. Outcomes of pregnancies in women with type 1 diabetes in Scotland: a national population-based study. *BJOG* 110:315–18.
26. Guerin, A., Nisenbaum, R., and Ray, J.G. 2007. Use of maternal GHb concentration to estimate the risk of congenital anomalies in the offspring of women with prepregnancy diabetes. *Diabetes Care* 30:1920–25.
27. Balsells, M., Garcia-Patterson, A., Gich, I., and Corcoy, R. 2012. Major congenital malformations in women with gestational diabetes mellitus: a systematic review and meta-analysis. *Diabetes Metab Res Rev* 28:252–57.
28. Wendland, E.M., Torloni, M.R., Falavigna, M., et al. 2012. Gestational diabetes and pregnancy outcomes—a systematic review of the World Health Organization (WHO) and the International Association of Diabetes in Pregnancy Study Groups (IADPSG) diagnostic criteria. *BMC Pregnancy Childbirth* 12:23.
29. **HAPO Study Cooperative Research Group. 2009. Hyperglycemia and Adverse Pregnancy Outcome (HAPO) study: associations with neonatal anthropometrics. Diabetes 58:453–59.** *Further data from HAPO showing links between maternal glucose and cord blood C-peptide concentrations in pregnancy, and offspring adiposity in newborns (thus being consistent with the Pederson hypothesis).*
30. Jensen, D.M., Damm, P., Ovesen, P., et al. 2010. Microalbuminuria, preeclampsia, and preterm delivery in pregnant women with type 1 diabetes: results from a nationwide Danish study. *Diabetes Care* 33:90–94.
31. Sermer, M., Naylor, C.D., Gare, D.J., et al. 1995. Impact of increasing carbohydrate intolerance on maternal-fetal outcomes in 3637 women without gestational diabetes. The Toronto Tri-Hospital Gestational Diabetes Project. *Am J Obstet Gynecol* 173:146–56.
32. Robert, M.F., Nett, R.K., Hubbell, J.P., Taeusch, H.W., and Avery, M.E. 1976. Association between maternal diabetes and the respiratory-distress syndrome in the newborn. *N Engl J Med* 294:357–60.

33. Mimouni, F., Tsang, R.C., Hertzberg, V.S., and Miodovnik, M. 1986. Polycythemia, hypomagnesemia, and hypocalcemia in infants of diabetic mothers. *Am J Dis Child* 140:798–800.
34. Wendland, E.M., Duncan, B.B., Mengue, S.S., and Schmidt, M.I. 2011. Lesser than diabetes hyperglycemia in pregnancy is related to perinatal mortality: a cohort study in Brazil. *BMC Pregnancy Childbirth* 11:92.
35. Ullmo, S., Vial, Y., Di Bernardo, S., et al. 2007. Pathologic ventricular hypertrophy in the offspring of diabetic mothers: a retrospective study. *Eur Heart J* 28:1319–25.
36. Way, G.L., Wolfe, R.R., Eshaghpour, E., Bender, R.L., Jaffe, R.B., and Ruttenberg, H.D. 1979. The natural history of hypertrophic cardiomyopathy in infants of diabetic mothers. *J Pediatr* 95:1020–25.
37. Rasmussen, K.L., Laugesen, C.S., Ringholm, L., Vestgaard, M., Damm, P., and Mathiesen, E.R. 2010. Progression of diabetic retinopathy during pregnancy in women with type 2 diabetes. *Diabetologia* 53:1076–83.
38. Pettitt, D.J., Baird, H.R., Aleck, K.A., Bennett, P.H., and Knowler, W.C. 1983. Excessive obesity in offspring of Pima Indian women with diabetes during pregnancy. *N Engl J Med* 308:242–45.
39. Pettitt, D.J., Aleck, K.A., Baird, H.R., Carraher, M.J., Bennett, P.H., and Knowler, W.C. 1988. Congenital susceptibility to NIDDM. Role of intrauterine environment. *Diabetes* 37:622–28.
40. Lindsay, R.S., Nelson, S.M., Walker, J.D., Greene, S.A., Milne, G., Sattar, N., and Pearson, D.W. 2010. Programming of adiposity in offspring of mothers with type 1 diabetes at age 7 years. *Diabetes Care* 33:1080–85.
41. Clausen, T.D., Mathiesen, E.R., Hansen, T., Pedersen, O., Jensen, D.M., Lauenborg, J., and Damm, P. 2008. High prevalence of type 2 diabetes and pre-diabetes in adult offspring of women with gestational diabetes mellitus or type 1 diabetes: the role of intrauterine hyperglycemia. *Diabetes Care* 31:340–46.
42. Pettitt, D.J., McKenna, S., McLaughlin, C., Patterson, C.C., Hadden, D.R., and McCance, D.R. 2010. Maternal glucose at 28 weeks of gestation is not associated with obesity in 2-year-old offspring: the Belfast Hyperglycemia and Adverse Pregnancy Outcome (HAPO) family study. *Diabetes Care* 33:1219–23.
43. Gillman, M.W., Oakey, H., Baghurst, P.A., Volkmer, R.E., Robinson, J.S., and Crowther, C.A. 2010. Effect of treatment of gestational diabetes mellitus on obesity in the next generation. *Diabetes Care* 33:964–68.
44. Metzger, B.E., Persson, B., Lowe, L.P., et al. 2010. Hyperglycemia and Adverse Pregnancy Outcome study: neonatal glycemia. *Pediatrics* 126:e1545–52.
45. Moynihan, R. 2011. Medicalization. A new deal on disease definition. *Br Med J* 342:d2548.
46. Buckley, B.S., Harreiter, J., Damm, P., et al. 2012. Gestational diabetes mellitus in Europe: prevalence, current screening practice and barriers to screening. A review. *Diabet Med* 29:844–54.
47. **Catalano, P.M., McIntyre, H.D., Cruickshank, J.K., et al. 2012. The Hyperglycemia and Adverse Pregnancy Outcome study: associations of GDM and obesity with pregnancy outcomes.** *Diabetes Care* **35:780–86.** *An additional paper from the HAPO study showing that maternal gestational diabetes and obesity are independently associated with adverse pregnancy outcomes, and that combined, the association is stronger than with that of either factor alone.*

Section II

Origins

3 Environmental Risk Factors for Gestational Diabetes

Eran Hadar and Moshe Hod
Helen Schneider Hospital for Women, Rabin Medical
Center, Petah Tikva, Israel, The Sackler Faculty of
Medicine, Tel Aviv University, Tel Aviv, Israel

CONTENTS

3.1 INTRODUCTION

Gestational diabetes mellitus (GDM) affects approximately 3–5% of pregnancies, and has a substantial impact on maternal, foetal, and neonatal short- and long-term health. Risk factors for GDM may be genetic or nongenetic and may exist prior to gestation or develop during pregnancy. The knowledge of risk factors for GDM is of importance to the clinician. Identifying patients at risk for GDM may impact the mode and timing of screening and diagnosis for GDM. More importantly, identifying modifiable risk factors may assist in introducing preemptive measures to prevent, or at least minimise, the occurrence of GDM for those at risk.

Previous studies have shown that positive screen results increase from 12% in women with no reported risk factors to 23–37.5% in women with a single risk factor (depending on the specific risk factor) to as high as 40% for those with multiple (≥3) risk factors.[1] The accumulation of several risk factors contributes exponentially to a higher frequency of diabetes—from 0.6% in risk-free women to as high as 33% for women with more than four risk factors accounted together.[2] Taking these facts into account may allow the treating physician to recommend a gravid woman at high risk for GDM to skip screening by the 50 g glucose challenge test (GCT), due the high probability of a positive screen result. Such women may undergo only a 75 or 100 g oral glucose challenge test (OGTT), and do so earlier in pregnancy. Better yet, some risk factors may even exist prior to pregnancy and, as such, may facilitate potential measures for risk reduction even before a woman becomes pregnant, and to be included in preconceptional recommendations.

Utilising protective and predictive factors, several authors have suggested the use of scoring systems and prediction models, in order to quantify GDM risk early in pregnancy.[3] Selective screening for GDM using four risk factors (age > 25, body mass index (BMI) > 27 kg/m^2, GDM family history, race) yields a 99.4% accuracy for diagnosis and would save screening 17% of women.[4] Other studies have constructed a prediction model using ethnicity, family history, history of GDM, and body mass index. The model had an area under the receiver operating characteristic curve of 0.77 (95% confidence interval (CI) 0.69–0.85). If an OGTT was performed in all women with a predicted probability of 2% or more, 43% of all women would be tested and 75% of the women with GDM would be identified.[5] Current American Diabetes Association (ADA) recommendations, as established at The Fifth International Workshop on GDM, recommend selective screening based on risk assessment. Low-risk women are considered those that are positive for all of the following: member of an ethnic group with a low prevalence of GDM, no known diabetes in first-degree relatives, age < 25 years, normal prepregnancy weight, normal birth weight, no history of abnormal glucose metabolism, and no history of poor obstetrical outcome. For these low-risk women no glucose testing is recommended, either by GCT, OGTT, or fasting plasma glucose. For high-risk women, blood glucose testing (either by GCT followed by OGTT or OGTT only) should be performed as soon as feasible during pregnancy. Women considered at high risk are those with severe obesity, strong family history of type 2 diabetes or previous history of GDM, impaired glucose metabolism, or glycosuria. If GDM is not diagnosed, blood glucose testing should be repeated at 24 to 28 weeks or at any time there are symptoms or signs suggestive of hyperglycaemia. Average-risk women— i.e., not low or high—should perform blood glucose testing at 24–28 weeks using either a GCT or OGTT.[6]

An important aspect of any discussion on risk factors for GDM is the risk for recurrence. McNeill et al.[7] in a retrospective longitudinal study of 651 women with GDM reported a recurrence rate of 35.6%. However, previous studies demonstrated a higher recurrence rate of 68–70%.[8–10] Contributing risk factors for GDM recurring

were parity ≥ 1,[8] BMI ≥ 30,[8,10] GDM diagnosed at ≤24 weeks,[8,9] insulin requirements,[8,9] weight gain,[8,10] interpregnancy interval of ≤24 months,[8] hospital admissions,[9] and older age.[10]

Therefore, our aim in this chapter is to discuss the environmental, nongenetic
risk factors associated with GDM. Special focus will be on maternal weight as a risk
factor for GDM and the intrauterine environment as a risk factor for future onset of
GDM, afflicting the foetus years later, as entering adulthood. It is beyond the scope
of this chapter to discuss the racial distribution of GDM, as well as familial and personal recurrence of GDM and the association between polycystic ovary syndrome
and GDM. Genetic risk factors are detailed in Chapter 4.

3.2 NONGENETIC RISK FACTORS FOR GESTATIONAL DIABETES MELLITUS

In one of the earliest, most comprehensive, and among the few prospective trials on
determinants and risk factors for GDM, Solomon et al.[11] conducted a prospective
cohort study, within the framework of the Nurses' Health Study II. They studied
14,613 nurses, aged 25–42 years, without previous diabetes. Out of the total cohort
only 722 had GDM, with a prevalence of 4.9%. The risk factors reported for GDM
included prepregnancy BMI of 25–29.9 kg/m^2 (odds ratio (OR) 2.13, 95% confidence
interval (CI) 1.65–2.74) and prepregnancy BMI ≥ 30 kg/m^2 (OR 2.90, 95% CI 2.15–
3.91). Other reported risk factors were greater weight gain in early adulthood, non-
Caucasian women, and smoking.

Since their report, multiple studies suggested the following factors to be associated with a higher risk of GDM (as summarised in Figure 3.1):

1. Older maternal age
2. Higher parity
3. Saturated fatty acid-rich diet
4. Vitamin D deficiency
5. Previous pregnancy complications:
    • Previous congenital malformations
    • Previous stillbirth
    • Previous macrosomia
    • Previous caesarean section
6. Multiple pregnancies
7. Lifestyle factors
8. Short stature
9. Maternal weight:
    • Higher prepregnancy weight
    • Higher prepregnancy BMI
    • Gestational weight gain
    • Adulthood weight gain
10. Infant of a diabetic mother
11. Foetal growth restriction

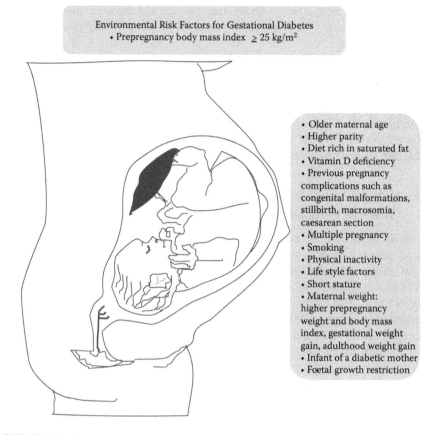

Environmental Risk Factors for Gestational Diabetes
• Prepregnancy body mass index ≥ 25 kg/m²

• Older maternal age
• Higher parity
• Diet rich in saturated fat
• Vitamin D deficiency
• Previous pregnancy complications such as congenital malformations, stillbirth, macrosomia, caesarean section
• Multiple pregnancy
• Smoking
• Physical inactivity
• Life style factors
• Short stature
• Maternal weight: higher prepregnancy weight and body mass index, gestational weight gain, adulthood weight gain
• Infant of a diabetic mother
• Foetal growth restriction

FIGURE 3.1 Summary diagram of the currently established environmental risk factors for gestational diabetes, emphasising the importance of a raised prepregnancy body mass index.

3.2.1 OLDER MATERNAL AGE

One of the best-studied and well-documented risk factors for GDM is older maternal age. Multiple studies[1,12–17] have shown that older maternal age is a risk factor for GDM, with age cutoffs ranging from 30 to 35, and up to 40 years of age. The average age gap between a gravid diabetic and a nondiabetic pregnant woman is approximately 2.2 years.[12,13,16] However, there is no one true age cutoff, but rather a linear continued association between maternal age and occurrence of GDM. Bo et al.[15] clearly demonstrated such a relationship in the company of an increasing prevalence of GDM with higher maternal age, starting from 0.15% in women under 20, to a 4.2% prevalence in women older than 30 (OR 2.8, 95% CI 1.9–4.3).

Jang et al.[12] studied 80 patients with GDM and 3,432 normal controls and reported that the mean age of patients with GDM was 31.7 + 4 versus 28.9 + 3.3 years in women without GDM ($p < 0.001$). In a later study[13] of 9,005 women, the same researchers similarly demonstrated a mean age of 31.1 ± 4.2 years in GDM patients versus 28.5 ± 3.4 years in normoglycaemic pregnancies. In the largest cohort to date, Jolly et al.[16] retrospectively analysed more than 385,000 singleton pregnancies and found the mean age of GDM patients to be 33.0 ± 4.8 versus 31.8 ± 4.4 years in the nondiabetic controls.

In a retrospective study of 2,574 pregnant women Jiménez-Moleón et al.[1] were able to demonstrate that 41.8% of the women with GDM were older than 30 years, and only 26.2% were younger than 25. Xiong at al.,[14] in a retrospective analysis of 111,563 deliveries in Canada, found that 22.4% of patients with GDM were older than 35, compared to only 10.3% in nondiabetic controls (OR 2.34, 95% CI 2.13–2.58). Similar results were also reported by Lao et al.[17] Pregnant women aged 35–40 are at an increased risk for GDM compared to younger women (OR 2.63, 95% CI 2.4–2.89).

3.2.2   HIGH PARITY

Several studies have shown that increasing parity is an independent risk factor for GDM, not age related.[12,13,18] As for the age factor, parity is a continuum, as shown by Egeland et al.[18] They demonstrated that the age-adjusted risks for women with two, three, or more deliveries were 1.5 (95% CI 1.2–1.9), 1.9 (95% CI 1.4–2.5), and 3.3 (95% CI 2.1–5.1), respectively, compared to women having only one delivery. Jang et al.,[12,13] in two large retrospective studies, previously described, have demonstrated that the mean parities of GDM and normal controls were 0.6 ± 0.9 and 0.4 ± 0.5, respectively ($p < 0.05$). Also, their studies demonstrated that 9.8% of women with GDM had given birth at least twice, compared to only 2.6% of the nondiabetic controls ($p < 0.001$).

3.2.3   SATURATED FATTY ACID-RICH DIET

Wijendran et al.[19] reported in a small study of 25 women lower erythrocyte polyunsaturated phospholipids in the umbilical cord vein of babies born to women with GDM. Also, women consuming a fat-rich diet, especially saturated fatty acids, are at an increased risk for deviation in glucose metabolism.[20] Fasting plasma phospholipid fatty acids are altered in women with GDM, with lower n-6 long-chain polyunsaturated fatty acids in patients with GDM, as well as lower concentrations of linoleic acid and precursors of docosahexaenoic acid (DHA).[21] Thus, the hypothesis is bidirectional and the involved mechanisms are still unclear. Insulin resistance, as in GDM, may impair the foetal metabolism of arachidonic acid (AA; 20:4n-6) and DHA (22:6n-3). Vice versa, a diet with a ratio favouring saturated fatty acids over polyunsaturated fatty acids is a predisposing factor for the onset of insulin resistance, and hence GDM. Another important aspect of this risk factor, still not elucidated, is whether intervention by a compatible diet, with or without dietary supplements, may decrease the risk. In the largest study to date, Bo et al.[15] studied 210 Caucasian women and reported that a saturated fat-rich diet is a risk factor for GDM (OR 2.0, 95% CI 1.2–3.2), as was a polyunsaturated fat-rich diet a protective factor (OR 0.85, 95% CI 0.77–0.92).

Although data are scarce and limited, it seems prudent to include recommendations for a long-chain polyunsaturated fatty acid properly balanced diet, with possible inclusion of food supplementation in women at risk or diagnosed with GDM.[22,23]

3.2.4 Vitamin D Deficiency

Available evidence, although limited and inconclusive, supports an important role of vitamin D in the glucose metabolism. Zhang et al.[24] prospectively measured vitamin D concentrations of maternal plasma in early pregnancy (16 weeks on average) in 953 pregnant women. Among the 57 women diagnosed with GDM, vitamin D levels were significantly lower than in controls (24.2 versus 30.1 ng/ml; $p < 0.001$). Approximately 33% of GDM cases, compared with 14% of controls ($p < 0.001$), had vitamin D concentrations consistent with vitamin D deficiency (defined as vitamin D lower than 20 ng/ml). The adjusted odds ratio for GDM, in the presence of vitamin D deficit, was 2.66 (95% CI 1.01–7.02), and each 5 ng/ml decrease contributed to a 1.29-fold increase in the risk (95% CI 1.05–1.60). Similar trends were reported by Parela et al.[25] in 116 women diagnosed with GDM versus 219 controls. Women with GDM had significantly lower first trimester vitamin D concentrations than normoglycaemic controls (56.3 versus 62.0 nmol/L; $p = 0.018$). After adjustment for confounders, vitamin D below the top quartile (< 73.5 nmol/L) was associated with a twofold greater likelihood of GDM (OR 2.21, 95% CI 1.19–4.13). However, other studies did not find similar associations,[26–28] suggesting that first trimester vitamin D deficiency and low first trimester vitamin D are not associated with GDM.

3.2.5 Previous Pregnancy Complications

The occurrence of pregnancy complications such as congenital malformation, intrauterine foetal death (IUFD), macrosomia, and caesarean section is also related to the risk of GDM in the following pregnancies.[2]

Jang et al.[12] reported that in patients with congenital malformations in their previous pregnancy the prevalence of GDM was 20.7%, versus only 2.4% in patients without an anomalous foetus (OR 22.5, 95% CI 4.1–21.1). In the same cohort, Jang et al.[12] also reported that a previous stillbirth is associated with a higher risk for GDM in the following pregnancy (OR 8.5, 95% CI 2.35–30.78). Similar results were also demonstrated Xiong et al.,[14] who reported that a previous neonatal death also increases the risk for GDM (OR 2.09 95% CI 1.06–1.34).

Jang et al.[12] also reported that a previous birth of a macrosomic baby is a risk factor for GDM. They found that 9.3% of GDM patients had a macrosomic baby in their previous pregnancy, compared to only 2.5% of patients who gave birth to an appropriate for age baby in their previous delivery (OR 5.8, 95% CI 1.98–17.02). Jiménez-Moleón et al.[1] also reported an odds ratio of 5.8 for GDM in women with previous delivery of a macrosomic baby. A previous caesarean section was also reported as a risk factor for GDM by Xiong et al.[14] Previous caesarean section was found in 14.8% of GDM patients and 10.1% of controls (OR 1.55, 95% CI 1.11–1.25).

3.2.6 Multiple Pregnancies

A larger placental mass is considered an important factor in the pathogenesis of GDM; however, the facts supporting this assumption are inconclusive, as can be seen in studies of multiple pregnancies. Wein et al., in a study of 61,914 singleton and

789 twin pregnancies, reported that the prevalence of GDM is 7.4% in twins versus 5.6% in singletons.[29] Schwartz et al.[30] found similar results, with a 7.7% prevalence of GDM in twins versus 4.1% in singletons. Hoskins[31] found a higher proportion of GDM in different sex twins compared to same sex twins (3,458 twin deliveries, 3.5% versus 1.6%, OR for dizygotic (DZ) compared to monozygotic (MZ) 8.6, 95% CI 3.5–21.0). Sivan et al.[32] found supporting evidence from studies in feotal reduction—103 women with triplet pregnancies versus 85 women who underwent foetal reduction from triplets to twins. Foetal reduction for triplets to twins reduced the incidence of GDM from 22.3% to 5.8%. However, other studies[33–35] have failed to demonstrate a similar association between GDM and multiple pregnancies.

3.2.7 LIFESTYLE FACTORS

Lifestyle factors, such as physical activity and inactivity, smoking, and as previously mentioned, dietary factors, are all associated with risk and protection of GDM. Zhang et al.[36] conducted a prospective cohort study amongst the participants of the Nurses' Health Study II, to assess the role of physical activity and sedentary behaviours in the development of GDM. After controlling for BMI and diet, they found a significant inverse association between vigorous activity and the risk of GDM (relative risk (RR) 0.77, 95% CI 0.69–0.94). Even among women who did not perform vigorous activity, brisk walking was associated with significant risk reduction for GDM (RR 0.66, 95% CI 0.46–0.95) compared with an easy pacing. Women who spent at least 20 h per week watching television, without physical activity, had a significantly higher GDM risk than women performing physical activity and who spent less than 2 h per week watching television (RR 2.30, 95% CI, 1.06–4.97).

In other lifestyle studies, smoking was also reported as a determinant of the occurrence of GDM.[11] These factors, as well as weight-related issues (to be discussed later in this chapter), emphasise the need to implement public health efforts to promote weight reduction, physical activity, smoking cessation, and healthy eating among all reproductive-aged women.

3.2.8 SHORT STATURE

Short stature is a risk factor for GDM, as observed in several studies, and remains an independent risk factor after adjustment for confounders. Jang et al.[12,13] demonstrated that the mean height of GDM patients is 158.1 ± 4.8 versus 159.7 ± 4.2 cm in nondiabetics. For women shorter than 157 cm the risk for developing GDM is three times greater than for women over 163 cm, corrected for age and BMI (Figure 3.2). Kousta et al.[37] have shown that women with previous GDM were shorter than women with normal gestational glucose tolerance: 162.9 ± 6.1 versus 165.3 ± 6.8 cm for European women ($p < 0.0001$) and 155.2 ± 5.4 versus 158.2 ± 6.3cm for South Asian women ($p < 0.003$). Similar results were also demonstrated by Branchtein et al.[38] in a study of 5,564 Brazilian women; a height under 150 cm was associated with a 60% increase in the risk for GDM. Ogonowski and Miazgowski[39] analysed the medical records of 1,830 Caucasian women with GDM and 1,011 healthy pregnant women. Women with GDM were significantly shorter than the healthy controls (165.7 ± 5.6

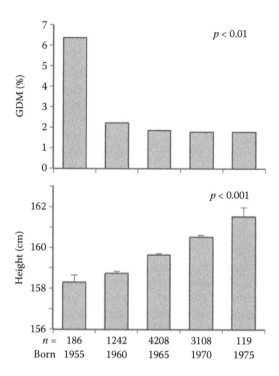

FIGURE 3.2   Age-adjusted prevalence of GDM and heights (means ± SEM) of each 5-year birth cohort. The age-adjusted prevalence of GDM was highest in the women born in 1955 (where the heights were least) and decreased rapidly as birth cohort (and women's heights) increased. (Reproduced from Jang, H.C. et al., *Diabetologia,* 41, 778–783, 1998. With kind permission from Springer Science and Business Media.)

versus 163.8 ± 6.6 cm; $p < 0.001$). The adjusted odds ratio for height was found significant, although the absolute added risk is petite (OR 0.958, 95% CI 0.94–0.97). In conclusion, women with GDM, regardless of ethnicity and BMI, are shorter than those without GDM. Although height is an independent predictor for GDM, its predictive value for identifying women at risk is relatively low and is usually not considered in the risk assessment for selective screening.

3.2.9   MATERNAL WEIGHT

The epidemic of the developed world is, without a doubt, obesity. More than one-third of the population is inflicted. Other than obesity itself, there is an outbreak of the metabolic syndrome, combining obesity with comorbidities such as diabetes, hypertension, dyslipidaemia, and insulin resistance as the underlining mechanism.[40] These are not only occurring in alarming numbers, but the onset occurs at a younger age, thus having a major impact on fertility-aged women and pregnancy.

Abundant studies have linked maternal weight to a significantly increased risk for various antepartum, intrapartum, and postpartum complications—one of which is GDM. The studies may diverge in the allocation of BMI categories, the exact definition of obesity by BMI categories, absolute weight, waist circumference, and other parameters. Also, the timing of which weight gain is addressed may be in several different time points, such as prepregnancy weight gain, gestational weight gain, adulthood weight gain, and even the prospective mother's birth weight. Still, generally speaking, the rule of thumb holds: obesity is a risk factor for diabetes, as well as other adverse pregnancy outcomes.

This information is highly important when planning a pregnancy, since the rate of GDM in obese women may be 2 to 10 times higher than in normal weight women.[41] Therefore, proper counselling for weight reduction should be offered for any women seeking pregnancy, especially for women with other concurrent risk factors for GDM.

3.2.9.1 Prepregnancy Weight as a Risk Factor for GDM

Multiple studies have linked absolute maternal weight to the risk for GDM. In two of their previously described studies, Jang et al.[12,13] have shown that the mean weight prior to pregnancy of future GDM patients was 56.4 ± 9.2 versus 51.6 ± 6.4 kg in nondiabetic controls ($p < 0.001$). In another study, Xiong et al.[14] found that 15.8% of women with GDM were obese prior to pregnancy (defined as weight ≥ 91 kg), compared to only 7.3% of normal controls (OR 2.4, 95% CI 2.06–2.98). Isaacs et al.,[42] in a retrospective study from 1994, showed that women weighing over 300 pounds have a significantly higher incidence of GDM versus a nonobese control group (mean weight 160 ± 21 pounds). Therefore, it seems that weight reduction prior to pregnancy may be beneficial.[43,44] This is indeed supported by Deitel et al.,[45] who studied 139 morbidly obese women who lost at least half of their weight via post-bariatric surgical procedures. The prevalence of GDM in these women decreased from 7% in past pregnancies to no GDM in the pregnancies that followed the weight reduction.

3.2.9.2 Gestational Weight Gain as a Risk Factor for GDM

High rates of gestational weight gain, especially during early pregnancy, may increase a woman's risk for GDM. As prepregnancy weight, it represents an important modifiable risk factor. Gestational weight gain is a significant risk factor for GDM, in all weight classes, but the association is stronger for obese patient.[46,47]

Gibson et al.[46] retrospectively assessed maternal weight gain before 24 weeks in 163 women who later developed GDM, versus 489 normoglycaemic controls. Obese and overweight women with diet-controlled and insulin-treated GDM gained significantly more weight by 24 weeks of gestation versus controls (15.6, 14.6, and 11.2 pounds, respectively). Hedderson et al.[47] estimated the relationship between gestational weight gain and the subsequent risk of GDM in 345 women with GDM and 800 controls. They concluded that the risk rises with increasing rates of gestational weight gain. Compared with the lowest tertile of gestational weight gain rate (<270 g/week), weight gains of 270–400 g/week and >400 g/week were associated with increased risk of GDM (OR 1.43, 95% CI 0.96–2.14 and OR 1.74, 95% CI 1.16–2.60, respectively).

3.2.9.3 Prepregnancy BMI as a Risk Factor for GDM

The most studied factor in the issue of maternal weight and its relation to GDM is the prepregnancy BMI (Table 3.1). Jang et al.[12,13] found that the prevalence of

TABLE 3.1

Impact of Maternal Obesity, in Various BMI Categories, on the Risk for Gestational Diabetes Mellitus

Study Reference	Year	Study Design	n	Definition of Obesity, BMI (kg/m²)	Risk for GDM
Seibre et al.[52]	2001	Retrospective	287,213	25–30	1.68
				>30	3.6
Weiss et al.[49]	2004	Prospective	16,102	30–35	2.6
				>35	4.0
Kumari et al.[50]	2001	Retrospective	188	>40	11.1
Schrauwers and Dekker[51]	2009	Retrospective	370	30–40	8.82
				>40	27.38
Solomon et al.[11]	1997	Prospective	14,613	25–30	2.13
				>30	2.9
Baeten et al.[48]	2001	Retrospective	96,801	25–30	2.4
				>30	5
Ogonowski et al.[54]	2009	Retrospective	2132	>22.85	1.91
Chu et al.[55]	2007	Meta-analysis	>500,000	25–30	2.14
				30–40	3.56
				>40	8.56
Torloni et al.[56]	2009	Meta-analysis	672,000	<20	0.75
				25–30	1.94
				30–35	3.01
				>35	5.55

GDM increases with rising BMI; 8.8% of the GDM patients were overweight (BMI > 27 kg/m²), compared to only 1.1% of controls ($p < 0.001$). Bo et al.[15] described the mean BMIs in GDM and normal controls to be 25.4 ± 5.3 and 23.6 ± 4.6 kg/m², respectively ($p < 0.02$). As previously discussed, Solomon et al.[11] found that prepregnancy BMIs 25–30 kg/m² and ≥30 kg/m² are associated with an increased risk for GDM (OR 2.13, 95% CI 1.65–2.74 and OR 2.90, 95% CI 2.15–3.91, respectively). Baeten et al.,[48] in a large population-based cohort study of 96,801 singleton nulliparous women, also found that not only obese women (BMI > 30 kg/m²) but also overweight women (BMI = 25.0–29.9 kg/m²) had a markedly increased risk for GDM (ORs 5.0 and 2.4, respectively). Weiss et al.,[49] in a large prospective study of 16,102 women, showed that obesity (BMI 30–35 kg/m²) and morbid obesity (BMI > 35 kg/m²) had a statistically significant association with GDM (ORs 2.6 and 4.0, respectively). Kumari et al.[50] studied a subgroup of morbidly obese women (BMI > 40 kg/m²) and found that the prevalence of GDM rises from 2.2% to 24.5% ($p < 0.0001$). In one of the recent studies of obesity outcomes Schrauwers and Dekker[51] retrospectively studied 370 Australian women with all BMI subclasses—overweight (BMI 25.1–30 kg/m²), obese (BMI 30.1–40 kg/m²), and morbidly obese women (BMI > 40 kg/m²). GDM occurred significantly more in classes

III and IV (ORs 8.82 and 27.38, respectively). To date, Sebire et al.[52] presented one of the largest studies of obesity's impact on pregnancy. In a study of 287,213 Londoner gravid women, overweight (BMI 25–30 kg/m^2) and obese women (BMI > 30 kg/m^2) were found to be at an increased risk for GDM (OR 1.68, 95% CI 1.53–1.84 and OR 3.6, 95% CI 3.25–3.98, respectively) as well as for several other pregnancy complications, compared to normal weight women (BMI 20–24.9 kg/m^2). Kim et al.[53] demonstrated rising prevalence of GDM by BMI category: 0.7% in underweight women (13–18.4 kg/m^2), 2.3% in normal weight women (18.5–24.9 kg/m^2), 4.8% in overweight women (25–29.9 kg/m^2), 5.5% in obese women (30–34.9 kg/m^2), and 11.5% in morbidly obese women. They calculated that the percentages of GDM attributable to overweight, obesity, and extreme obesity were 15.4% (95% CI 8.6–22.2), 9.7% (95% CI 5.2–14.3), and 21.1% (CI = 15.2–26.9), respectively. The overall population-attributable fraction was 46.2% (95% CI 36.1–56.3), suggesting that if all overweight and obese women had a GDM risk equal to that of normal weight women (BMI > 25 kg/m^2), nearly half of GDM cases could be prevented. Ogonowski et al.[54] analysed records of 1,121 GDM patients and 1,011 healthy controls. A BMI cutoff of 22.85 kg/m^2 has an odds ratio of 1.91 (95% CI 1.5–2.1), with a 47.8% sensitivity and 65.9% specificity. This implies that even for normal weight women, the risk for GDM increases with higher pregravid BMI.

Most of the above-mentioned studies were summarised in two large meta-analyses. In a 2007 meta-analysis of 20 studies incorporating more than half a million women, the risks for GDM were 2.14 (95% CI 1.82–2.53), 3.56 (3.05–4.21), and 8.56 (5.07–16.04) among overweight, obese, and severely obese women compared with normal weight pregnant women, respectively.[55] In a later meta-analysis from 2009, with approximately 672,000 women and 70 studies, the calculated odds ratio for GDM was 0.75 for underweight women (95% CI 0.69–0.82), 1.97 for overweight obese women (95% CI 1.77–2.19), 3.01 for moderately obese women (95% CI 2.34–3.87), and 5.55 for morbidly obese women (95% CI 4.27–7.21), against normal weight women. For every 1 kg/m^2 increase in BMI, the prevalence of GDM increases by 0.92%[56] (Figure 3.3).

3.2.10 Intrauterine Environment/Intergenerational Transmission of GDM

Foetal exposure to an intrauterine environment of hyperglycaemia has well-established short-term consequences. However, in recent years it has become evident that adverse outcomes may be sustained well into adulthood, and that the infants of diabetic mothers may carry a higher risk of overweight, obesity, impaired glucose tolerance, and diabetes, all associated with insulin resistance.[57] The underlying mechanisms leading to these adverse outcomes may be genetic, environmental, or due to epigenetic programming.

Environmental effects related to a higher risk of GDM include maternal hyperglycaemia, foetal growth restriction, and foetal macrosomia. Macrosomic and growth restricted foetuses are at an increased risk for future long-term onset of the metabolic syndrome, including impaired glucose tolerance and diabetes.[58–60]

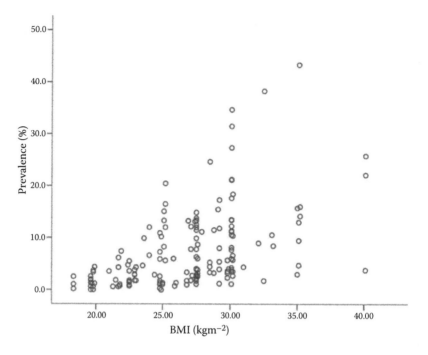

FIGURE 3.3   Prevalence of GDM according to initial maternal BMI. Fifty-six cohort studies that provided data for unadjusted odds ratio calculations (totalling inclusion of data from 631,763 women) were used to construct this graph. For each change in BMI category (corresponding to 5 kg/m^2), there was an increase of approximately 4.6% in the GDM prevalence. (Reproduced from Torloni, M.R. et al., *Obes. Rev.*, 10, 194–203, 2009. With permission.)

3.2.11   INFANT OF DIABETIC MOTHER

Freinkel, in the Banting Lecture of 1980,[61] was among the first to introduce the notion that a foetus exposed to a hyperglycaemic environment, as seen in GDM, may suffer long-term consequences and be at risk for impaired glucose tolerance, diabetes, and obesity. Crucial support to this hypothesis came in later years from several longitudinal epidemiological studies held among two populations: the Pima Indians from Arizona[62–68] and the ethnically diverse population followed at the pregnancy centre of Chicago, at the Northwesternn University.[69,70] The series of studies held on the Pima Indians population demonstrated that infants of diabetic mothers exhibit long-term consequences, such as large for gestational age (LGA), childhood obesity, adulthood obesity, and diabetes. This special population has an extremely high incidence of type 2 diabetes. The prevalence of diabetes reaches approximately 80% in offspring of diabetic mothers, compared to a lesser prevalence in infants of prediabetic mothers (i.e., mothers who will be diabetic in their following pregnancies) and nondiabetic mothers. This difference in prevalence implies that the intrauterine diabetic environment, and not merely the gene pool transferred to the foetus, is responsible for the high prevalence of diabetes to appear in childhood and adolescence. However, the intergenerational transmission of diabetes may be a combination of both inheritance of "diabetogenic genes" and the intrauterine environment. To elucidate this point, Dabelea et al.[71] studied discordant sibling pairs, i.e., one sibling born after a normoglycaemic pregnancy and the other following a pregnancy with maternal type 2 diabetes. Out of 28 compatible sibling pairs, in 21 of the pairs the diabetic sibling was born after the onset of maternal diabetes, compared to only 7 from the remaining pairs, where the diabetic sibling was born before the mother's diabetes developed (OR 3, $p < 0.01$). Thus, since siblings born before and after the onset of diabetes carry the same risk to inherit diabetogenic genes, it seems that the risk for diabetes is carried through the intrauterine hyperglycaemic environment. Studies from the Northwestern University added an important aspect to the issue. During their follow-up of diabetic women they collected third trimester amniotic fluid samples and measured concentrations of insulin. It was found that there is a correlation between insulin levels and childhood obesity. Thus, this cohort supports that the intrauterine hazardous environment is mediated through foetal hyperinsulinaemia, which is the consequence of maternal hyperglycaemia—as hypothesised by Pedersen[72] and supported by the HAPO study.[73] Suggested mechanisms speculate that foetal hyperinsulinism programs the hypothalamic centres of appetite, satiety, and energy.[74] These intrauterine alterations may lead to enhanced glucose sensitivity,[75,76] pancreatic beta-cell hyperplasia,[77,78] or impaired insulin secretion.[79,80]

3.2.12 FOETAL GROWTH RESTRICTION

Another important aspect of the intrauterine environment involves babies born growth restricted. Approximately 10% of all babies are born small for gestational age (SGA), a poorly understood and ill-defined aetiological phenomenon that remains unexplained.

Barker, in his novel hypothesis, suggested from epidemiological data that foetal growth restriction is a risk factor for the future development of type 2 diabetes, hypertension, and other insulin resistance-dependent complications.[81–83] Barker studied 407 men born between 1920 to 1930 and 266 men born between 1935 and 1943, with known birth weight and weight at 1 year of age. He found a higher prevalence of the metabolic syndrome with lower birth weight. This finding, as well as other publications, was later supported by a large meta-analysis by Newsome et al.,[84] who found that asymmetric offspring with foetal growth restriction, a larger abdominal circumference, and a brain sparing effect are more prone to long-term diabetes.

The pathogenesis is largely unknown, but it is assumed that foetal adaptation that is meant to ensure the short-term intrauterine survival of the foetus is achieved at the expense of endocrine and metabolic changes that have long-term adverse outcomes. One hypothesis is related to permanent alteration in the hypothalamic-pituitary-adrenal axis, with possible extension to the ovaries. Clark et al.[85] reported that urinary glucocorticoid excretion was higher in SGA and LGA babies versus approximately grown foetuses. This was revalidated at age 9, suggesting that the changes in the hypothalamic-pituitary-adrenal axis are long term and possibly irreversible. In contrast, Dahlgren et al.[86] did not find such a correlation between cortisol secretion at age 9 to birth weight; however, dehydroepiandrosterone sulphate (DHEAS) was inversely correlated to birth weight, suggesting a role for the adrenal gland.

REFERENCES

Key references are in bold.

1. Jiménez-Moleón, J.J., Bueno-Cavanillas, A., Luna-del-Castillo, J.D., Lardelli-Claret, P., García-Martín, M., and Gálvez-Vargas, R. 2000. Predictive value of a screen for gestational diabetes mellitus: influence of associated risk factors. *Acta Obstet Gynecol Scand* 79:991–98.
2. King, H. 1998. Epidemiology of glucose intolerance and gestational diabetes in women of childbearing age. *Diabetes Care* 21(Suppl 2):B9–13.
3. **Teede, H.J., Harrison, C.L., Teh, W.T., Paul, E., and Allan, C.A. 2011. Gestational diabetes: development of an early risk prediction tool to facilitate opportunities for prevention.** *Aust N Z J Obstet Gynaecol* **51:499–504.** *An original article developing and testing the utility of an early risk prediction tool capable of predicting those women in their first trimester of pregnancy who are most at risk of subsequently developing GDM.*
4. Davey, R.X., and Hamblin, P.S. 2001. Selective versus universal screening for gestational diabetes mellitus: an evaluation of predictive risk factors. *Med J Aust* 174:118–21.
5. **van Leeuwen, M., Opmeer, B.C., Zweers, E.J., et al. 2010. Estimating the risk of gestational diabetes mellitus: a clinical prediction model based on patient characteristics and medical history.** *BJOG* **117:69–75.** *Another clinical prediction tool for GDM based on the ethnicity, family history, history of GDM, and body mass index of pregnant women.*
6. Metzger, B.E., Buchanan, T.A., Coustan, D.R., et al. 2007. Summary and recommendations of the Fifth International Workshop—Conference on Gestational Diabetes Mellitus. *Diabetes Care* 30(Suppl 2):S251–60.
7. MacNeill, S., Dodds, L., Hamilton, D.C., Armson, B.A., and VandenHof, M. 2001. Rates and risk factors for recurrence of gestational diabetes. *Diabetes Care* 24:659–62.
8. Major, C.A., deVeciana, M., Weeks, J., and Morgan, M.A. 1998. Recurrence of gestational diabetes: who is at risk? *Am J Obstet Gynecol* 179:1038–42.
9. Spong, C.Y., Guillermo, L., Kuboshige, J., and Cabalum, T. 1998. Recurrence of gestational diabetes mellitus: identification of risk factors. *Am J Perinatol* 15:29–33.
10. Foster-Powell, K.A., and Cheung, N.W. 1998. Recurrence of gestational diabetes. *Aust N Z J Obstet Gynaecol* 38:384–87.
11. Solomon, C.G., Willett, W.C., Carey, V.J., et al. 1997. A prospective study of pregravid determinants of gestational diabetes mellitus. *JAMA* 278:1078–83.
12. Jang, H.C., Cho, N.H., Jung, K.B., Oh, K.S., Dooley, S.L., and Metzger, B.E. 1995. Screening for gestational diabetes mellitus in Korea. *Int J Gynaecol Obstet* 51:115–22.
13. Jang, H.C., Min, H.K., Lee, H.K., Cho, N.H., and Metzger, B.E. 1998. Short stature in Korean women: a contribution to the multifactorial predisposition to gestational diabetes mellitus. *Diabetologia* 41:778–83.
14. Xiong, X., Saunders, L.D., Wang, F.L., and Demianczuk, N.N. 2001. Gestational diabetes mellitus: prevalence, risk factors, maternal and infant outcomes. *Int J Gynaecol Obstet* 75:221–28.
15. Bo, S., Menato, G., Lezo, A., et al. 2001. Dietary fat and gestational hyperglycaemia. *Diabetologia* 44:972–78.
16. Jolly, M., Sebire, N., Harris, J., Robinson, S., and Regan, L. 2000. The risks associated with pregnancy in women aged 35 years or older. *Hum Reprod* 15:2433–37.
17. Lao, T.T., Chan, P.L., and Tam, K.F. 2001. Gestational diabetes mellitus in the last trimester—a feature of maternal iron excess? *Diabet Med* 18:218–23.
18. Egeland, G.M., Skjaerven, R., and Irgens, L.M. 2000. Birth characteristics of women who develop gestational diabetes: population based study. *BMJ* 321:546–47.

19. Wijendran, V., Bendel, R.B., Couch, S.C., Philipson, E.H., Cheruku, S., and Lammi-Keefe, C.J. 2000. Fetal erythrocyte phospholipid polyunsaturated fatty acids are altered in pregnancy complicated with gestational diabetes mellitus. *Lipids* 35:927–31.
20. Lichtenstein, A.H., and Schwab, U.S. 2000. Relationship of dietary fat to glucose metabolism. *Atherosclerosis* 150:227–43.
21. Wijendran, V., Bendel, R.B., Couch, S.C., et al. 1999. Maternal plasma phospholipid polyunsaturated fatty acids in pregnancy with and without gestational diabetes mellitus: relations with maternal factors. *Am J Clin Nutr* 70:53–61.
22. Loosemore, E.D., Judge, M.P., and Lammi-Keefe, C.J. 2004. Dietary intake of essential and long-chain polyunsaturated fatty acids in pregnancy. *Lipids* 39:421–24.
23. Thomas, B., Ghebremeskel, K., Lowy, C., Crawford, M., and Offley-Shore, B. 2006. Nutrient intake of women with and without gestational diabetes with a specific focus on fatty acids. *Nutrition* 22:230–36.
24. Zhang, C., Qiu, C., Hu, F.B., David, R.M., van Dam, R.M., Bralley, A., and Williams, M.A. 2008. Maternal plasma 25-hydroxyvitamin D concentrations and the risk for gestational diabetes mellitus. *PLoS One* 3:e3753.
25. Parlea, L., Bromberg, I.L., Feig, D.S., Vieth, R., Merman, E., and Lipscombe, L.L. 2012. Association between serum 25-hydroxyvitamin D in early pregnancy and risk of gestational diabetes mellitus. *Diabet Med* 29:e25–32.
26. Baker, A.M., Haeri, S., Camargo, C.A., Jr., Stuebe, A.M., and Boggess, K.A. 2012. First-trimester maternal vitamin D status and risk for gestational diabetes (GDM) a nested case-control study. *Diabetes Metab Res Rev* 28:164–68.
27. Savvidou, M.D., Akolekar, R., Samaha, R.B., Masconi, A.P., and Nicolaides, K.H. 2011. Maternal serum 25-hydroxyvitamin D levels at 11(+0)–13(+6) weeks in pregnant women with diabetes mellitus and in those with macrosomic neonates. *BJOG* 118:951–55.
28. Makgoba, M., Nelson, S.M., Savvidou, M., Messow, C.M., Nicolaides, K., and Sattar, N. 2011. First-trimester circulating 25-hydroxyvitamin D levels and development of gestational diabetes mellitus. *Diabetes Care* 34:1091–93.
29. Wein, P., Warwick, M.M., and Beischer, N.A. 1992. Gestational diabetes in twin pregnancy: prevalence and long-term implications. *Aust N Z J Obstet Gynaecol* 32:325–27.
30. Schwartz, D.B., Daoud, Y., Zazula, P., et al. 1999. Gestational diabetes mellitus: metabolic and blood glucose parameters in singleton versus twin pregnancies. *Am J Obstet Gynecol* 181:912–14.
31. Hoskins, R.E. 1995. Zygosity as a risk factor for complications and outcomes of twin pregnancy. *Acta Genet Med Gemellol (Roma)* 44:11–23.
32. Sivan, E., Maman, E., Homko, C.J., Lipitz, S., Cohen, S., and Schiff, E. 2002. Impact of fetal reduction on the incidence of gestational diabetes. *Obstet Gynecol* 99:91–94.
33. Egeland, G.M., and Irgens, L.M. 2001. Is a multiple birth pregnancy a risk factor for gestational diabetes? *Am J Obstet Gynecol* 185:1275–76.
34. Fitzsimmons, B.P., Bebbington, M.W., and Fluker, M.R. 1998. Perinatal and neonatal outcomes in multiple gestations: assisted reproduction versus spontaneous conception. *Am J Obstet Gynecol* 179:1162–67.
35. Henderson, C.E., Scarpelli, S., LaRosa, D., and Divon, M.Y. 1995. Assessing the risk of gestational diabetes in twin gestation. *J Natl Med Assoc* 87:757–58.
36. Zhang, C., Solomon, C.G., Manson, J.E., and Hu, F.B. 2006. A prospective study of pregravid physical activity and sedentary behaviors in relation to the risk for gestational diabetes mellitus. *Arch Intern Med* 166:543–48.
37. Kousta, E., Lawrence, N.J., Penny, A., Millauer, B.A., Robinson, S., Johnston, D.G., and McCarthy, M.I. 2000. Women with a history of gestational diabetes of European and South Asian origin are shorter than women with normal glucose tolerance in pregnancy. *Diabet Med* 17:792–97.

38. Branchtein, L., Schmidt, M.I., Matos, M.C., Yamashita, T., Pousada, J.M., and Duncan, B.B. 2000. Short stature and gestational diabetes in Brazil. Brazilian Gestational Diabetes Study Group. *Diabetologia* 43:848–51.

39. Ogonowski, J., and Miazgowski, T. 2010. Are short women at risk for gestational diabetes mellitus? *Eur J Endocrinol* 162:491–97.

40. World Health Organisation. 2000. Obesity: preventing and managing a global epidemic. *World Health Organization Tech Report* 894:1–4.

41. Yogev, Y., and Visser, G.H.A. 2009. Obesity, gestational diabetes and pregnancy outcome. *Semin Fetal Neonatal Med* 14:77–84.

42. Isaacs, J.D., Magann, E.F., and Martin, R.W. 1994. Obstetric challenges of massive obesity complicating pregnancy. *J Perinatol* 14:10–14.

43. American College of Obstetricians and Gynecologists. 2005. *Obesity in pregnancy*. ACOG Committee Opinion 315.

44. Galtier-Dereure, F., Boegner, C., and Bringer, J. 2000. Obesity and pregnancy: complications and cost. *Am J Clin Nutr* 71(5 Suppl):1242S–48S.

45. Deitel, M., Stone, E., Kassam, H.A., Wilk, E.J., and Sutherland, D.J. 1988. Gynecologic-obstetric changes after loss of massive excess weight following bariatric surgery. *J Am Coll Nutr* 7:147–53.

46. Gibson, K.S., Waters, T.P., and Catalano, P.M. 2012. Maternal weight gain in women who develop gestational diabetes mellitus. *Obstet Gynecol* 119:560–65.

47. Hedderson, M.M., Gunderson, E.P., and Ferrara, A. 2010. Gestational weight gain and risk of gestational diabetes mellitus. *Obstet Gynecol* 115:597–604.

48. Baeten, J.M., Bukusi, E.A., and Lambe, M. 2001. Pregnancy complications and outcomes among overweight and obese nulliparous women. *Am J Public Health* 91:436–40.

49. Weiss, J.L., Malone, F.D., Emig, D., et al. 2004. Obesity, obstetric complications and cesarean delivery rate—a population-based screening study. *Am J Obstet Gynecol* 190:1091–97.

50. Kumari, A.S. 2001. Pregnancy outcome in women with morbid obesity. *Int J Gynaecol Obstet* 73:101–7.

51. Schrauwers, C., and Dekker, G. 2009. Maternal and perinatal outcome in obese pregnant patients. *J Matern Fetal Neonatal Med* 22:218–26.

52. Sebire, N.J., Jolly, M., Harris, J.P., et al. 2001. Maternal obesity and pregnancy outcome: a study of 287,213 pregnancies in London. *Int J Obes Relat Metab Disord* 25:1175–82.

53. **Kim, S.Y., England, L., Wilson, H.G., Bish, C., Satten, G.A., and Dietz, P. 2010. Percentage of gestational diabetes mellitus attributable to overweight and obesity. *Am J Public Health* 100:1047–52.** *An original article charting the percentage of GDM attributable to overweight and obesity and showing that if the risk for GDM in overweight and obese women could be lowered to that of normal weight women, the prevalence of GDM could be almost halved.*

54. Ogonowski, J., Miazgowski, T., Kuczyńska, M., Krzyzanowska-Swiniarska, B., and Celewicz, Z. 2009. Pregravid body mass index as a predictor of gestational diabetes mellitus. *Diabet Med* 26:334–38.

55. **Chu, S.Y., Callaghan, W.M., Kim, S.Y., et al. 2007. Maternal obesity and risk of gestational diabetes mellitus. *Diabetes Care* 30:2070–76.** *A meta-analysis including more than 500,000 pregnant women, testing the association between maternal obesity and GDM.*

56. **Torloni, M.R., Betrán, A.P., Horta, B.L., et al. 2009. Prepregnancy BMI and the risk of gestational diabetes: a systematic review of the literature with meta-analysis. *Obes Rev* 10:194–203.** *An ever-larger meta-analysis including 672,000 pregnant women, testing the association between maternal obesity and GDM.*

57. Reaven, G.M. 1988. Banting Lecture 1988. Role of insulin resistance in human disease. *Diabetes* 37:1595–607.

58. Hales, C.N., and Barker, D.J. 2001. The thrifty phenotype hypothesis. *Br Med Bull* 60:5–20.
59. Barker, D.J., Eriksson, J.G., Forsen, T., and Osmond, C. 2002. Fetal origins of adult disease: strength of effects and biological basis. *Int J Epidemiol* 31:1235–39.
60. Barker, D.J., Hales, C.N., Fall, C.H., Osmond, C., Phillips, K., and Clark, P.M. 1993. Type 2 (non-insulin dependent) diabetes mellitus, hypertension and hyperlipidaemia (syndrome X): relation to reduced fetal growth. *Diabetologia* 36:62–67.
61. Freinkel, N. 1980. Banting Lecture 1980. Of pregnancy and progeny. *Diabetes* 29:1023–35.
62. Pettitt, D.J., Baird, H.R., Aleck, K.A., Bennett, P.H., and W.C. Knowler. 1983. Excessive obesity in offspring of Pima Indian women with diabetes during pregnancy. *N Engl J Med* 308:242–45.
63. Petitt, D.J., Bennett, P.H., Knowler, W.C., Baird, H.R., and Aleck, K.A. 1985. Gestational diabetes mellitus and impaired glucose tolerance during pregnancy. Long-term effects on obesity and glucose tolerance in the offspring. *Diabetes* 34(Suppl 2):119–22.
64. Pettitt, D.J., Knowler, W.C., Bennett, P.H., Aleck, K.A., and Baird, H.R. 1987. Obesity in offspring of diabetic Pima Indian women despite normal birth weight. *Diabetes Care* 10:76–80.
65. Dabelea, D., Pettitt, D.J., Hanson, R.L., Imperatore, G., Bennett, P.H., and Knowler, W.C. 1999. Birth weight, type 2 diabetes, and insulin resistance in Pima Indian children and young adults. *Diabetes Care* 22:944–50.
66. Pettitt, D.J., Bennett, P.H., Saad, M.F., Charles, M.A., Nelson, R.G., and Knowler, W.C. 1991. Abnormal glucose tolerance during pregnancy in Pima Indian women. Long-term effects on offspring. *Diabetes* 40(Suppl 2):126–30.
67. Dabelea, D., and Pettitt, D.J. 2001. Intrauterine diabetic environment confers risks for type 2 diabetes mellitus and obesity in the offspring, in addition to genetic susceptibility. *J Pediatr Endocrinol Metab* 14:1085–91.
68. Dabelea, D., Knowler, W.C., and Pettitt, D.J. 2000. Effect of diabetes in pregnancy on offspring: follow-up research in the Pima Indians. *J Matern Fetal Med* 9:83–88.
69. Metzger, B.E., Silverman, B.L., Freinkel, N., Dooley, S.L., Ogata, E.S., and Green, O.C. 1990. Amniotic fluid insulin concentration as a predictor of obesity. *Arch Dis Child* 65:1050–52.
70. Silverman, B.L., Rizzo, T., Green, O.C., et al. 1991. Long-term prospective evaluation of offspring of diabetic mothers. *Diabetes* 40(Suppl 2):121–25.
71. Dabelea, D., Hanson, R.L., Lindsay, R.S., et al. 2000. Intrauterine exposure to diabetes conveys risks for type 2 diabetes and obesity: a study of discordant sibships. *Diabetes* 49:2208–11.
72. Pedersen, J. 1952. Diabetes and pregnancy. Blood sugar of newborn infants (PhD thesis), 230. Copenhagen: Danish Science Press.
73. HAPO Study Cooperative Research Group, Metzger, B.E., Lowe, L.P., et al. 2008. Hyperglycemia and adverse pregnancy outcomes. *N Engl J Med* 358:1991–2002.
74. Metzger, B.E. 2007. Long-term outcomes in mothers diagnosed with gestational diabetes mellitus and their offspring. *Clin Obstet Gynecol* 50:972–79.
75. Gentz, J., Lunell, N.O., Olin, P., Persson, B., and Sterky, G. 1967. Glucose tolerance in overweight babies and infants of diabetic mothers. *Acta Paediatr Scand* 56:228–29.
76. Pildes, R.S., Hart, R.J., Warrner, R., and Cornblath, M. 1969. Plasma insulin response during oral glucose tolerance tests in newborns of normal and gestational diabetic mothers. *Pediatrics* 44:76–83.
77. Van Assche, F.A., and Gepts, W. 1971. The cytological composition of the foetal endocrine pancreas in normal and pathological conditions. *Diabetologia* 7:434–44.
78. Heding, L.G., Persson, B., and Stangenberg, M. 1980. B-cell function in newborn infants of diabetic mothers. *Diabetologia* 19:427–32.

79. Hultquist, G.T., and Olding, L.B. 1975. Pancreatic-islet fibrosis in young infants of diabetic mothers. *Lancet* 2(7943):1015–16.

80. Gautier, J.F., Wilson, C., Weyer, C., et al. 1992. Low acute insulin secretory responses in adult offspring of people with early onset type 2 diabetes. *Diabetes* 50:1828–33.

81. Hales, C.N., and Barker, D.J. 1992. Type 2 (non-insulin-dependent) diabetes mellitus; the thrifty phenotype hypothesis. *Diabetologia* 35:595–601.

82. Jornayvaz, F.R., Selz, R., Tappy, L., and Theinz, G.E. 2004. Metabolism of oral glucose in children born small for gestational age: evidence for an impaired whole body glucose oxidation. *Metabolism* 53:847–51.

83. Eriksson, J.G., Forsen, T., Tuomilehto, J., Osmond, C., and Barker, D.J. 2003. Early adiposity rebound in childhood and risk of type 2 diabetes in adult life. *Diabetologia* 46:190–94.

84. Newsome, C.A., Shiell, A.W., Fall, C.H., et al. 2003. Is birth weight related to later glucose and insulin metabolism? A systematic review. *Diabet Med* 20:339–48.

85. Clark, P.M., Hindsmarch, P.C., Shiel, A.W., Law, C.M., Honour, J.W., and Barker, D.J. 1996. Size at birth and adrenocortical function in childhood. *Clin Endocrinol (Oxf)* 45:721–26.

86. Dahlgren, J., Boguszewski, M., Rosberg, S., and Albertson-Wikland, K. 1998. Adrenal steroid hormones in short children born small for gestational age. *Clin Endocrinol (Oxf)* 49:353–61.

4 Genetic Risk Factors for Gestational Diabetes

Clive J. Petry
Department of Paediatrics, University of Cambridge,
Addenbrooke's Hospital Cambridge, United Kingdom

CONTENTS

4.1   INTRODUCTION

Gestational diabetes mellitus (GDM) aggregates in families. The cause of this clustering with first-degree relatives who have previously had either GDM or another form of diabetes is likely to have genetic, epigenetic, and environmental components, especially given that in females both low and high birth weights are associated with the future development of GDM.[1] Therefore, a woman who is pregnant and has poorly controlled, preexisting type 1 diabetes has an increased risk of delivering a macrosomic offspring due to her increased blood glucose concentrations crossing the placenta and stimulating the release of insulin, which then acts as a foetal growth factor. The high birth weight offspring, if female, is herself at increased risk of subsequently developing GDM or type 2 diabetes[2] in the reproductive years and beyond. In addition to such metabolic programming effects, common genetic variation also regulates size at birth,[3] and therefore future GDM risk in babies born with high or low birth weights.

In recent years the establishment of large case-control and population cohorts, combined with improvements in DNA and bioinformatic technologies, particularly in the field of genome-wide association studies (GWASs) that are not limited by the need for a priori hypotheses, has driven rapid increases in knowledge about genetic risk variants for all major forms of diabetes. This is important when considering genetic risk for GDM. Some observers believe that GDM is actually the same condition as type 2 diabetes, just developing earlier than it otherwise might have done due mainly to the physiological insulin resistance of the later stages of pregnancy.[4] Indeed, the links between GDM, maternal obesity, and insulin resistance and the increased risk for type 2 diabetes that a woman has once she has experienced GDM[5] support this theory. Whilst this may be true for the majority of women who develop GDM, a subset of women with GDM have an autoimmune- or human leucocyte antigen (HLA)-related condition that more closely resembles type 1 than type 2 diabetes.[6] Indeed, this may hold true for around 10% of the women with GDM.[6] GDM is traditionally defined as any form of glucose intolerance that first presents itself in pregnancy,[7] so any form of diabetes detected in pregnancy that was not diagnosed previously could be labelled as GDM. Given this and the links between GDM and other forms of diabetes, it is vital to think about the genetics of all forms of diabetes when considering the genetics of GDM. Indeed, it is from genetic risk factors for other forms of diabetes that new markers of GDM risk are most likely to be drawn. The gene abbreviations used in this chapter are given in Table 4.1.

4.2 GENETIC RISK FACTORS FOR TYPE 1 DIABETES AND GESTATIONAL DIABETES

Studies of the familial clustering of diabetes have shown an increased prevalence of type 1 diabetes in people exposed to maternal GDM in utero.[8] Genetic precedents may therefore share some commonality between GDM, type 1 diabetes, and latent autoimmune diabetes in adults (LADA).[6] Much of the risk of an individual developing type 1 diabetes is genetic in nature,[9] and almost a quarter of the gene-related threat of developing this condition (in terms of sibling relative risk) is attributable to polymorphic variation in the HLA genes of the major histocompatibility complex (MHC).[10] The highest susceptibility for type 1 diabetes in this 3.6 Mb segment on chromosome 6p21 is in loci in HLA class II DR and DQ genes, especially in genes encoding their β-chains.[9,11] Indeed, HLA-related risk of type 1 diabetes is established by haplotypes composed from DRB1, DQA1, and DQB1 alleles.[12] Specifically, the transdimer coded by *DRB*301-DQB*201* and *DRB*401-DQA*301-DQB*302* confers the greatest risk of developing type 1 diabetes with background population prevalences of 1–2% in Europeans and over 30% in people with type 1 diabetes.[12,13] This leads to an apparent increased risk of type 1 diabetes amongst DR3/4 heterozygotes in comparison to either DR3/3 or DR4/4 homozygotes.[14] Some HLA haplotypes are protective for type 1 diabetes, especially the *DQB*602* allele, which is present in people with type 1 diabetes around 15 times less commonly than in the general population of people with European descent.[13] Indeed, this protective allele was also found to be at a lower prevalence than in the general population in one study of women with nonautoimmune GDM, with an odds ratio of 0.64 (0.51–0.80).[15] In contrast, the same study found no increased risk of GDM associated with the type 1 diabetes high risk HLA-DQ alleles DQB1*201 and DQB1*302. Some other studies have shown no linkage or association between GDM and HLA markers.[16–19] Due to the modestly sized, ethnically mixed study groups that have been used to date,[6] linkage to HLA has proved to be inconsistent; however, other studies have found positive relationships. This includes positive relationships with markers such as HLA-DR3 or

TABLE 4.1
Gene Abbreviations Used in This Chapter

Abbreviation	Gene
ABCC8	ATP-binding cassette, subfamily C, member 8
ACE	Angiotensin I-converting enzyme
ADIPOQ	Adipocyte, C1q, and collagen domain containing (adiponectin)
ADRB3	Beta-3-adrenergic receptor
BLK	Tyrosine kinase, B-lymphocyte specific
BMAL1	Brain and muscle ARNT-like protein 1 (aryl hydrocarbon receptor nuclear translocator-like protein)
CACHD1	Cache domain containing 1
CALB2	Calbindin 2
CAPN10	Calpain 10
CDKAL1	CDK5 regulatory subunit-associated protein 1-like 1
CDKN2A	Cyclin-dependent kinase inhibitor 2A
CDKN2B	Cyclin-dependent kinase inhibitor 2B
CEL	Carboxyl-ester lipase
FTO	Fat mass- and obesity-associated gene
FTSJD1	FtsJ methyltransferase domain containing 1
GCK	Glucokinase
GCKR	Glucokinase regulator
GHRL	Ghrelin
H19	H19 gene (adult skeletal muscle gene)
HHEX	Haematopoietically expressed homeobox
HLA	Human leucocyte antigen
HNF1A	HNF1 homeobox A (hepatocyte nuclear factor 1-alpha)
HNF1B	HNF1 homeobox B (hepatocyte nuclear factor 1-beta)
HNF4A	Hepatocyte nuclear factor 4-alpha
IDE	Insulin-degrading enzyme
IGF2	Insulin-like growth factor 2
IGF2BP2	Insulin-like growth factor 2 mRNA-binding protein 2
INS	Insulin
INSR	Insulin receptor
IL10	Interleukin 10
IPF1	Insulin promoter factor 1 (pancreas/duodenum homeobox protein 1)
IRS1	Insulin receptor substrate 1
JAZF1	Juxtaposed with another zinc finger gene 1
KCNJ11	Potassium channel, inwardly rectifying, subfamily J, member 11
KCNQ1	Potassium channel, voltage-gated, KQT-like subfamily, member 1
KLF11	Kruppel-like factor 11
LBXCOR1	LBX1 corepressor 1, mouse, homologue of
LRRC3B	Leucine-rich repeat containing 3B
MB1	B-lymphocyte-specific mb1 protein (CD79A antigen)

Continued

TABLE 4.1 (*Continued*)
Gene Abbreviations Used in This Chapter

Abbreviation	Gene
MTNR1B	Melatonin receptor 1B
NEUROD3	Neurogenic differentiation 3 (neurogenin 1)
PAI1	Plasminogen activator inhibitor 1 (serpin peptidase inhibitor, clade E (nexin, plasminogen activator inhibitor type 1), member 1)
PAX4	Paired box gene 4
PGR	Progesterone receptor
PLD1	Phospholipase D1, phosphatidylcholine specific
PPARG	Peroxisome proliferator-activated receptor-gamma
PTPN22	Protein tyrosine phosphatase, nonreceptor type, 22
SLC30A8	Solute carrier family 30 (zinc transporter), member 8
SRR	Serine racemase
SUR1	Sulphonylurea receptor (ATP-binding cassette, subfamily c, member 8); see *ABCC8*
TCF7L2	Transcription factor 7-like 2
TINAG	Tubulointerstitial nephritis antigen
TNF	Tumour necrosis factor alpha
TRPM6	Transient receptor potential cation channel, subfamily m, member 6
TSPAN8	Tetraspanin 8
tRNALeu(UUA)	Mitochondrial transfer RNA for leucine 1
VNTR	Variable number of tandem repeats

HLA DR4 in women with GDM,[20–22] HLA Cw7,[23] and HLA DR3-DQ2, DR4-DQ8, and MHC class I chain-related gene A (MICA) 5·0/5·1 in autoantibody-positive women with GDM and HLA DR7-DQ2, DR9-DQ9, DR14-DQ5, and MICA5·0 in women with GDM who were not autoantibody positive.[24]

Given the autoimmune aetiology of type 1 diabetes,[13] it is perhaps surprising that the only type 1 diabetes risk gene known to date that encodes a protein that is an autoantigen is the insulin (*INS*) gene, which encodes pre-proinsulin. The risk loci for type 1 diabetes actually maps to the variable number of tandem repeats (VNTR) located slightly upstream of the *INS* gene,[9] with the class I (26 to 63 repeats) alleles conferring risk and class III alleles (140 to 210 repeats) being dominantly protective. In a study of 161 Greek women with GDM and 111 pregnant women with normal glucose tolerance, *INS* VNTR class III homozygosity was more prevalent in GDM than in the controls, with an odds ratio of 3.97 (1.1–14.29).[25] Another study found no such association between GDM and *INS* VNTR in Arabian and Scandinavian women, however.[19] The lack of reproducibility in different populations and the fact that any association appears to be with *INS* VNTR class III alleles, rather than the class I alleles that confer the risk for type 1 diabetes, reflect the associations between this loci and type 2 diabetes where class III alleles have appeared to confer risk in some studies[26,27] but not others.[28–30]

In addition to HLA and *INS* genes, more than 45 other genetic loci appear to be associated with type 1 diabetes (Figure 4.1)[9,13] (curated in the type 1 database:

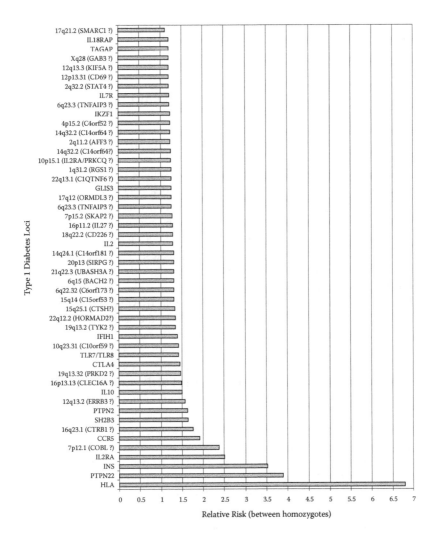

FIGURE 4.1 Genetic variants that are currently thought to be associated with type 1 diabetes. Where loci are listed twice, this is because two variants at the same loci are independently associated with it. (Reprinted from Todd, J.A., *Immunity,* 32, 457–67, 2010. With permission from Elsevier.)

http://www.t1dbase.org[31]). With the exception of *PTPN22*, they were nearly all found through using multiple, very large cohorts (to increase statistical power), association rather than linkage (to further increase power where there is linkage disequilibrium between the genetic loci and type 1 diabetes[32]), and high-throughput genome-wide techniques (analyses of which are not dependent on having a priori hypotheses). Few of the other genetic variants associated with type 1 diabetes have also been reported in relation to gestational diabetes. However, a single-nucleotide polymorphism (SNP) in the promoter of one such gene, *IL10*, was found to be associated with gestational diabetes in one study of women from Malaysia.[33] It is likely that as larger, better-powered cohorts are studied using more sophisticated techniques, additional type 1 diabetes variants will prove to also be genetic risk factors for gestational diabetes, albeit with likely modest effect sizes.

4.3   GENETIC RISK FACTORS OF TYPE 2 DIABETES AND GESTATIONAL DIABETES

As already stated, whilst around 10% of women with GDM have a condition that is autoimmune or HLA related resembling type 1 diabetes,[6] the vast majority of women with GDM have traits that more closely resemble those of type 2 diabetes. Being anthropometrically, metabolically, and genetically (as far as has been tested) matched,[4,34] these women have a condition that strongly resembles type 2 diabetes, but have some of their insulin resistance caused by pregnancy hormones. Indeed, in a subset of GDM women the glucose intolerance does not resolve postpartum, at which point they are considered to have type 2 diabetes.[35] Even those women whose glucose tolerance does normalise postpartum are at greatly increased risk of developing type 2 diabetes at some point in the future.[36]

Given these similarities, it is not surprising that trawling the genetic risk factors for type 2 diabetes is so far proving fruitful in the search for GDM risk factors.[4,34,37–40] Like for type 1 diabetes, more than 50 common genetic variants have been confirmed as risk factors for type 2 diabetes[41–52] (Figure 4.2), generally in multiple large case-control populations. This has been possible due to technological advancements, including relatively automated SNP genotyping in GWAS, and increased cohort sizes and international collaborations allowing meta-analyses to be performed, which have greatly increased the available statistical power. This contrasts with the situation 10 years ago, when only two loci, which were found through linkage or candidate genetic association studies, were robustly associated with type 2 diabetes. These loci corresponded to variants in the peroxisome proliferator-activated receptor-γ (*PPARG*) and K channel, inwardly rectifying, subfamily J, member 11 (*KCNJ11*) genes.[41] Since this time and the emergence of GWAS, it has become apparent that most of the variants associated with type 2 diabetes relate to pancreatic β-cell function rather than insulin resistance.[53]

Candidate gene association studies using mainly Caucasian and Asian populations have so far found associations between GDM and 14 of the genetic variants found to be associated with type 2 diabetes in GWAS studies (*CDKAL1, CDKN2A/CDKN2B, FTO, GCK, HHEX/IDE, HNF1A, HNF1B, IGF2BP2, IRS1, KCNJ11, KCNQ1, MTNR1B, SLC30A8,* and *TCF7L2*).[34,37–39,54–66] In addition, in the European and Asian parts of the multinational Hyperglycemia and Adverse Pregnancy Outcome (HAPO) study containing over 5,000 pregnant women, variants in both *GCK* and *TCF7L2* were associated with fasting and post-challenge glucose concentrations.[67] A recent meta-analysis of GDM genetic studies, performed using 22 studies that passed the eligibility criteria and included a total of 10,336 GDM cases and 17,445 controls, found 8 variants to be significantly associated with GDM[68] (Table 4.2). Overall, these studies again confirm the link between GDM and type 2 diabetes, although as a note of caution such a link could also be established if a high proportion of the women diagnosed with GDM actually had

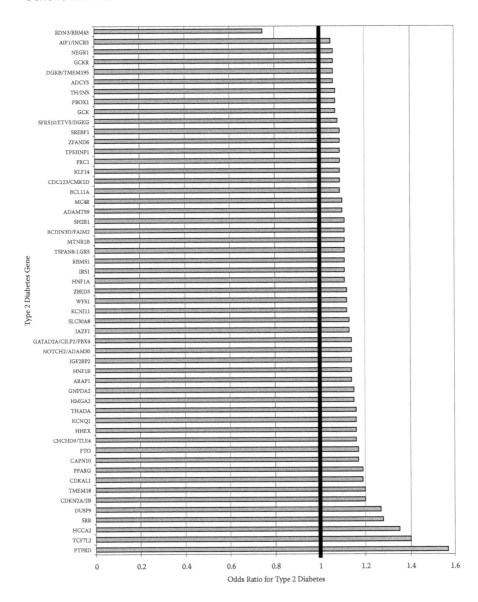

FIGURE 4.2 Genetic variants that are currently thought to be associated with type 2 diabetes. (Data are taken from a number of different study populations.)[41–58]

undiagnosed type 2 diabetes at conception (which may have occurred prior to the acceptance of the new International Association of the Diabetes and Pregnancy Study Groups' guidelines for the diagnosis of GDM[69]). Clearly, though, further studies of the remaining type 2 diabetes risk variants may provide additional genetic variants for GDM. Additional genetic variants, which were not found in type 2 diabetes GWAS studies, have also been found to be associated with GDM in some candidate gene studies (and even some meta-analyses), although on the

TABLE 4.2

Genetic Variants Shown to Be Associated with GDM Using a Random Effects Meta-Analysis of 22 Studies That Met the Selection Criteria and Included a Total of 10,336 Women with GDM and 17,445 Pregnant Women without It

Gene and Variant	Risk Allele	Odds Ratio (95% confidence interval) for GDM	p
TCF7L2 rs7903146	T	1.51 (1.39–1.65)	$< 1 \times 10^{-5}$
CDKAL1 rs775484	C	1.43 (1.12–1.71)	$< 1 \times 10^{-4}$
MTNR1B rs10830963	G	1.34 (1.18–1.52)	$< 1 \times 10^{-5}$
IGF2BP2 rs4402960	T	1.21 (1.08–1.36)	0.001
KCNQ1 rs2237892	C	1.20 (1.09–1.31)	$< 1 \times 10^{-4}$
KCNQ1 rs2237895	C	1.20 (1.09–1.31)	0.0001
KCNJ11 rs5219	T	1.15 (1.06–1.24)	0.0004
GCK rs4607517	A	1.12 (1.02–1.23)	0.01

Source: Mao, H. et al., *PLoS One,* 7:e45882, 2012.

whole they tend to be smaller studies with less robust findings that require confirmation in other populations. These include variants in or close to the following genes: *ADIPOQ,*[70] *ADRB3,*[71] *BMAL1,*[72] *CAPN10,*[73,74] *GCKR,*[65] *IGF2,*[75] *IL10,*[33] *INSR,*[75] *JAZF1,*[65] *MBL,*[76] *PAI1,*[77] *PPARG,*[66,78] *SLC30A8,*[70] *SRR,*[60] *SUR1 (ABCC8),*[79] *TNF,*[80] *TSPAN8,*[65] *GHRL,*[81] and *tRNALeu(UUA).*[82] In addition, a variant in *TRPM6* was recently found to be associated with glycated haemoglobin concentrations in pregnancy and therefore GDM risk.[83]

The first GDM GWAS was published in 2012,[84] thereby fulfilling a great need.[85] Here 468 Korean women with GDM were recruited for stage 1 of the genome scan, where their results were compared with those from 1,242 women without diabetes. The second stage of the genome scan was performed on a further 931 women with GDM and 783 women without diabetes. Eleven variants independent (pairwise linkage disequilibrium, $r^2 < 0.5$) were assessed in both stages, based on either suggestive genome-wide significance ($p < 2.0 \times 10^{-5}$) or markers near known type 2 diabetes risk loci ($p < 1 \times 10^{-3}$). These variants were in or near the following genes: *CACHD1, CDKAL1, CDKN2A/CDKN2B, FTSJD1/CALB2, HHEX/IDE, IGF2BP2, LBXCOR1, LRRC3B, MTNR1B, PLD1,* and *TINAG.* This list shows limited (4/11) similarity with those genes associated with GDM in candidate association studies, and almost the same for genes also associated with type 2 diabetes (5/11). Although *IDE* ($p = 0.035$) and *IGF2BP2* ($p = 0.0042$) showed nominal significance at stage 2 of the genome scan, only *CDKAL1* ($p = 2.9 \times 10^{-7}$) and *MTNR1B* ($p = 6.95 \times 10^{-8}$) achieved genome-wide significance. Combining results from both genome scan stages, genome-wide significance was achieved with variants in *CDKAL1* ($p = 6.65 \times 10^{-16}$) and near *MTNR1B* ($p = 2.49 \times 10^{-13}$), both having previously been found to be associated with GDM in candidate gene studies.[34,53,59,60] In addition to these markers *IGF2BP2* ($p = 1.67 \times 10^{-7}$) almost reached the study's overall cutoff for overall genome-wide significance ($p < 5 \times 10^{-8}$).

Performing bioinformatic pathway analysis (using the DAVID bioinformatic annotation tool[86,87]) on the 14 genetic variants that have thus far been found to be associated with both type 2 diabetes (by GWAS) and GDM (by candidate gene studies), there is an enrichment of genes associated with type 2 diabetes (enrichment score 12.7), with such a high score being expected by definition. However, there is also an enrichment score of 4.5 for a cluster of genes that included those associated, amongst other processes, with the regulation of insulin secretion ($p = 2.45 \times 10^{-5}$), the regulation of cellular localisation ($p = 3.02 \times 10^{-4}$), and glucose homeostasis ($p = 8.29 \times 10^{-4}$) (Petry, unpublished; all p values adjusted using the Benjamini method to reduce the false discovery rate). Therefore, it is not surprising that just like with the genetics of type 2 diabetes,[53] for GDM a genetic deficit in pancreatic β-cell function appears to be more important than those that contribute toward insulin resistance. This would be because of the complex nature of the pancreatic β-cell adaptation to pregnancy that exists to overcome the physiological insulin resistance that occurs during the second half of pregnancy.[88]

Both low and high birth weight females are at increased risk of subsequently developing GDM (in their own pregnancies)[1,89] or type 2 diabetes (especially in populations with a high prevalence of maternal diabetes[90]). Consequently, it is not surprising that some of the genetic variants associated with GDM are also associated with variation in birth weight. In the HAPO study maternal *TCF7L2* and *GCK* were both strongly associated with birth weight.[62] *TCF7L2* was also associated with birth weight in one[91] but not all[92–95] other studies. The evidence for an association between *GCK* and birth weight is more compelling, with associations found in all four studies that tested and reported it.[96–99] Other studies have found associations between birth weight and both *CDKAL1* and *HHEX/IDE*,[94,100–102] although such associations did not always reach statistical significance.[93] A polymorphism near *CDKN2A* and *CDKN2B* was associated with birth weight in two populations,[93,94] but not in all populations.[100] A meta-analysis found that *FTO* is only nominally associated with birth weight,[103] but a further study showed that its relationship with offspring body weight does not develop postnatally until the child reaches 2 weeks of age.[104] Genetic variation in *IRS1* has been associated with birth weight in some populations,[105,106] but not others.[107,108] *IGF2BP2* was not associated with birth weight in any of three different populations[93,94,100] or *SLC30A8* in any of four.[93,94,100,102] *KCNJ11* was found to be associated with being small for gestational age in one study,[109] but was not associated with birth weight in three further studies.[93,94,110] *KCNQ1* and *MTNR1B* appear not to have been studied in relation to associations with size at birth.

In summary, of the genetic variants that are associated with both GDM and type 2 diabetes, many of them show variable associations with offspring birth weight. *GCK* appears to be strongly associated with size at birth, and *IGF2BP2* and *SLC30A8* appear not to be associated with it. As more genetic variants are found to be associated with either GDM or birth weight, however, there is a fair chance that they will also be associated with the other clinical correlate as well. For future hypothesis-driven candidate gene studies, however, the richest source of new GDM genetic variants is still likely to come from those variants already shown to be associated with type 2 diabetes risk. As for the genetic risk of type 1 diabetes and GDM, however, it is likely that the common variants with the largest effect sizes have already been found, and as gene technology increases, newer genetic risk common variants with very modest effects (as well as rarer ones with larger effect sizes) will emerge.

4.4   GENETIC RISK FACTORS OF OTHER FORMS OF DIABETES AND GESTATIONAL DIABETES

Although type 1 and 2 diabetes and GDM are undoubtedly the major forms of diabetes, they are not the only subtypes. One group of rarer forms, collectively known as maturity-onset diabetes of the young (MODY), is the cause for around 1–2% of people with diabetes.[111] As it can emerge more insidiously than other forms of diabetes, if it presents in pregnancy, it can be wrongly diagnosed as GDM or even type 2 diabetes once the glucose intolerance continues postpartum. So far 12 genes have been shown to contain mutations in some individuals that can lead to MODY (*HNF4A, GCK, HNF1A, IPF1, HNF1B, NEUROD1, KLF11, CEL, PAX4, INS, BLK,* and *ABCC8*), although the first four genes in the list account for the vast majority of cases.[112,113] Mutations in *KCNJ11* and *ABCC8* can lead to permanent neonatal diabetes, and other *ABCC8* mutations can cause transient neonatal diabetes.[114] These conditions share many of the characteristics of MODY, not least of which is their autosomal dominant inheritance. Genetic variants in at least four of these genes (*HNF1A, HNF1B, GCK,* and *KCNJ11*, plus possibly *ABCC8*[74]) are also associated with GDM, the high degree of concordance perhaps not being surprising given that all the MODY and neonatal diabetes genes relate to impaired pancreatic β-cell function.[58] The other form of diabetes that some people consider a subtype is LADA.[115] This apparent form of the condition results from the autoimmune destruction of pancreatic β-cells, like in type 1 diabetes, but presents in adults and often does not require insulin treatment at diagnosis, like in type 2 diabetes. The similarities between LADA and both major forms of diabetes lead some investigators to term the condition type 1.5 diabetes,[116] but the idea that LADA is actually just a form of type 1 diabetes that presents in adult life more insidiously than that which presents in childhood means that it is not recognised as a separate form of diabetes by either the World Health Organisation[117] or the American Diabetes Association.[7] Nevertheless, the genetic risk factors for LADA do not appear to be exactly the same as those confirmed for type 1 diabetes.[118] Thus, whilst both LADA and type 1 diabetes are associated with HLA-DQB1 *0201/*0302,[119] they appear to be able to be differentiated by *MICA* gene 5.1,[120] which appears to be a risk factor for LADA but not for type 1 diabetes. Polymorphic variation in MICA 5.1 therefore seems to be a risk factor for both LADA[120] and GDM.[24] Interestingly, polymorphic variation in *TCF7L2*, which confers a relatively strong (at least for SNPs) risk for type 2 diabetes[41–52] and GDM,[34,38,39,54,62,63,67] was also found to be associated with LADA in one study.[119] Therefore, LADA and GDM do seem to share some genetic risk. Unlike other forms of diabetes, though, LADA is unlikely to provide many new markers of GDM risk, as they would probably emerge from studies of the more common type 1 (and potentially type 2) diabetes. Finally, other forms of diabetes, that have not been mentioned so far, exist,[7] but are unlikely to share genetic risk factors with GDM, as their cause may be chromosomal or not transmitted genetically (e.g., iatrogenic diabetes).

4.5 GESTATIONAL DIABETES-SPECIFIC GENETIC RISK

Unlike genetic risk factors that GDM shares with other forms of diabetes, GDM-specific genetic risk factors have thus far remained somewhat elusive.[121] A mother carrying an unborn baby is the one situation in human life where two individuals with two different genomes might be able to influence each other's metabolism and physiology. To look for GDM-specific genetic risk factors, the most fruitful search might therefore involve studying the foetus. Indeed, an emerging area in the field of GDM genetics is the suggestion that the foetus is able to modify its mother's risk of developing GDM.[122] Evidence of this has been observed in several indirect studies. First, in a large observational study stratifying maternal glucose concentrations in pregnancy by the sex of their offspring, a small increase in glucose concentrations was found in mothers carrying boys when comparing them to those of mothers carrying girls,[123] a finding that was subsequently confirmed in a different population.[124] Such observations could be caused by increased energy intakes in such women when compared to women carrying girls.[125] Offspring sex has also been shown to modify associations between maternal glucose concentrations in pregnancy and polymorphic variation in various maternal genes, including *PGR*,[126] *PPARG*,[127] and *ACE*.[128] In a Chinese study the risk for GDM according to the mother's *PPARG* gene was modified by the foetal *PPARG* gene.[129] In another large observational study, higher maternal glucose concentrations were found in pregnant women carrying twins than in those carrying only one foetus.[130] A nonsignificant trend for an increased incidence of GDM was observed in women carrying offspring with Beckwith Wiedemann syndrome (BWS), in comparison to when the same women carried unaffected offspring in an underpowered case-control study using a BWS registry.[131] Using a contemporary birth cohort, we found that in first pregnancies a common polymorphism in the imprinted gene *H19* was associated with maternal glucose concentrations in the third trimester of pregnancy when transmitted to the foetus.[132] The foetus, whether through genetic means or otherwise, therefore appears to be able to influence maternal glucose concentrations (and GDM risk) in pregnancy.

Given that polymorphic variation in maternal genes such as *TCF7L2* and *GCK* is associated with both GDM risk[67] and offspring birth weight,[62] there is a clear link between the genetic risk of GDM and alterations in offspring size at birth. Following an earlier suggestion by Haig,[133] we suggested that polymorphic variation in *foetal* growth genes[3] could be associated with changes in *maternal* glucose concentrations in pregnancy, and therefore maternal GDM risk.[122] Haig's kinship or conflict hypothesis suggests that to suit the needs of each parent, maternal genes will tend to limit foetal growth and paternal genes will tend to boost it,[134,135] potentially through modulating foetal nutritional supply. Such effects could be mediated by imprinted genes, where only one copy of a gene is expressed (the copy from the other parent being imprinted or "turned off"), depending on its parent of origin, tissue specificity, and developmental stage. Alternatively, maternal effects could be mediated by mitochondrial DNA, which is exclusively maternally transmitted as long as there is no paternal leakage, heteroplasmy, or recombination.[136]

Given that in our previous *H19* study[132] cord blood IGF-II concentrations were raised in those pregnancies with the *H19* genotype that was associated with higher maternal glucose concentrations, we chose to concentrate on *IGF2* variation to test the hypothesis that polymorphic variation in a foetal growth gene is associated with alterations in maternal glucose concentrations and GDM risk. Initial studies used a mouse model where a 13 kb genetic region containing the *H19* gene and *Igf2* control element was disrupted. In this model, when offspring inherit the disrupted gene region from their mothers, the resulting biallelic *Igf2* expression (this gene usually being imprinted in foetal life) leads to increased offspring weights (of around 30% at birth) and placentomegaly.[137,138] In our studies we found that phenotypically wild-type pregnant mice carrying such offspring had higher circulating glucose concentrations in the last week of pregnancy, such that on day 16 areas under intraperitoneal glucose tolerance test curves were nearly 30% higher than those of genetically matched controls.[139] Subsequent studies of haplotype tag SNPs in humans found an association between paternally transmitted foetal *IGF2* genotype and maternal glucose concentrations in week 28 of pregnancy in two birth cohorts.[140] Four SNPs reached statistical significance, the strongest of which (rs10770125) was associated with an effect size of 0.4 mmol/L (7.2 mg/dl) glucose, which is modest but appropriate for what is probably caused by a single SNP effect. Consistent with imprinting, there were no such associations with maternally transmitted foetal *IGF2* SNP alleles. (Foetally derived) placentas from pregnancies with all four of the paternally transmitted foetal *IGF2* SNPs that were significantly associated with maternal glucose concentrations had increased IGF-II contents compared with placentas from pregnancies with none of the risk SNP alleles. Whilst mechanistic studies are ongoing, we propose that the link between polymorphic variation in foetal growth genes and maternal glucose concentrations may be mediated by either a change in placental hormone concentrations (such as human placental lactogen or placental growth hormone) that cause alterations in maternal insulin secretion or sensitivity, or a placental inflammatory reaction that leads to changes in maternal circulating cytokine concentrations (Figure 4.3).[40,122] Our findings in relation to *IGF2* are the only ones that we know of relating common polymorphic variation in a foetal growth gene with maternal glucose concentrations in pregnancy, but in studies of the *H19* gene we found an association between a relatively uncommon maternally transmitted foetal SNP (rs3741216) and maternal glucose concentrations at week 28 of pregnancy (*p* = 0.01 for only 8 pregnancies with the risk allele and 885 without it).[141] Whilst for this analysis the study was clearly underpowered, the findings suggest associations between parentally transmitted foetal SNPs in growth genes, and maternal glucose concentrations are not limited to *IGF2* and may be a more general phenomenon. All

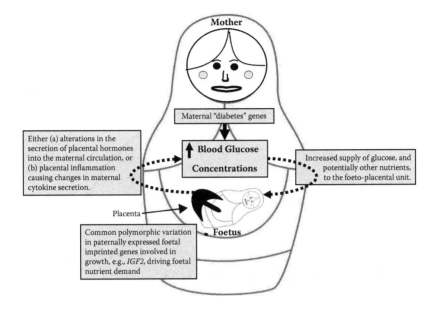

FIGURE 4.3 Schematic diagram of how variation in the foetal genotype can potentially affect maternal GDM risk in pregnancy. Changes in maternal circulating placental hormone concentrations may reduce insulin sensitivity or secretion (perhaps through reducing the pancreatic β-cell expansion that occurs during pregnancy). Changes in maternal (adipo)cytokine concentrations could also lead to changes in insulin sensitivity or secretion.

the findings relating foetal genetics with maternal GDM risk require confirmation in other populations and more detailed mechanistic studies, but foetal genes may include the one set of genetic risk factors that distinguish GDM from all other forms of diabetes.

4.6 FUTURE PROSPECTS

Like for type 1 and 2 diabetes,[42,142,143] the overall genetic risk for GDM looks like it is made up from the sum of relatively small contributions from a number of different genes[34]—and perhaps different genes in different populations, depending on population prevalences of the various risk alleles and the tendency for maternal obesity. Given that GDM in pregnant women tends to reveal a genetic predisposition to other types of diabetes (Figure 4.4), it is not surprising that most commonly the form in question is type 2 diabetes, especially if other risk factors such as obesity are also present. For type 2 diabetes there have now been so many genome-wide association studies and meta-analyses of these that apart from studies of underrepresented ethnicities (such as sub-Saharan Africans), we are now almost in a post-GWAS era when searching for new genetic susceptibility variants. The large cohort sizes investigated so far and which have then been combined in meta-analyses,[144] and the low odds ratios for type 2 diabetes associated with the discovered susceptibility markers, suggest that not many more new markers will emerge using current

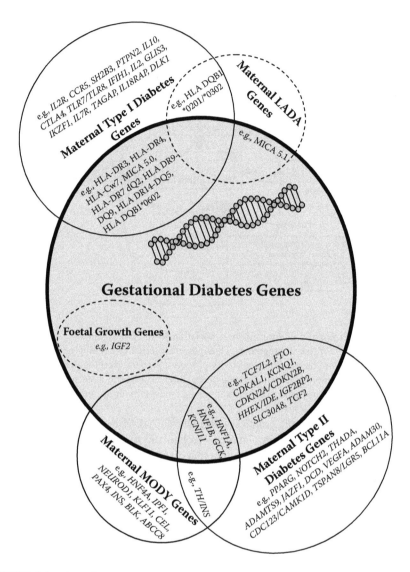

FIGURE 4.4 Venn diagram to summarise the genetic variants that are associated with the development of gestational diabetes, and the contribution by variants associated with other forms of diabetes (and potentially foetal growth). As knowledge increases the genes may move from one section of the diagram to another.

GWAS techniques, even with the increased statistical power available from testing even larger cohorts. Yet it has been estimated that even combining all the current genetic risk markers only accounts for only around 10% of the familial clustering risk for type 2 diabetes in people with European ancestry.[45,145] It is likely that further markers will emerge when using alternative techniques to detect changes in epigenetics, copy number variation, and relatively rare variants with large effect sizes (which may emerge using next-generation sequencing techniques[146]). Given its somewhat temporary nature, it is difficult to collect large GDM cohorts over a relatively short period of time, so due to the strong genetic links between GDM and type 2 diabetes,[4,34] these type 2 diabetes studies are likely to prove the most fruitful of any type of study for candidate (epi-)genetic markers of GDM risk. Slightly less fruitful for this will probably be studies of these type of (epi-)genetic variants as risk factors for type 1 diabetes, because although combining the known genetic susceptibility markers for a similar familial clustering variance has been explained, as for type 2 diabetes,[145] a smaller proportion of the GDM population is affected by type 1 diabetes variants. The promising nature of foetal genetic variants of maternal GDM risk suggests that more of these susceptibility variants will emerge with time. The limiting factor of cohort studies for their discovery, however, is the requirement for mother-father-offspring DNA triads when parent of origin becomes important, although as a spin-off, transmission disequilibrium testing can then also be performed to add linkage to the association and remove the possible effects of population stratification.

Ultimately genetic susceptibility may only account for a relatively small portion of total GDM risk. The cost relative to benefit of large-scale genotyping of individual patients for GDM risk may therefore be legitimately questioned. However, it has already been shown that producing a risk score having genotyped women with diagnosed GDM for variants associated with type 2 diabetes is able to predict those women most at risk of having diabetes postpartum.[147] This strategy could be used to target resources to women with a high genetic risk score. Similar genetic panels could also be used early in pregnancy to predict risk of developing GDM per se. Genetic studies are also important to help ascertain mechanisms of GDM development and potentially discover therapeutic targets. For type 2 diabetes, the biggest potential use of genetics for GDM is likely to be pharmacogenetics.[121,148-150] For the treatment of GDM in the short term, potential teratogenic effects have to be avoided, along with long-term metabolic programming effects on the offspring and toxic effects on the mother. However, these have to be considered alongside the fact that if no treatment is given, there will already be negative effects on both the mother and her unborn offspring. So far treatments tried for GDM include insulin, sulphonylureas, and biguanides,[40] and the last two groups of drugs on the list have variable efficacy, depending on the drug in question and the patient genotype.[148,149] Genetics may therefore ultimately be used to help tailor treatments to individual women with GDM, potentially improving both pregnancy outcomes[151] and transgenerational risk.

ACKNOWLEDGEMENTS

The studies that I have been involved in described in this manuscript have been funded by the Evelyn Trust, the Medical Research Council, the Wellcome Trust, and the Wellbeing of Women and Diabetes UK.

REFERENCES

Key references are in bold.

1. Innes, K.E., Byers, T.E., Marshall, J.A., Barón, A., Orleans, M., and Hamman, R.F. 2002. Association of a woman's own birth weight with subsequent risk for gestational diabetes. *JAMA* 287:2534–41. Erratum in *JAMA* 287:3212.
2. Sobngwi, E., Boudou, P., Mauvais-Jarvis, F., et al. 2003. Effect of a diabetic environment in utero on predisposition to type 2 diabetes. *Lancet* 361:1861–65.
3. Dunger, D.B., Petry, C.J., and Ong, K.K. 2007. Genetics of size at birth. *Diabetes Care* 30(Suppl 2):S150–55.
4. Robitaille, J., and Grant, A.M. 2008. The genetics of gestational diabetes mellitus: evidence for relationship with type 2 diabetes mellitus. *Genet Med* 10:240–50.
5. Verier-Mine, O. 2010. Outcomes in women with a history of gestational diabetes. Screening and prevention of type 2 diabetes. *Diabetes Metab* 36:595–616.
6. Lapolla, A., Dalfrà, M.G., and Fedele, D. 2009. Diabetes related autoimmunity in gestational diabetes mellitus: is it important? *Nutr Metab Cardiovasc Dis* 19:674–82.
7. American Diabetes Association. 2012. Diagnosis and classification of diabetes mellitus. *Diabetes Care* 35:S64–71.
8. Dörner, G., Plagemann, A., and Reinagel, H. 1987. Familial diabetes aggregation in type I diabetics: gestational diabetes an apparent risk factor for increased diabetes susceptibility in the offspring. *Exp Clin Endocrinol* 1987; 89:84–90.
9. Polychronakos, C., and Li, Q. 2011. Understanding type 1 diabetes through genetics: advances and prospects. *Nat Rev Genet* 12:781–92.
10. Risch, N. 1987. Assessing the role of HLA-linked and unlinked determinants of disease. *Am J Hum Genet* 40:1–14.
11. Melanitou, E., Fain, P., and Eisenbarth, G.S. 2003. Genetics of type 1A (immune mediated) diabetes. *J Autoimmun* 21:93–98.
12. Erlich, H., Valdes, A.M., Noble, J., et al. 2008. HLA DR-DQ haplotypes and genotypes and type 1 diabetes risk: analysis of the type 1 diabetes genetics consortium families. *Diabetes* 57:1084–92.
13. Todd, J.A. 2010. Etiology of type 1 diabetes. *Immunity* 32:457–67.
14. Rotter, J.I., Anderson, C.E., Rubin, R., Congleton, J.E., Terasaki, P.I., and Rimoin, D.L. 1983. HLA genotypic study of insulin-dependent diabetes: the excess of DR3/DR4 heterozygotes allows rejection of the recessive hypothesis. *Diabetes* 32:169–74.
15. Papadopoulou, A., Lynch, K.F., Shaat, N., et al. 2009. The type 1 diabetes protective HLA DQB1*0602 allele is less frequent in gestational diabetes mellitus. *Diabetologia* 52:1339–42.
16. Bell, D.S., Barger, B.O., Go, R.C., et al. 1990. Risk factors for gestational diabetes in black population. *Diabetes Care* 13:1196–201.
17. Stangenberg, M., Agarwal, N., Rahman, F., Sheth, K., al Sedeiry, S., and De Vol, E. 1990. Frequency of HLA genes and islet cell antibodies (ICA) and result of postpartum oral glucose tolerance tests (OGTT) in Saudi Arabian women with abnormal OGTT during pregnancy. *Diabetes Res* 14:9–13.
18. Vambergue, A., Fajardy, I., Bianchi, F., et al. 1997. Gestational diabetes mellitus and HLA class II (-DQ, -DR) association: the Digest Study. *Eur J Immunogenet* 24:385–94.
19. Shaat, N., Ekelund, M., Lernmark, A., et al. 2004. Genotypic and phenotypic differences between Arabian and Scandinavian women with gestational diabetes mellitus. *Diabetologia* 47:878–84.
20. Rubinstein, P., Walker, M., Krassner, J., et al. 1981. HLA antigens and islet cell antibodies in gestational diabetes. *Hum Immunol* 3:271–75.
21. Freinkel, N., Metzger, B.E., Phelps, R.L., et al. 1985. Gestational diabetes mellitus. Heterogeneity of maternal age, weight, insulin secretion, HLA antigens, and islet cell antibodies and the impact of maternal metabolism on pancreatic B-cell and somatic development in the offspring. *Diabetes* 34(Suppl 2):1–7.

22. Ferber, K.M., Keller, E., Albert, E.D., and Ziegler, A.G. 1999. Predictive value of human leukocyte antigen class II typing for the development of islet autoantibodies and insulin-dependent diabetes postpartum in women with gestational diabetes. *J Clin Endocrinol Metab* 84:2342–48.

23. Lapolla, A., Betterle, C., Sanzari, M., et al. 1996. An immunological and genetic study of patients with gestational diabetes mellitus. *Acta Diabetol* 33:139–44.

24. Törn, C., Gupta, M., Sanjeevi, C.B., Aberg, A., Frid, A., and Landin-Olsson, M. 2004. Different HLA-DR-DQ and MHC class I chain-related gene A (MICA) genotypes in autoimmune and nonautoimmune gestational diabetes in a Swedish population. *Hum Immunol* 65:1443–50.

25. Litou, H., Anastasiou, E., Thalassinou, L., Sarika, H.L., Philippou, G., and Alevizaki, M. 2007. Increased prevalence of VNTR III of the insulin gene in women with gestational diabetes mellitus (GDM). *Diabetes Res Clin Pract* 76:223–28.

26. Ong, K.K., Phillips, D.I., Fall, C., et al. 1999. The insulin gene VNTR, type 2 diabetes and birth weight. *Nat Genet* 21:262–63.

27. Huxtable, S.J., Saker, P.J., Haddad, L., et al. 2000. Analysis of parent-offspring trios provides evidence for linkage and association between the insulin gene and type 2 diabetes mediated exclusively through paternally transmitted class III variable number tandem repeat alleles. *Diabetes* 49:126–30.

28. Mitchell, S.M., Hattersley, A.T., Knight, B., et al. 2004. Lack of support for a role of the insulin gene variable number of tandem repeats minisatellite (INS-VNTR) locus in fetal growth or type 2 diabetes-related intermediate traits in United Kingdom populations. *J Clin Endocrinol Metab* 89:310–17.

29. Lindsay, R.S., Hanson, R.L., Wiedrich, C., Knowler, W.C., Bennett, P.H., and Baier, L.J. 2003. The insulin gene variable number tandem repeat class I/III polymorphism is in linkage disequilibrium with birth weight but not type 2 diabetes in the Pima population. *Diabetes* 52:187–93.

30. Hansen, S.K., Gjesing, A.P., Rasmussen, S.K., et al. 2004. Large-scale studies of the HphI insulin gene variable-number-of-tandem-repeats polymorphism in relation to type 2 diabetes mellitus and insulin release. *Diabetologia* 47:1079–87.

31. Burren, O.S., Adlem, E.C., Achuthan, P., Christensen, M., Coulson, R.M., and Todd, J.A. 2011. T1DBase: update 2011, organization and presentation of large-scale data sets for type 1 diabetes research. *Nucleic Acids Res* 39:D997–1001.

32. Elston, R.C. 1995. Linkage and association to genetic markers. *Exp Clin Immunogenet* 12:129–40.

33. Montazeri, S., Nalliah, S., and Radhakrishnan, A.K. 2010. Is there a genetic variation association in the IL-10 and TNF alpha promoter gene with gestational diabetes mellitus? *Hereditas* 147:94–102.

34. **Lauenborg, J., Grarup, N., Damm, P., et al. 2009. Common type 2 diabetes risk gene variants associate with gestational diabetes. *J Clin Endocrinol Metab* 94:145–50.** *A study showing that several of the newly discovered type 2 diabetes genetic risk variants are also risk factors for gestational diabetes.*

35. Buchanan, T.A., Xiang, A., Kjos, S.L., and Watanabe, R. 2007. What is gestational diabetes? *Diabetes Care* 30(Suppl 2):S105–11.

36. Kim, C., Newton, K.M., and Knopp, R.H. 2002. Gestational diabetes and the incidence of type 2 diabetes: a systematic review. *Diabetes Care* 25:1862–68.

37. Shaat, N., Ekelund, M., Lernmark, A., et al. 2005. Association of the E23K polymorphism in the KCNJ11 gene with gestational diabetes mellitus. *Diabetologia* 48:2544–51.

38. Watanabe, R.M., Allayee, H., Xiang, A.H., et al. 2007. Transcription factor 7-like 2 (TCF7L2) is associated with gestational diabetes mellitus and interacts with adiposity to alter insulin secretion in Mexican Americans. *Diabetes* 56:1481–85.

39. Shaat, N., Lernmark, A., Karlsson, E., et al. 2007. A variant in the transcription factor 7-like 2 (TCF7L2) gene is associated with an increased risk of gestational diabetes mellitus. *Diabetologia* 50:972–79.

40. Petry, C.J. 2010. Gestational diabetes: risk factors and recent advances in its genetics and treatment. *Br J Nutr* 104:775–87.

41. Frayling, T.M. 2007. Genome-wide association studies provide new insights into type 2 diabetes aetiology. *Nat Rev Genet* 8:657–62.

42. Weedon, M.N., McCarthy, M.I., Hitman, G., et al. 2006. Combining information from common type 2 diabetes risk polymorphisms improves disease prediction. *PLoS Med* 3:e374.

43. Doria, A., Patti, M.E., and Kahn, C.R. 2008. The emerging genetic architecture of type 2 diabetes. *Cell Metab* 8:186–200.

44. Zeggini, E., Scott, L.J., Saxena, R., et al. 2008. Meta-analysis of genome-wide association data and large-scale replication identifies additional susceptibility loci for type 2 diabetes. *Nat Genet* 40:638–45.

45. Wheeler, E., and Barroso, I. 2011. Genome-wide association studies and type 2 diabetes. *Brief Funct Genomics* 10:52–60.

46. Tsai, F.J., Yang, C.F., Chen, C.C., et al. 2010. A genome-wide association study identifies susceptibility variants for type 2 diabetes in Han Chinese. *PLoS Genet* 6:e1000847.

47. Palmer, N.D., McDonough, C.W., Hicks, et al. 2012. A genome-wide association search for type 2 diabetes genes in African Americans. *PLoS One* 7:e29202.

48. Ahlqvist, E., Ahluwalia, T.S., and Groop, L. 2011. Genetics of type 2 diabetes. *Clin Chem* 57:241–54.

49. Voight, B.F., Scott, L.J., Steinthorsdottir, V., et al. 2010. Twelve type 2 diabetes susceptibility loci identified through large-scale association analysis. *Nat Genet* 42:579–89.

50. Sladek, R., Rocheleau, G., Rung, J., et al. 2007. A genome-wide association study identifies novel risk loci for type 2 diabetes. *Nature* 445:881–85.

51. Dupuis, J., Langenberg, C., Prokopenko, I., et al. 2010. New genetic loci implicated in fasting glucose homeostasis and their impact on type 2 diabetes risk. *Nat Genet* 42:105–16.

52. Saxena, R., Elbers, C.C., Guo, Y., et al. 2012. Large-scale gene-centric meta-analysis across 39 studies identifies type 2 diabetes loci. *Am J Hum Genet* 90:410–25.

53. Imamura, M., and Maeda, S. 2011. Genetics of type 2 diabetes: the GWAS era and future perspectives. *Endocrinol J* 58:723–39.

54. **Cho, Y.M., Kim, T.H., Lim, S., et al. 2009. Type 2 diabetes-associated genetic variants discovered in the recent genome-wide association studies are related to gestational diabetes mellitus in the Korean population.** *Diabetologia* **52:253–61.** *Another study showing that several of the newly discovered type 2 diabetes genetic risk variants are also risk factors for gestational diabetes.*

55. Zhou, Q., Zhang, K., Li, W., et al. 2009. Association of KCNQ1 gene polymorphism with gestational diabetes mellitus in a Chinese population. *Diabetologia* 52:2466–68.

56. Shin, H.D., Park, B.L., Shin, H.J., et al. 2010. Association of KCNQ1 polymorphisms with the gestational diabetes mellitus in Korean women. *J Clin Endocrinol Metab* 95:445–49.

57. Fallucca, F., Dalfrà, M.G., Sciullo, E., et al. 2006. Polymorphisms of insulin receptor substrate 1 and beta3-adrenergic receptor genes in gestational diabetes and normal pregnancy. *Metabolism* 55:1451–56.

58. **Shaat, N., Karlsson, E., Lernmark, A., et al. 2006. Common variants in MODY genes increase the risk of gestational diabetes mellitus.** *Diabetologia* **49:1545–51. Erratum in** *Diabetologia* **49:2226–27.** *A study showing that several of the genes that are risk factors for MODY contain variants that are risk factors for gestational diabetes.*

59. Kim, J.Y., Cheong, H.S., Park, B.L., et al. 2011. Melatonin receptor 1 B polymorphisms associated with the risk of gestational diabetes mellitus. *BMC Med Genet* 12:82.

60. Wang, Y., Nie, M., Li, W., et al. 2011. Association of six single nucleotide polymorphisms with gestational diabetes mellitus in a Chinese population. *PLoS One* 6:e26953.

61. Kwak, S.H., Kim, T.H., Cho, Y.M., Choi, S.H., Jang, H.C., and Park, K.S. 2010. Polymorphisms in KCNQ1 are associated with gestational diabetes in a Korean population. *Horm Res Paediatr* 74:333–38.

62. Pappa, K.I., Gazouli, M., Economou, K., et al. 2011. Gestational diabetes mellitus shares polymorphisms of genes associated with insulin resistance and type 2 diabetes in the Greek population. *Gynecol Endocrinol* 27:267–72.

63. Papadopoulou, A., Lynch, K.F., Shaat, N., et al. 2011. Gestational diabetes mellitus is associated with TCF7L2 gene polymorphisms independent of HLA-DQB1*0602 genotypes and islet cell autoantibodies. *Diabet Med* 28:1018–27.

64. Klein, K., Haslinger, P., Bancher-Todesca, D., et al. 2012. Transcription factor 7-like 2 gene polymorphisms and gestational diabetes mellitus. *J Matern Fetal Neonatal Med* 25:1783–86.

65. Stuebe, A.M., Wise, A., Nguyen, T., Herring, A., North, K.E., and Siega-Riz, A.M. 2013. Maternal genotype and gestational diabetes. *Am J Perinatol* DOI: 10.1055/s-0033-1334451.

66. Chon, S.J., Kim, S.Y., Cho, N.R., Min, D.L., Hwang, Y.J., and Mamura, M. 2013. Association of variants in PPARγ2, IGF2BP2, and KCNQ1 with a susceptibility to gestational diabetes mellitus in a Korean population. *Yonsei Med J* 54:352–57.

67. **Freathy, R.M, Hayes, M.G., Urbanek, M., et al. 2010. Hyperglycemia and Adverse Pregnancy Outcome (HAPO) study: common genetic variants in GCK and TCF7L2 are associated with fasting and postchallenge glucose levels in pregnancy and with the new consensus definition of gestational diabetes mellitus from the International Association of Diabetes and Pregnancy Study Groups. *Diabetes* 59:2682–89.** *The first genetics manuscript to be published from the international HAPO study, the largest single-study resource available for the study of the genetics of gestational diabetes.*

68. **Mao, H., Li, Q., and Gao, S. 2012. Meta-analysis of the relationship between common type 2 diabetes risk gene variants with gestational diabetes mellitus. *PLoS One* 7:e45882.** *A recent meta-analysis of the genetic variants associated with GDM.*

69. International Association of Diabetes and Pregnancy Study Groups Consensus Panel, Metzger, B.E., Gabbe, S.G., et al. 2010. International association of diabetes and pregnancy study groups recommendations on the diagnosis and classification of hyperglycemia in pregnancy. *Diabetes Care* 33:676–82.

70. Liang, Z., Dong, M., Cheng, Q., and Chen, D. 2010. Gestational diabetes mellitus screening based on the gene chip technique. *Diabetes Res Clin Pract* 89:167–73.

71. Festa, A., Krugluger, W., Shnawa, N., Hopmeier, P., Haffner, S.M., and Schernthaner, G. 1999. Trp64Arg polymorphism of the beta3-adrenergic receptor gene in pregnancy: association with mild gestational diabetes mellitus. *J Clin Endocrinol Metab* 84:1695–99.

72. Pappa, K.I., Gazouli, M., Anastasiou, E., Iliodromiti, Z., Antsaklis, A., and Anagnou, N.P. 2013. The major circadian pacemaker ARNT-like protein-1 (BMAL1) is associated with susceptibility to gestational diabetes mellitus. *Diabetes Res Clin Pract* 99:151–57.

73. Leipold, H., Knöfler, M., Gruber, C., Haslinger, P., Bancher-Todesca, D., and Worda, C. 2004. Calpain-10 haplotype combination and association with gestational diabetes mellitus. *Obstet Gynecol* 103:1235–40.

74. Wu, H.R., and Yang, H.X. 2009. Association of the calpain-10 gene polymorphism with glucose metabolism disorder in pregnant women. *Zhonghua Fu Chan Ke Za Zhi* 44:183–87.

75. Ober, C., Xiang, K.S., Thisted, R.A., Indovina, K.A., Wason, C.J., and Dooley, S. 1989. Increased risk for gestational diabetes mellitus associated with insulin receptor and insulin-like growth factor II restriction fragment length polymorphisms. *Genet Epidemiol* 6:559–69.

76. Megia, A., Gallart, L., Fernández-Real, J.M., et al. 2004. Mannose-binding lectin gene polymorphisms are associated with gestational diabetes mellitus. *J Clin Endocrinol Metab* 89:5081–87.

77. Leipold, H., Knöfler, M., Gruber, C., Klein, K., Haslinger, P., and Worda, C. 2006. Plasminogen activator inhibitor 1 gene polymorphism and gestational diabetes mellitus. *Obstet Gynecol* 107:651–56.

78. Wang, C., Li, X., Huang, Z., and Qian, J. 2013. Quantitative assessment of the influence of PPARG P12A polymorphism on gestational diabetes mellitus risk. *Mol Biol Rep* 40:811–17.

79. Rissanen, J., Markkanen, A., Kärkkäinen, P., et al. 2000. Sulfonylurea receptor 1 gene variants are associated with gestational diabetes and type 2 diabetes but not with altered secretion of insulin. *Diabetes Care* 23:70–73.

80. Guzmán-Flores, J.M., Escalante, M., Sánchez-Corona, J., et al. 2013. Association analysis between –308G/A and –238G/A TNF-alpha gene promoter polymorphisms and insulin resistance in Mexican women with gestational diabetes mellitus. *J Investig Med* 61:265–69.

81. dos Santos, I.C., Frigeri, H.R., Daga, D.R., et al. 2010. The ghrelin gene allele 51Q (rs34911341) is a protective factor against the development of gestational diabetes. *Clin Chim Acta* 411:886–87.

82. Chen, Y., Liao, W.X., Roy, A.C., Loganath, A., and Ng, S.C. 2000. Mitochondrial gene mutations in gestational diabetes mellitus. *Diabetes Res Clin Pract* 48:29–35.

83. Nair, A.V., Hocher, B., Verkaart, S., et al. 2012. Loss of insulin-induced activation of TRPM6 magnesium channels results in impaired glucose tolerance during pregnancy. *Proc Natl Acad Sci U S A* 109:11324–29.

84. **Kwak, S.H., Kim, S.H., Cho, Y.M., et al. 2012. A genome-wide association study of gestational diabetes mellitus in Korean women.** *Diabetes* **61:531–41.** *The first genome wide association study directly relating to gestational diabetes.*

85. Watanabe, R.M., Black, M.H., Xiang, A.H., Allayee, H., Lawrence, J.M., and Buchanan, T.A. 2007. Genetics of gestational diabetes mellitus and type 2 diabetes. *Diabetes Care* 30(Suppl 2):S134–40.

86. Huang, D.W., Sherman, B.T., and Lempicki, R.A. 2009. Systematic and integrative analysis of large gene lists using DAVID Bioinformatics Resources. *Nature Protoc* 4:44–57.

87. Huang, D.W., Sherman, B.T., and Lempicki, R.A. 2009. Bioinformatics enrichment tools: paths toward the comprehensive functional analysis of large gene lists. *Nucleic Acids Res* 37:1–13.

88. Ernst, S., Demirci, C., Valle, S., Velazquez-Garcia, S., and Garcia-Ocaña, A. 2011. Mechanisms in the adaptation of maternal β-cells during pregnancy. *Diabetes Manag (Lond)* 1:239–48.

89. Seghieri, G., Anichini, R., De Bellis, A., Alviggi, L., Franconi, F., and Breschi, M.C. 2002. Relationship between gestational diabetes mellitus and low maternal birth weight. *Diabetes Care* 25:1761–65.

90. Whincup, P.H., Kaye, S.J., Owen, C.G., et al. 2008. Birth weight and risk of type 2 diabetes: a systematic review. *JAMA* 300:2886–97.

91. Freathy, R.M., Weedon, M.N., Bennett, A., et al. 2007. Type 2 diabetes TCF7L2 risk genotypes alter birth weight: a study of 24,053 individuals. *Am J Hum Genet* 80:1150–61.

92. Cauchi, S., Meyre, D., Choquet, H., et al. 2007. TCF7L2 rs7903146 variant does not associate with smallness for gestational age in the French population. *BMC Med Genet* 8:37.

93. Pulizzi, N., Lyssenko, V., Jonsson, A., et al. 2009. Interaction between prenatal growth and high-risk genotypes in the development of type 2 diabetes. *Diabetologia* 52:825–29.

94. Zhao, J., Li, M., Bradfield, J.P., et al. 2009. Examination of type 2 diabetes loci implicates CDKAL1 as a birth weight gene. *Diabetes* 58:2414–18.

95. Mook-Kanamori, D.O., de Kort, S.W., van Duijn, C.M., et al. 2009. Type 2 diabetes gene TCF7L2 polymorphism is not associated with fetal and postnatal growth in two birth cohort studies. *BMC Med Genet* 10:67.

96. Weedon, M.N., Frayling, T.M., Shields, B., et al. 2005. Genetic regulation of birth weight and fasting glucose by a common polymorphism in the islet cell promoter of the glucokinase gene. *Diabetes* 54:576–81.

97. Weedon, M.N., Clark, V.J., Qian, Y., et al. 2006. A common haplotype of the glucokinase gene alters fasting glucose and birth weight: association in six studies and population-genetics analyses. *Am J Hum Genet* 79:991–1001.

98. Singh, R., Pearson, E.R., Clark, P.M., and Hattersley, A.T. 2007. The long-term impact on offspring of exposure to hyperglycaemia in utero due to maternal glucokinase gene mutations. *Diabetologia* 50:620–24.

99. Shields, B.M., Spyer, G., Slingerland, A.S., et al. 2008. Mutations in the glucokinase gene of the fetus result in reduced placental weight. *Diabetes Care* 31:753–57.

100. Freathy, R.M., Bennett, A.J., Ring, S.M., et al. 2009. Type 2 diabetes risk alleles are associated with reduced size at birth. *Diabetes* 58:1428–33.

101. Andersson, E.A., Pilgaard, K., Pisinger, C., et al. 2010. Type 2 diabetes risk alleles near ADCY5, CDKAL1 and HHEX-IDE are associated with reduced birthweight. *Diabetologia* 53:1908–16.

102. Winkler, C., Illig, T., Koczwara, K., Bonifacio, E., and Ziegler, A.G. 2009. HHEX-IDE polymorphism is associated with low birth weight in offspring with a family history of type 1 diabetes. *J Clin Endocrinol Metab* 94:4113–15.

103. Kilpeläinen, T.O., den Hoed, M., Ong, K.K., et al. 2011. Obesity-susceptibility loci have a limited influence on birth weight: a meta-analysis of up to 28,219 individuals. *Am J Clin Nutr* 93:851–60.

104. López-Bermejo, A., Petry, C.J., Díaz, M., et al. 2008. The association between the FTO gene and fat mass in humans develops by the postnatal age of two weeks. *J Clin Endocrinol Metab* 93:1501–5.

105. Simońska-Cichocka, E., Gumprecht, J., Zychma, M., et al. 2008. The polymorphism in insulin receptor substrate-1 gene and birth weight in neonates at term. *Endokrynol Pol* 59:212–16.

106. Bezerra, R.M., de Castro, V., Sales, T., et al. 2002. The Gly972Arg polymorphism in insulin receptor substrate-1 is associated with decreased birth weight in a population-based sample of Brazilian newborns. *Diabetes Care* 25:550–53.

107. Mason, S., Ong, K.K., Pembrey, M.E., Woods, K.A., and Dunger, D.B. 2000. The Gly972Arg variant in insulin receptor substrate-1 is not associated with birth weight in contemporary English children. The ALSPAC Study Team. Avon Longitudinal Study of Pregnancy and Childhood. *Diabetologia* 43:1201–2.

108. Rasmussen, S.K., Urhammer, S.A., Hansen, T., et al. 2000. Variability of the insulin receptor substrate-1, hepatocyte nuclear factor-1alpha (HNF-1alpha), HNF-4alpha, and HNF-6 genes and size at birth in a population-based sample of young Danish subjects. *J Clin Endocrinol Metab* 85:2951–53.

109. Morgan, A.R., Thompson, J.M., Murphy, R., et al. 2010. Obesity and diabetes genes are associated with being born small for gestational age: results from the Auckland Birthweight Collaborative Study. *BMC Med Genet* 11:125.

110. Bennett, A.J., Sovio, U., Ruokonen, A., et al. 2008. No evidence that established type 2 diabetes susceptibility variants in the PPARG and KCNJ11 genes have pleiotropic effects on early growth. *Diabetologia* 51:82–85.

111. Thanabalasingham, G., and Owen, K.R. 2011. Diagnosis and management of maturity onset diabetes of the young (MODY). *BMJ* 343:d6044.
112. Fajans, S.S., and Bell, G.I. 2011. MODY: history, genetics, pathophysiology, and clinical decision making. *Diabetes Care* 34:1878–84.
113. Bowman, P., Flanagan, S.E., Edghill, E.L., et al. 2012. Heterozygous ABCC8 mutations are a cause of MODY. *Diabetologia* 55:123–27.
114. Greeley, S.A., Tucker, S.E., Naylor, R.N., Bell, G.I., and Philipson, L.H. 2010. Neonatal diabetes mellitus: a model for personalized medicine. *Trends Endocrinol Metab* 21:464–72.
115. Tuomi, T., Groop, L.C., Zimmet, P.Z., Rowley, M.J., Knowles, W., and Mackay, I.R. 1993. Antibodies to glutamic acid decarboxylase reveal latent autoimmune diabetes mellitus in adults with a non-insulin-dependent onset of disease. *Diabetes* 42:359–62.
116. Schernthaner, G., Hink, S., Kopp, H.P., Muzyka, B., Streit, G., and Kroiss, A. 2001. Progress in the characterization of slowly progressive autoimmune diabetes in adult patients (LADA or type 1.5 diabetes). *Exp Clin Endocrinol Diabetes* 109(Suppl 2):S94–108.
117. World Health Organisation and International Diabetes Federation Technical Advisory Group. 2006. *Definition and diagnosis of diabetes mellitus and intermediate hyperglycaemia: Report of a WHO/IDF consultation*. Geneva: World Health Organisation. Available from http://www.who.int/diabetes/publications/diagnosis_diabetes2006/en/index.html.
118. Grant, S.F., Hakonarson, H., and Schwartz, S. 2010. Can the genetics of type 1 and type 2 diabetes shed light on the genetics of latent autoimmune diabetes in adults? *Endocrinol Rev* 31:183–93.
119. Cervin, C., Lyssenko, V., Bakhtadze, E., et al. 2008. Genetic similarities between latent autoimmune diabetes in adults, type 1 diabetes, and type 2 diabetes. *Diabetes* 57:1433–37.
120. Gambelunghe, G., Ghaderi, M., Tortoioli, C., et al. 2001. Two distinct MICA gene markers discriminate major autoimmune diabetes types. *J Clin Endocrinol Metab* 86:3754–60.
121. **Watanabe, R.M. 2011. Inherited destiny? Genetics and gestational diabetes mellitus.** ***Genome Med* 3:18.** *A well-written review outlining the evidence that risk for gestational diabetes has a genetic component.*
122. Petry, C.J., Ong, K.K., and Dunger, D.B. 2007. Does the fetal genotype affect maternal physiology during pregnancy? *Trends Mol Med* 13:414–21.
123, Sheiner, E., Levy, A., Katz, M., Hershkovitz, R., Leron, E., and Mazor, M. 2004. Gender does matter in perinatal medicine. *Fetal Diagn Ther* 19:366–69.
124. Di Renzo, G.C., Rosati, A., Sarti, R.D., Cruciani, L., and Cutuli, A.M. 2007. Does fetal sex affect pregnancy outcome? *Gend Med* 4:19–30.
125. Tamimi, R.M., Lagiou, P., Mucci, L.A., Hsieh, C.C., Adami, H.O., and Trichopoulos, D. 2003. Average energy intake among pregnant women carrying a boy compared with a girl. *BMJ* 326:1245–46.
126. Hocher, B., Chen, Y.P., Schlemm, L., et al. 2009. Fetal sex determines the impact of maternal PROGINS progesterone receptor polymorphism on maternal physiology during pregnancy. *Pharmacogenet Genomics* 19:710–18.
127. Hocher, B., Schlemm, L., Haumann, H., et al. 2010. Interaction of maternal peroxisome proliferator-activated receptor gamma2 Pro12Ala polymorphism with fetal sex affects maternal glycemic control during pregnancy. *Pharmacogenet Genomics* 20:139–42.
128. Hocher, B., Schlemm, L., Haumann, H., et al. 2011. Offspring sex determines the impact of the maternal ACE I/D polymorphism on maternal glycaemic control during the last weeks of pregnancy. *J Renin Angiotensin Aldosterone Syst* 12:254–61.

129. Cheng, Y., Ma, Y., Peng, T., Wang, J., Lin, R., and Cheng, H.D. 2010. Genotype dis-crepancy between maternal and fetal Pro12Ala polymorphism of PPARG2 gene and its association with gestational diabetes mellitus. *Zhonghua Fu Chan Ke Za Zhi* 45:170–73.

130. Schwartz, D.B., Daoud, Y., Zazula, P., et al. 1999. Gestational diabetes mellitus: meta-bolic and blood glucose parameters in singleton versus twin pregnancies. *Am J Obstet Gynecol* 181:912–14.

131. Wangler, M.F., Chang, A.S., Moley, K.H., Feinberg, A.P., and Debaun, M.R. 2005. Factors associated with preterm delivery in mothers of children with Beckwith-Wiedemann syndrome: a case cohort study from the BWS registry. *Am J Med Genet A* 134A:187–91.

132. Petry, C.J., Ong, K.K., Barratt, B.J., et al. 2005. Common polymorphism in H19 associ-ated with birthweight and cord blood IGF-II levels in humans. *BMC Genet* 6:22.

133. Haig, D. 1996. Placental hormones, genomic imprinting, and maternal–fetal communi-cation. *J Evol Biol* 9:357–80.

134. Haig, D., and Westoby, M. 1989. Parent-specific gene expression and the triploid endo-sperm. *Am Nat* 134:147–55.

135. Haig, D. 1993. Genetic conflicts in human pregnancy. *Q Rev Biol* 68:495–532.

136. White, D.J., Wolff, J.N., Pierson, M., and Gemmell, N.J. 2008. Revealing the hidden complexities of mtDNA inheritance. *Mol Ecol* 17:4925–42.

137. Leighton, P.A., Ingram, R.S., Eggenschwiler, J., Efstratiadis, A., and Tilghman, S.M. 1995. Disruption of imprinting caused by deletion of the H19 gene region in mice. *Nature* 375:34–39.

138. Chiao, E., Fisher, P., Crisponi, L., et al. 2002. Overgrowth of a mouse model of the Simpson-Golabi-Behmel syndrome is independent of IGF signaling. *Dev Biol* 243:185–206.

139. Petry, C.J., Evans, M.L., Wingate, D.L., et al. 2010. Raised late pregnancy glucose concentrations in mice carrying pups with targeted disruption of H19delta13. *Diabetes* 59:282–86.

140. **Petry, C.J., Seear, R.V., Wingate, D.L., et al. 2011. Associations between paternally transmitted fetal IGF2 variants and maternal circulating glucose concentrations in pregnancy. *Diabetes* 50:3090–96.** *The first study showing an association between polymorphic variation in a foetal growth gene and maternal gestational diabetes risk.*

141. Petry, C.J., Seear, R.V., Wingate, D.L., et al. 2011. Maternally transmitted foetal H19 variants and associations with birth weight. *Hum Genet* 130:663–70.

142. Lango, H., UK Type 2 Diabetes Genetics Consortium, Palmer, C.N., et al. 2008. Assessing the combined impact of 18 common genetic variants of modest effect sizes on type 2 diabetes risk. *Diabetes* 57:3129–35.

143. van Hoek, M., Dehghan, A., Witteman, J.C., et al. 2008. Predicting type 2 diabetes based on polymorphisms from genome-wide association studies: a population-based study. *Diabetes* 57:3122–28.

144. Visscher, P.M., Brown, M.A., McCarthy, M.I., and Yang, J. 2012. Five years of GWAS discovery. *Am J Hum Genet* 90:7–24.

145. So, H.C., Gui, A.H., Cherny, S.S., and Sham, P.C. 2011. Evaluating the heritability explained by known susceptibility variants: a survey of ten complex diseases. *Genet Epidemiol* 35:310–17.

146. Kwak, S.H., Jang, H.C., and Park, K.S. 2012. Finding genetic risk factors of gestational diabetes. *Genomics Inform* 10:239–43.

147. Ekelund, M., Shaat, N., Almgren, P., et al. 2012. Genetic prediction of postpartum dia-betes in women with gestational diabetes mellitus. *Diabetes Res Clin Pract* 97:394–98.

148. Distefano, J.K., and Watanabe, R.M. 2010. Pharmacogenetics of anti-diabetes drugs. *Pharmaceuticals (Basel)* 3:2610–46.

149. Pearson, E.R. 2009. Pharmacogenetics in diabetes. *Curr Diab Rep* 9:172–81.

150. Lambrinoudaki, I., Vlachou, S.A., and Creatsas, G. 2010. Genetics in gestational diabetes mellitus: association with incidence, severity, pregnancy outcome and response to treatment. *Curr Diabetes Rev* 6:393–99.
151. HAPO Study Cooperative Research Group, Metzger, B.E., Lowe, L.P., et al. 2008. Hyperglycemia and adverse pregnancy outcomes. *N Engl J Med* 358:1991–2002.

Section III

Complications

5 Complications of Gestational Diabetes

Liat Salzer and Yariv Yogev
Helen Schneider Hospital for Women, Rabin Medical
Center, Petah Tikva, Israel, The Sackler Faculty of
Medicine, Tel Aviv University, Tel Aviv, Israel

CONTENTS

5.1 INTRODUCTION: OBESITY, GLUCOSE INTOLERANCE, AND THE METABOLIC SYNDROME—A VICIOUS CYCLE COMPLICATING PREGNANCY

In 1988, Reaven[1] proposed that resistance to insulin-stimulated glucose uptake (insulin resistance) and secondary hyperinsulinaemia are involved in the aetiology of three major related diseases: cardiovascular disease, type 2 diabetes mellitus, and hypertension. He coined the term *syndrome X*, which was later modified to metabolic syndrome. Metabolic syndrome describes a group of abnormalities that increase the risk for cardiovascular disease: resistance to insulin-stimulated glucose uptake, glucose intolerance, hyperinsulinaemia, increased triglyceride, decreased HDL cholesterol, and hypertension. Obesity is the most important risk factor for metabolic syndrome. In the National Health and Nutrition Examination Survey (NHANES) metabolic syndrome was present in 4.6, 22.4, and 59.6% of normal weight, overweight, and obese men, respectively.[2] Insulin resistance and hyperinsulinaemia may be the basic common ground of elevated blood pressure and type 2 diabetes mellitus. Both diseases predispose to long-term cardiovascular complications.

Pregnancy is normally attended by progressive insulin resistance that begins near mid-pregnancy and progresses through the third trimester to levels that approximate insulin resistance seen in individuals with type 2 diabetes mellitus. It is estimated that insulin resistance increases by 40–50% in comparison to pregravid condition.[3] The insulin resistance appears to result from a combination of increased maternal adiposity and the insulin-desensitising effects of hormonal products of the placenta. The fact that insulin resistance rapidly abates following delivery suggests that the major contributor to this state is resistance, caused by placental hormones.

Pregnant patients may develop components resembling metabolic syndrome preceding or along the duration of pregnancy, with some of the elements existing prior to conception, while others develop during gestation. As such, obesity, along with hypertensive disorders and gestational diabetes mellitus (GDM), is a central attribute of the metabolic syndrome that may occur whilst pregnant. Different studies have estimated that about 3–15% of women develop GDM during pregnancy. Many factors are related to this risk, including ethnicity, previous occurrence of GDM, advanced maternal age, parity, family history of diabetes, and degree of hyperglycaemia in pregnancy and obesity. Obesity is an independent risk for developing GDM, with a risk of about 20%.[4] It has been shown that even minor degrees of carbohydrate intolerance are related to obesity and pregnancy outcome.[5,6] Sebire et al.[7] conducted a retrospective analysis of 287,213 pregnancies, comparing women with normal body mass indices (BMIs) and obese pregnant women and found a mean of twofold increase in the rate of GDM. Kumari,[8] comparing obese and non-obese patients, found a rate of GDM of 24.5% for the obese and 2.2% for the non-obese. Bianco et al.[9] reported a threefold increase in GDM for obese patients. A population based cohort study of 96,801 singleton births found that not only obese women but also overweight women had a markedly increased risk for GDM (odds ratios (ORs) 5.0 and 2.4, respectively).[10] Yogev et al.,[11] in a study of 6,857 women, found a direct association between glucose screening categories, obesity, and rate of GDM. For patients with 50 g glucose challenge test (GCT) screening results from

130 to 189 mg/dl (7.2–10.5 mmol/L), the rate of obesity was approximately 24–30%. Thereafter, at GCT results > 190 mg/dl (10.6 mmol/L) the rate of obesity increased twofold. These data demonstrate that the degree of obesity and glucose tolerance are both independently associated with the development of GDM.

The impact of obesity and GDM on both the foetus and the mother often becomes circular, as the majority of women with GDM are obese, and a significant proportion of those who are obese have GDM.

5.2 MATERNAL, FOETAL, AND NEONATAL COMPLICATIONS OF GESTATIONAL DIABETES MELLITUS

GDM poses a risk to mother and child. The separation of these risks and outcomes to maternal and foetal is sometimes artificial, as some of the maternal complications have a direct effect upon the foetus. Also, it is not always possible to differentiate the risks into short- and long-term ones, since some of the complications pose a continuous risk for either the mother or her offspring, and moreover, some of the outcomes complicate both the mother and her child.

For the purpose of this chapter, we categorised most of the important maternal, foetal, and neonatal complications of GDM.

5.2.1 Maternal Complications: Short-Term Outcomes

Even mild hyperglycaemia during pregnancy can adversely impact maternal health and is associated with a significantly higher risk of hypertensive disorders,[12,13] caesarean delivery,[12,13] and later metabolic disorder.[14]

5.2.1.1 The Association between Obesity, Diabetes, and Hypertension

Insulin resistance with secondary hyperinsulinaemia is suspected to be the link between hypertension and diabetes. The hypertensive effect of hyperinsulinaemia is postulated to be due to weight gain, extracellular fluid volume expansion due to renal sodium retention, and increased sympathetic activity.[15] Another theory linking insulin resistance, obesity, and type 2 diabetes mellitus is a process of low-grade inflammation. Obesity is associated with high adiposity and hyperlipidaemia, and it appears that inflammation, mediated by adipokines and cytokines,[16] especially tumour necrosis factor-alpha (TNF-α) and interleukin-6 (IL-6),[16–18] may modulate insulin resistance in GDM.

Several studies deal with the association between GDM and gestational hypertensive disorders. Some have suggested that gestational hypertension, but not preeclampsia, is associated with insulin resistance,[19,20] while others illustrated that the association is true for the entire spectrum of hypertensive disorders.[5,21–23] A study by Barden et al. examined 184 women with GDM and found that preeclampsia was more frequent among women with diabetes (approximately 12%) versus the nondiabetic population (8%).[24] The significant independent predictors for developing preeclampsia in those pregnancies were fasting glucose, elevated C-reactive protein, a family history of hypertension, and the proband's mother having gestational diabetes. Another study done by Bryson et al.[25] examined the relationship between GDM and hypertension by conducting a case-control analysis of birth records of mothers delivering infants in Washington State between 1992 and 1998. Diagnoses of pregnancy-induced hypertension were identified by *International Classification of Diseases, ninth revision* (ICD-9) codes and divided into populations with gestational hypertension ($n = 8,943$), mild preeclampsia ($n = 5,468$), severe preeclampsia ($n = 1,180$), and eclampsia ($n = 154$). GDM was also identified by ICD-9 code, and a control population ($n = 47, 237$) was selected by random sampling. The women with pregnancy-induced hypertension were younger, had lower BMI, were more often primigravid, and had improved prenatal care compared with those of the control women. The data revealed that after adjusting for BMI, age, race/ethnicity, parity, and adequate prenatal care, GDM was significantly associated with mild and severe preeclampsia, as well as gestational hypertension with ORs of 1.50, 1.53, and 1.40, respectively.

The rate of preeclampsia has been found to correlate with the level of glycaemic control: in a study by Yogev et al., when fasting plasma glucose (FPG) was <105 mg/dl (5.8 mmol/L), the rate of preeclampsia was 7.8%; with an FPG >105 mg/dl, the rate of preeclampsia was 13.8%.[26] In this same study, pregravid BMI was also significantly related to the development of preeclampsia. Moreover, mid-pregnancy postprandial glycaemia has been noted to be positively associated with odds of subsequent gestational hypertension and preeclampsia. The Toronto Tri-Hospital Project cohort study[5] of 4,274 screened gravidas with singleton pregnancies examined 3,836 women who went on to have a 3 h 100 g oral glucose tolerance test. Postprandial glucose but not fasting glucose values showed an association with the probability for subsequent preeclampsia, with the most significant being the 2 h value. Among those with values of <100 mg/dl (5.6 mmol/L), 3.3% had preeclampsia, with rates rising to 4.7, 6.5, and 6.4% among those in the 101–116 mg/dl (5.6–6.4 mmol/L), 117–131 mg/dl (6.5–7.3 mmol/L), and > 131 mg/dl (7.3 mmol/L) strata. A retrospective case-control study[27] compared 97 women with new-onset hypertension in late pregnancy and 77 normotensive control gravidas. The study demonstrated that after adjustment of BMI and baseline systolic and diastolic blood pressures, the post-50 g challenge 1 h glucose value at 24–28 weeks was significantly higher among those developing hypertension.

A secondary analysis of the Calcium for Preeclampsia Prevention multicenter calcium prophylaxis preeclampsia trial[28] examined the association between glucose tolerance and subsequent gestational hypertension or preeclampsia among 3,381 screened nulliparous gravidas. The adjusted (by study centre) relative risks of gestational hypertension and preeclampsia of those with GDM compared with those with 50 g 1 h values of <140 mg/dl (7.8 mmol/L) were 1.48 (95% confidence interval (CI) 0.99– 2.22) and 1.67 (0.92–3.05), respectively, and reached statistical significance when the two hypertensive outcomes were combined: OR 1.54 (1.28–2.11). When the 227 gravidas with screening test values of ≥140 mg/dl (7.8 mmol/L) but without GDM were compared with those with values < 140 mg/dl, no difference in hypertension incidence could be detected. However, as in earlier studies, the 1 h 50 g glucose value among all gravidas correlated strongly ($p < 0.0001$) with preeclampsia risk after adjustment for clinical centre, race, and BMI.

In patients who have chronic hypertension coexisting with diabetes, preeclampsia may be difficult to distinguish. Patients with chronic hypertension and diabetes are at increased risk of intrauterine growth restriction, superimposed preeclampsia, placental abruption, and maternal stroke.

5.2.1.2 Mode of Delivery

An increased rate of caesarean (C) section has been observed among women affected by GDM. Studies have shown that these C-sections are mostly unjustified.[29,30] Recent studies identified a C-section rate among women with this condition as high as 35%,[31] and indicated a probability of undertaking a C-section in this group around 1.5 times the probability among non-GDM women[32] (Figure 5.1).

Furthermore, babies born to women with GDM are significantly more exposed to perinatal risk, mostly related to foetal macrosomia. This clinical condition is associated with an increased risk of intrapartum traumatic lesions and asphyxia. These newborns are characterised by a trunk mass larger than the head, and consequently are more exposed to shoulder dystocia, bone fractures, and brachial plexus injury, possibly with permanent outcomes. Vaginal delivery of macrosomic babies also exposes the mother to further trauma by increasing the rates of operative vaginal delivery and episiotomy.[33] Still, the question regarding active management protocol for early elective delivery is debatable. Several studies[34,35] have demonstrated an advantage for an induction of labour based on the estimated foetal weight. Pregnancy prolongation beyond 38 weeks was found to increase the prevalence of large for gestational

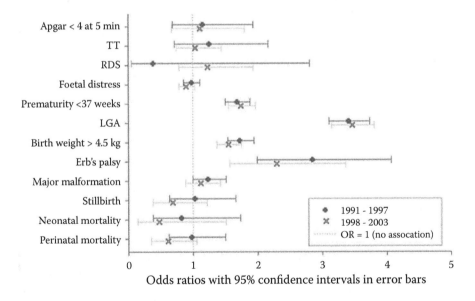

FIGURE 5.1 Maternal and neonatal outcomes and time trends of gestational diabetes mellitus in Sweden from 1991 to 2003 (n = 1,260,297 women), split into 1991–1997 and 1998–2003. Results from logistic regression models adjusted for maternal age, body mass index, coronary heart disease, ethnicity, parity, and smoking. LGA, large for gestational age; PE, preeclampsia; PIH, pregnancy-induced hypertension; RDS, respiratory distress syndrome; TT, transient tachypnoea; VE, vacuum extraction. (From Fadl, H.E. et al., *Diabet. Med., 27,* 436–41, 2010. Reproduced with permission.)

age newborns, foetal macrosomia, and shoulder dystocia.[36,37] On the other hand, a retrospective analysis of 124 women with GDM revealed no significant differences in perinatal outcomes, including shoulder dystocia and C-section rate.[38]

To date, there is only one prospective randomised controlled trial (RCT) that compared active induction of labour at 38 weeks of gestation with expectant management in 187 insulin-requiring GDM mothers.[37] The results showed a nonsignificant difference in C-section rate, but an increased number of large for gestational age (LGA) babies (23% versus 10%) and shoulder dystocia (3% versus none).

5.2.2 Maternal Complications: Long-Term Outcomes

5.2.2.1 Metabolic Syndrome, Obesity, and Type 2 Diabetes

Though most women with GDM return to normal glucose tolerance after delivery, they have an increased risk of developing type 2 diabetes mellitus as much as sevenfold over their lifetime.[39] Studies have also found that having GDM is a definitive risk factor, a predictor, or even an early manifestation of the metabolic syndrome. Vohr and Boney[40] found that women with a prior history of GDM and obesity had a significantly greater risk of developing metabolic syndrome than mothers with no history of GDM or obesity. The rate of metabolic syndrome in both the GDM women and controls increased between 4 and 11 years postdelivery to 27.2% in the GDM and 8.2% in the control group, and the incidence of metabolic syndrome was threefold higher in the GDM compared to control women at each follow-up visit. Vambergue et al.[41] found that the strongest predictors for developing type 2 diabetes mellitus in women was previous GDM, medical history of hypertension, being 33 years or older at age of delivery, a family history of diabetes, a fasting glucose concentration during pregnancy of 100 mg/dl (5.6 mmol/L), and severity level of hyperglycaemia during pregnancy. Noussitou et al.,[42] retrospectively studying 5,788 deliveries, identified 159 (2.7%) patients with GDM out of the total study population. In 26% of these women, some aspects of the metabolic syndrome were identified prior to the index pregnancy (obesity 84%, hypertension 38%, and dyslipidaemia 22%). In the postpartum follow-up, 11% had type 2 diabetes mellitus and 16% had impaired fasting glucose. Consequently, within pregnancy period, GDM was accompanied and preceded by metabolic abnormalities compatible with the metabolic syndrome. Noussitou's study also found that women with GDM and metabolic abnormalities were independently associated with a fivefold increase in the risk of developing an abnormal glucose tolerance in the close postpartum (average of 9.5 weeks).

Indeed, several studies have investigated the relationship between GDM and obesity to a future diagnosis of the metabolic syndrome. Bo et al.[43] reported that the prevalence of the metabolic syndrome and its components was 2- to 4-fold higher in women with prior gestational hyperglycaemia and 10-fold higher if prepregnancy obesity coexisted as well. These findings suggest that GDM, especially in combination with prepregnancy obesity, predicts a subsequent syndrome of high cardiovascular risk. Pallardo et al.[44] studied 788 Caucasian women with GDM 3–6 months postpartum where 3.7% were diagnosed with overt diabetes. The area under the postpartum glucose curve was positively associated with BMI, waist circumference, waist-to-hip ratio, circulating triglyceride concentrations, and systolic and diastolic blood pressures. It was concluded that postpartum glucose intolerance predicts a high-risk cardiovascular profile that includes risk factors besides type 2 diabetes mellitus.

5.2.2.2 Hypertension and Cardiovascular Disease

The association of glucose intolerance and insulin resistance in early and mid-pregnancy with subsequent gestational hypertension and preeclampsia suggests that patients with GDM may already have subclinical vasculopathy that results in later hypertension and vascular disease. Women with a previous history of GDM have been shown to have impaired markers of endothelial and cardiac function. Heitritter et al. found that women with a history of GDM had greater vascular resistance, lower stroke volume, and lower cardiac output than women without a history of GDM.[45] Postpartum GDM women also appear to have greater diastolic dysfunction upon echocardiography,[46] increased carotid intimal medial thickness,[47] and poorer brachial artery flow-mediated dilation compared with controls,[48] all of which are markers for vascular dysfunction.

Clinical studies regarding the association between GDM and cardiovascular disease are hard to conduct owing to the long lag time that follows between pregnancy and cardiovascular disease events, typically two to three decades later. Currently, no large prospective cohort studies of GDM and non-GDM women exist that ascertain cardiovascular disease events in a systematic fashion. Nevertheless, two studies did examine this relationship: Carr et al.[49] compared women with ($n = 332$) and without ($n = 663$) a history of GDM regarding (1) metabolic syndrome, (2) the prevalence of type 2 diabetes mellitus, and (3) self-reported cardiovascular disease. They found that among women with a family history of type 2 diabetes mellitus, those with prior GDM were more likely to not only have cardiovascular disease risk factors, including metabolic syndrome and type 2 diabetes mellitus, but also experience cardiovascular disease events, which occurred at a younger age. The authors concluded that women with both family history of type 2 diabetes mellitus and personal history of GDM may be especially suitable for early interventions aimed at preventing or reducing their risk of cardiovascular disease and diabetes. One of the limitations of the study was that all women in it had at least two first-degree relatives with type 2 diabetes and were participants in the Genetics of Non-Insulin Dependent Diabetes (GENNID) study, and thus were probably at preliminary higher risk. The second retrospective study, done by Shah et al.,[50] also found that a history of GDM was associated with a greater risk of coronary disease events. As in the study by Carr et al., much of this risk was attributed to the elevated type 2 diabetes risk of women with histories of GDM.

As for hypertensive disorders, women with GDM were found to be at a significantly higher risk of developing hypertension after the index pregnancy.[51] Volpe et al.[52] examined 28 women 2 to 5 years after a pregnancy complicated by GDM and found that these women had higher systolic blood pressures than those of women with normoglycaemic pregnancies. Patients with underlying renal or retinal vascular disease are at a substantially higher risk, with 40% having chronic hypertension.

5.2.3 Foetal and Neonatal Complications

Perinatal mortality (PNM) in diabetic pregnancies has decreased 30-fold since the discovery of insulin in 1922 and the introduction of intensive obstetrical and infant care in the 1970s. Nevertheless, current studies show a 1.5- to 3-fold higher risk of perinatal death of offspring of women with GDM compared to those of nondiabetic pregnancies.[53] Congenital malformations, respiratory distress syndrome (RDS), and extreme prematurity account for most perinatal deaths in diabetic pregnancies. Regarding PNM, most of the studies have been conducted in women with overt insulin-treated pregestational diabetes. The physiological basis of perinatal death in GDM is less understood and occurs mainly in advanced stages of pregnancy. The increased PNM rate in GDM has been correlated to early-onset diabetes, advanced maternal age, and obesity. These findings suggest the possibility of undetected pregestational diabetes. Bradley et al.[54] collected foetal cord samples by cordocentesis from 28 women with pregestational diabetes between 20 and 40 weeks of gestation. They found that some foetuses were significantly acidotic and hyperlacticaemic during the third trimester of pregnancy. This finding may suggest a possible mechanism for late foetal death in diabetic pregnancies caused mainly by metabolic acidosis rather than the hypoxic asphyxia mechanism that dominates in nondiabetic pregnancies.

In GDM, the correlation between congenital anomalies and PNM is not well established. Some studies demonstrated a slightly increased rate of congenital malformations close to that reported for pregestational diabetes,[55,56] but the majority documented a rate similar to that of the general population.[57,58] It seems reasonable to assume that studies reporting a higher prevalence of foetal malformation in GDM included patients with undiagnosed type 2 diabetes mellitus. Since obesity and diabetes tend to coexist, rates of congenital anomalies are probably influenced by obesity as well. Several studies report a significant increase in birth defects among obese woman. Studies documented an increased risk for neural tube defects,[59] heart defects,[60] and omphalocele.[61] Nevertheless, because these types of congenital anomalies are often seen with pregestational diabetes, some investigators suggest that again, many of these obese women may have had undiagnosed type 2 diabetes mellitus.[60]

5.2.3.1 Level of Glycaemic Control and Its Influence on Perinatal Morbidity and Mortality

Since glucose intolerance is characterised by a gradual continuum disorder in the carbohydrate metabolism, it will be reasonable to assume that higher mean blood glucose levels during pregnancy (reflecting either low treatment quality or higher severity of GDM) are related to an increase in PNM. For a few centuries, studies have shown the decrease in PNM according to the mean blood glucose levels.[62–64] Langer and Conway[65] postulated that different thresholds of mean glucose values are associated with different foetal complications, such as stillbirth, spontaneous abortion, congenital anomalies, foetal macrosomia, and metabolic and respiratory complications. For each complication, a different targeted threshold from normality is required to be achieved in order to eliminate the complication. This fundamental observation supplies an explanation for the controversy and differences in reported results of perinatal outcome obtained among different centres, usually demonstrating low congenital malformation rates on one hand, but high neonatal death rate on the other. Here also, most of the studies were done on pregestational diabetes.

In light of the information regarding tight glycaemic control, the American Diabetes Association (ADA) position statement suggests that a threshold of fasting

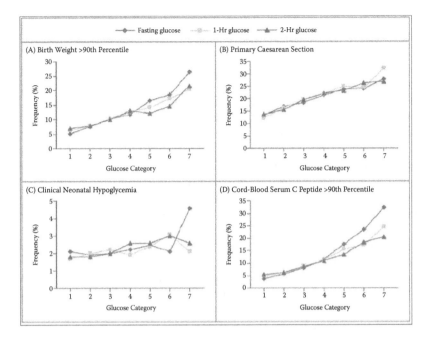

FIGURE 5.2   Hyperglycemia and Adverse Pregnancy Outcome study associations between maternal glucose concentrations (fasting, and 1 and 2 h postglucose load, expressed as septiles) in a 75 g oral glucose tolerance test between 24 and 32 weeks gestation and adverse pregnancy outcomes: (A) offspring birth weight above the 90th percentile, (B) primary caesarean section, (C) clinical neonatal hypoglycaemia, and (D) cord blood C-peptide concentrations above the 90th percentile. (From HAPO Study Cooperative Research Group, Metzger, B.E. et al., *N. Engl. J. Med.*, 358, 1991–2002, 2008. Reproduced with permission.)

hyperglycaemia (which objectively reflects level of disease severity) of >105 mg/dl (5.8 mmol/L) may be associated with an increased risk of late intrauterine foetal death in women with GDM.[36] Still, findings are not consistent regarding the threshold. The Hyperglycemia and Adverse Pregnancy Outcome (HAPO) research study group examined data from more than 25,000 women who underwent 75 g oral glucose tolerance testing at 24–32 weeks of gestation and found significant associations between elevated fasting plasma glucose and an elevation in cord blood serum C-peptide level above the 90th percentile, an increased risk of primary caesarean delivery, and an increased risk of neonatal hypoglycaemia (Figure 5.2). A more ominous finding was that there were no obvious thresholds at which these risks increased.[41] Nevertheless, it is now well established that rigorous control of diabetes during pregnancy significantly reduces the PNM rate.

5.2.4   Foetal and Neonatal Short-Term Outcomes

5.2.4.1   Foetal Overgrowth

During the early phases of organ embryogenesis, control of foetal growth is exercised primarily by the genome. Beyond this point, however, the ultimate growth of the foetus is controlled by a multitude of factors, such as nutrients, environmental considerations, and aberrant metabolic states, i.e., diabetes. Maternal diabetes results in an increased placental transport of glucose and other nutrients from the mother to the foetus, in addition to increased foetoplacental availability of nutrients in late gestation, resulting in macrosomia.

Macrosomia, the most commonly reported effect of maternal diabetes in newborns, has been variously defined as birth weight above either 4,000 or 4,500 g, as well as birth weight above the 90th or 95th percentile of the gestational age for population and sex-specific growth curves. Studies have shown that both pregestational diabetes and GDM are associated with macrosomia,[66,67] and it is 10 times more frequent for a diabetic mother to deliver an infant weighting greater than 4,500 g than a woman with normal glucose tolerance.[68] The reported rate of large for gestational age (LGA) infants reaches up to 30% of pregnancies in woman with diabetes mellitus, a threefold increase from normoglycaemic controls (assumed to be 10%). Many of the LGA foetuses, though born to diabetic mothers, fall into the Gaussian distribution and are constitutionally large but healthy.

Macrosomia is strongly associated with foetal death, prematurity, birth trauma, and respiratory distress syndrome.[69] These foetuses are less resistant to a hostile intrauterine environment, and hence more susceptible to in-labour insults. Large for gestational age and macrosomic infants face significantly increased risk for injury at the time of vaginal birth, such as shoulder dystocia and newborn asphyxia. Although delivery in a C-section in these infants offers the potential for avoiding birth trauma to the foetus, it can result in increased trauma to the mother when compared to vaginal delivery. Data from the Diabetes in Early Pregnancy Project indicated that foetal birth weight correlates best with second and third trimester postprandial blood sugar levels and not with fasting or mean glucose levels.[70] When postprandial glucose values average 120 mg/dl (6.7 mmol/L) or less, approximately 20% of infants can be expected to be macrosomic. When postprandial levels range as high as 160 mg/dl (8.9 mmol/L), macrosomia rates can reach 35%. Moreover, the foetal birth weight is largely determined by maternal factors other than hyperglycaemia. The most significant influences are gestational age at delivery, maternal prepregnancy BMI, weight gain through pregnancy, the presence of hypertension, and cigarette smoking. Obesity and overweight that frequently coexist with diabetes are independent risk factors for foetal macrosomia.[71,72]

5.2.4.2   Shoulder Dystocia and Brachial Plexus Injury

Shoulder dystocia has traditionally been strongly associated with macrosomia, but up to one-half of cases of shoulder dystocia occur in neonates weighing less than 4,000 g.[73] Neonates of diabetic mothers have a unique pattern of overgrowth, which involves larger shoulder and extremity circumference, a decreased head-to-shoulder ratio, significantly higher body fat, and thicker upper extremity skinfolds compared with nondiabetic control infants of similar weights.[74] Because foetal head size is not increased during poorly controlled diabetic pregnancy, but shoulder and abdominal girth can be markedly augmented, the risk of injury to the foetus after delivery of the head (e.g., Erb palsy) is significantly increased. Thus, birth injuries, including shoulder dystocia and brachial plexus trauma, are more common among infants of diabetic mothers, and macrosomic foetuses are at the highest risk. The risk for shoulder dystocia with a foetal weight over 4,000 g in a diabetic pregnant woman is reported to be up to 30%.[73] Recent data from the Australian Carbohydrate Intolerance Study in Pregnant Women (ACHOIS) trial demonstrated a positive relationship between severity of maternal fasting hyperglycaemia and risk of shoulder dystocia, with an 18 mg/dl (1 mmol/L) increase in fasting glucose concentrations leading to a 2.09 relative risk for shoulder dystocia.[75]

5.2.4.3 Respiratory Distress Syndrome

Neonates born to women with GDM are considered to have a greater risk of developing respiratory distress syndrome than neonates born to women without GDM. This syndrome is most often found in premature infants due to developmental insufficiency of surfactant production and structural immaturity in the lungs. The reason that respiratory distress syndrome is more prevalent in full-term infants born to women with GDM is not completely clear, although there is evidence that hyperglycaemia delays foetal lung maturity. Piper[76] claimed that poorly controlled maternal diabetes in pregnancy may delay foetal pulmonary maturation. However, diabetic women with good glycaemic control have foetal lung maturation at the same gestational age as nondiabetic women. Respiratory distress syndrome is rare in well-controlled diabetic pregnancies confirmed by early ultrasound to be at or beyond 37 weeks. Moore[77] found that foetal pulmonary maturation, measured by the onset of phosphatidylglycerol production, was delayed in diabetic pregnancies by 1–1.5 weeks.

Still, studies are inconclusive regarding lung maturity in diabetes patients. For example, Berkowitz et al.[78] found no clinical or statistical differences in lecithin/sphingomyelin (L/S) ratio between diabetic and nondiabetic patients, and that lung maturity strongly correlates with gestational age and not significantly with diabetes. Kjos et al.[79] found that the only independent predictor for RDS in term infants of diabetic mothers was caesarean delivery. Another study of 526 diabetic patients found that the majority of infants exhibiting signs of respiratory distress did not have immature lung development with insufficient surfactant production.[80] After reviewing the literature, Langer[81] concluded that although 10–20% of lung testing results will demonstrate immaturity (phosphatidylglycerol)—after the 37th week of gestation in the presence of well-controlled glucose—foetal morbidity will not be related to the lung testing results.

Since the 1970s, improved prenatal maternal management for diabetes and new techniques in obstetrics for timing and mode of delivery has resulted in a dramatic decline in respiratory distress syndrome incidence. Nevertheless, respiratory distress syndrome continues to be a relatively preventable complication.

5.2.4.4 Neonatal Hypoglycaemia

Up to 15–25% of neonates delivered from women with diabetes during gestation develop hypoglycaemia during the immediate newborn period. This effect results from the infant's insulin surge in response to maternal hyperglycaemia. The relationship between the maternal and neonatal glycaemia was also described by the HAPO study group that presented data from plasma glucose measurements of 17,000 infants of mothers without diabetes. The study found a strong continuous association between maternal OGTT glucose levels and cord blood C-peptide levels (Figure 5.2).[12] Cord blood C-peptide levels were associated with neonatal hypoglycaemia and excessive size at birth. Larger or fatter infants were more likely to develop hypoglycaemia and hyperinsulinaemia. The fact that these relationships extend across the entire range of maternal glycaemia suggests a physiologic relationship between maternal glycaemia and foetal insulin production.[82] Neonatal hypoglycaemia occurs less frequently when tight glycaemic control is maintained during pregnancy and in labour. Unrecognised postnatal hypoglycaemia may lead to neonatal seizures, coma, and brain damage.

5.2.4.5   Hyperbilirubinaemia and Jaundice

Hyperbilirubinaemia occurs in up to 38% of offspring of pregnancies with GDM.[68] The causes of hyperbilirubinaemia in infants of diabetic mothers are multiple, but prematurity and polycythaemia are the primary proposed contributing factors. Increased destruction of red blood cells contributes to the risk of jaundice and kernicterus. Treatment of this complication is usually with phototherapy, but exchange transfusions may be necessary if bilirubin levels are markedly elevated.

5.2.4.6   Polycythaemia

A central venous haemoglobin concentration greater than 20 g/dl or a haematocrit value greater than 65% (polycythaemia) is not uncommon in infants of diabetic mothers and is related to glycaemic control. Hyperglycaemia is a powerful stimulus to foetal erythropoietin production, mediated by decreased foetal oxygen tension. Untreated neonatal polycythaemia may promote vascular sludging, ischaemia, and infarction of vital tissues, including the kidneys and central nervous system.

5.2.4.7   Calcium and Magnesium Abnormalities

Infants of diabetic mothers may have low levels of serum calcium (<7 mg/dl or 1.75 mmol/L) even after exclusion of predisposing factors such as prematurity and birth asphyxia. These changes in calcium appear to be attributable to a functional hypoparathyroidism, though the exact pathophysiology is not well understood. With improved management of diabetes in pregnancy, the rate of neonatal hypocalcaemia has been reduced to 5% or less. Decreased serum magnesium levels have been also documented in pregnant diabetic woman as well as in their infants. These findings may be explained by reduced foetal magnesium urinary extraction. Magnesium deficiency may paradoxically inhibit foetal parathyroid hormone secretion.

5.2.4.8   Preterm Delivery

Some researchers have proposed an increased risk for preterm deliveries in GDM women, and that there is a higher incidence of preterm delivery in association with different levels of glucose intolerance. Yogev and Langer[83] followed 1,526 GDM patients and found that the rate of spontaneous preterm delivery in GDM was not increased in comparison to that in non-GDM patients. Still, reaching desired levels of glycaemic control may reduce the rate of spontaneous preterm delivery in GDM.

Reports regarding preterm deliveries in obesity as a sole risk factor are inconclusive. Most studies report a decreased risk of spontaneous preterm deliveries[84] and an increased risk for elective preterm deliveries with increasing BMI.[84]

5.2.5 FOETAL AND NEONATAL LONG-TERM OUTCOMES

5.2.5.1 The Concepts of Foetal Programming and Metabolic Memory

During the last decade and even before, evidence has raised the assumption that exposure to an adverse foetal or early postnatal environment may enhance susceptibility to a number of chronic diseases in the future life of offspring.[85] The thrifty phenotype hypothesis, proposed by Hales and Barker,[86] argues that poor foetal and infant growth results in the subsequent development of type 2 diabetes mellitus and the metabolic syndrome due to the effects of poor nutrition in early life, which produces permanent changes in glucose-insulin metabolism. At the critical and delicate period of foetal development, the process by which a stimulus induces long-term impacts on the foetus, previously described and established as "foetal programming" by Hales and Barker, creates a "metabolic memory." The metabolic abnormalities of diabetic pregnancies create an in utero environment around the foetus, which programs it to diseases during adulthood.

In diabetic pregnancies, this memory may result in type 2 diabetes mellitus and obesity associated with metabolic syndrome. Evidence for the phenomenon of metabolic memory is seen also in several studies on humans and animals. For example, maternal pregnancy hypercholesterolaemia is associated with atherosclerosis during childhood,[87] and there is a good correlation between maternal and foetal plasma cholesterol levels in 5- to 6-month-old human foetuses.[88] Another example is a study that shows that diabetic pregnancy in rats alters the differentiation of hypothalamic neurons of newborns.[89] These alterations may increase the risk of high food intake, overweight, obesity, and diabetogenic status in offspring at adulthood.

5.2.5.2 Metabolic Syndrome, Obesity, and Type 2 Diabetes

The epidemic of obesity and subsequent risk of diabetes and components of the metabolic syndrome clearly may begin in utero with foetal overgrowth and adiposity. The adverse downstream effects of abnormal maternal metabolism on the offspring have been documented well into puberty and later in adulthood. Recent studies have demonstrated that exposure to hyperglycaemia during pregnancy can significantly increase a child's risk for other long-term complications as well. After birth, these newborns often are left with possible lifelong increased risks of glucose intolerance and obesity, even though they are no longer being exposed to a high-glucose environment.

Evidence shows that children born to mothers with GDM have increased risk of developing childhood obesity or metabolic syndrome compared to children born to nondiabetic mothers. The childhood metabolic syndrome includes childhood obesity, hypertension, dyslipidaemia, and glucose intolerance. A growing body of literature supports a relationship between intrauterine exposure to maternal diabetes and risk of a metabolic syndrome later in life.[90,91] Foetuses of diabetic women that are born large for gestational age appear to be at the greatest risk. Verma et al.[92] confirmed this finding, while they reported that 27% of children born to mothers diagnosed with GDM and 8.2% born to controls developed features of insulin resistance by age 11 years. The cumulative hazard for developing the metabolic syndrome in the next 2 years was 26 times higher among children to GDM subjects with prepregnant obesity, compared with controls. Vohr and Boney[40] found that the development of metabolic syndrome in children is related to maternal GDM, level of glycaemia in the third trimester, maternal obesity, neonatal macrosomia, and childhood obesity. These authors concluded that prevalence of obesity in both adults and children and associated disorders of blood pressure and lipid metabolism suggests a vicious perpetuating cycle. This cycle of increasing obesity, insulin resistance, and abnormal lipid metabolism may have ominous consequences for next successive generations.

Untreated GDM may be associated with a twofold risk of increased weight in offspring at 5–7 years.[93] Moreover, some investigators have found that maternal weight gain during pregnancy increases the offspring's risk of obesity later in life, independently of genetic factors.[94] There is an increase in the risk of obesity in these children at ages 1–9 years and in adolescents ages 14–16 years. Silverman and colleagues[95] have reported that there is a solid correlation between amniotic fluid insulin levels and increased BMI in 14- to 17-year-old children, indicating an association between islet cell activation in utero and development of childhood obesity. This obesity present in childhood then predisposes to obesity in the adult.

Dabelea et al.[96] found that the offspring of Native American (Pima) women who had diabetes during pregnancy were more obese and had a higher prevalence of type 2 diabetes mellitus. Pettit et al.[97] similarly found in a population of Pima Indians that the metabolic abnormalities associated with diabetic pregnancies were associated with long-term effects on the offspring, including insulin resistance, obesity, and type 2 diabetes mellitus, which in turn may contribute to transmission of risk for developing the same problems in the next generation.

5.2.5.3 Cardiovascular Risk

Only a few studies have dealt with the effect of maternal diabetes in utero and future cardiovascular risk in offspring. An associational study[98] found that offspring born to mothers with diabetes exhibited higher levels of biomarkers for endothelial damage and inflammation, as well as higher leptin levels, BMI, waist circumference, and systolic blood pressure, and decreased adiponectin levels. The association remained significant when controlling for maternal prepregnancy BMI. However, this association is still inconclusive. Beyerlein et al.[99] examined 12,542 children ages 3–17 years with full information concerning GDM and maternal BMI (data were available from the German nationwide KiGGS study). They concluded that GDM did not appear to have a relevant effect on cardiovascular disease correlates such as blood pressure or cholesterol levels in children. Moreover, they postulated that the potential effect of GDM on body composition seems to be widely explainable by maternal BMI.

5.3 SUMMARY

Most women who have GDM deliver healthy babies. However, GDM that is undiagnosed or not carefully managed can lead to uncontrolled maternal blood sugar levels

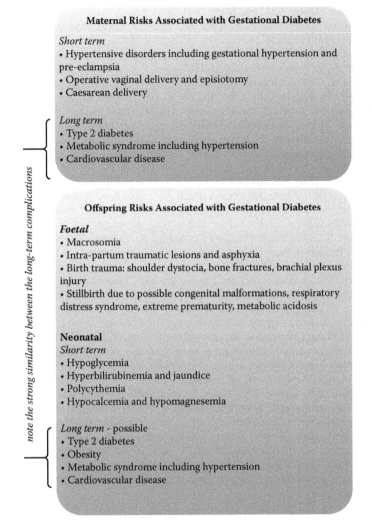

FIGURE 5.3   Schematic outlining the short- and long-term risks to the mother and her offspring associated with gestational diabetes.

and cause health complications for both the mother and her offspring. It is now clear that complications of GDM persist even later in life and pose a risk for further morbidity and mortality (Figure 5.3). Awareness and strict glycaemic control may allow primary prevention of many of the above-mentioned complications.

REFERENCES

Key references are in bold.

1. Reaven, G.M. 1988. Banting Lecture: Role of insulin resistance in human disease. *Diabetes* 37:1595–607.

2. Ford, E.S., Giles, W.H., and Dietz, W.H. 2002. Prevalence of the metabolic syndrome among US adults: findings from the third National Health and Nutrition Examination Survey. *JAMA* 287:356–59.

3. Catalano, P. 2003. Editorial: obesity and pregnancy—the propagation of a viscous cycle? *J Clin Endocrinol Metab* 88:3505–6.

4. Gabbe, S. 1986. Gestational diabetes mellitus. *N Engl J Med* 315:1025–26.

5. Sermer, M., Naylor, C.D., Gare, D.J., et al. 1995. Impact of increasing carbohydrate intolerance on maternal-fetal outcomes in 3637 women without gestational diabetes: the Toronto Tri-Hospital Gestational Diabetes Project. *Am J Obstet Gynecol* 173:146–56.

6. Jensen, D.M., Damm, P., Sørensen, B., et al. 2003. Pregnancy outcome and prepregnancy body mass index in 2459 glucose-tolerant Danish women. *Am J Obstet Gynecol* 189:239–44.

7. Sebire, N.J., Jolly, M., Harris, J.P., et al. 2001. Maternal obesity and pregnancy outcome: a study of 287,213 pregnancies in London. *Int J Obes Relat Metab Disord* 25:1175–82.

8. Kumari, A. 2001. Pregnancy outcome in women with morbid obesity. *Int J Gynaecol Obstet* 73:101–7.

9. Bianco, A.T., Smilen, S.W., Davis, Y., Lopez, S., Lapinski, R., and Lockwood, C.J. 1998. Pregnancy outcome and weight gain recommendations for the morbidly obese woman. *Obstet Gynecol* 91:97–102.

10. Baeten, J.M., Bukusi, E.A., and Lambe, M. 2001. Pregnancy complications and outcomes among overweight and obese nulliparous women. *Am J Public Health* 91:436–40.

11. Yogev, Y., Langer, O., Xenakis, E.M., and Rosenn, B. 2004. Glucose screening in Mexican-American women. *Obstet Gynecol* 103:1241–45.

12. **HAPO Study Cooperative Research Group, Metzger, B.E., Lowe, L.P., et al. 2008. Hyperglycemia and adverse pregnancy outcomes.** *N Engl J Med* **358:1991–2002.** *The study found significant associations between adverse outcomes and higher levels of maternal glucose even within a nondiabetic range.*

13. **Landon, M.B., Spong, C.Y., Thom, E., et al. 2009. A multicenter, randomized trial of treatment for mild gestational diabetes.** *N Engl J Med* **361:1339–48.** *Outcomes that were influenced by treatment of mild gestational diabetes mellitus were foetal overgrowth, shoulder dystocia, caesarean delivery, and hypertensive disorders.*

14. Gunderson, E.P., Jacobs, D.R., Chiang, V., et al. 2009. Childbearing is associated with higher incidence of the metabolic syndrome among women of reproductive age controlling for measurements before pregnancy: the CARDIA study. *Am J Obstet Gynecol* 201:177.e1–9.

15. Howard, G., O'Leary, D.H., Zaccaro, D., et al. 1996. Insulin sensitivity and atherosclerosis. *Circulation* 93:1809–17.

16. Atègbo, J.M., Grissa, O., Yessoufou, A., et al. 2006. Modulation of adipokines and cytokines in gestational diabetes and macrosomia. *J Clin Endocrinol Metab* 91:4137–43.

17. Dandona, P., Aljada, A., and Bandyopadhyay, A. 2004. Inflammation: the link between insulin resistance, obesity and diabetes. *Trends Immunol* 25:4–7.

18. Coppack, S.W. 2001. Pro-inflammatory cytokines and adipose tissue. *Proc Nutr Soc* 60:349–56.

19. Caruso, A., Ferrazzani, S., De Carolis, S., et al. 1999. Gestational hypertension but not pre-eclampsia is associated with insulin resistance syndrome characteristics. *Hum Reprod* 14:219–23.

20. Yasuhi, I., Hogan, J.W., Canick, J., Sosa, M.B., and Carpenter, M.W. 2001. Midpregnancy serum C-peptide concentration and subsequent pregnancy-induced hypertension. *Diabetes Care* 24:743–47.

21. Sierra-Laguado, J., García, R.G., Celedón, J., et al. 2007. Determination of insulin resistance using the homeostatic model assessment (HOMA) and its relation with the risk of developing pregnancy-induced hypertension. *Am J Hypertens* 20:437–42.

22. Wolf, M., Sandler, L., Munoz, K., Hsu, K., Ecker, J.L., and Thadhani, R. 2002. First trimester insulin resistance and subsequent preeclampsia: a prospective study. *J Clin Endocrinol Metab* 87:1563–68.

23. Solomon, C.G., Graves, S.W., Green, M.F., and Seely, E.W. 1994. Glucose intolerance as a predictor of hypertension in pregnancy. *Hypertension* 23:717–21.

24. Barden, A., Singh, R., Walters, B., Ritchie, J., Roberman, B., and Beilin, L. 2004. Factors predisposing to pre-eclampsia in women with gestational diabetes. *J Hypertens* 22:2371–78.

25. Bryson, C.L., Ioannou, G.N., Rulyak, S.J., and Critchlow, C. 2003. Association between gestational diabetes and pregnancy-induced hypertension. *Am J Epidemiol* 158:1148–53.

26. Yogev, Y., Xenakis, E.M., and Langer, O. 2004. The association between preeclampsia and the severity of gestational diabetes: the impact of glycemic control. *Am J Obstet Gynecol* 191:1655–60.

27. Solomon, C.G., Graves, S.W., Green, M.F., and Seely, E.W. 1994. Glucose intolerance as a predictor of hypertension in pregnancy. *Hypertension* 23:717–21.

28. Joffe G.M., Esterlitz, J.R., Levine, R.J., et al. 1998. The relationship between abnormal glucose tolerance and hypertensive disorders of pregnancy in healthy nulliparous women: Calcium for Preeclampsia Prevention (CPEP) study group. *Am J Obstet Gynecol* 179:1032–37.

29. Moses, R.G., Knights, S.J., Lucas, E.M., et al. 2000. Gestational diabetes: is a higher caesarean section rate inevitable? *Diabetes Care* 23:15–17.

30. Blackwell, S.C., Hassan, S.S., Wolfe, H.W., Michaelson, J., Berry, SM., and Sorokin, Y. 2000. Why are caesarean delivery rates so high in diabetic pregnancies? *J Perinat Med* 28:316–20.

31. Lapolla, A., Dalfrà, M.G., Bonomo, M., et al. 2009. Gestational diabetes mellitus in Italy: A multicenter study. *Eur J Obstet Gynecol Reprod Biol* 145:149–53.

32. Fadl, H.E., Östlund, I.K.M., Magnuson, A.F.K., and Hanson, U.S.B. 2010. Maternal and neonatal outcomes and time trends of gestational diabetes mellitus in Sweden from 1991 to 2003. *Diabet Med* 27:436–41.

33. Nassar, A.H., Usta, I.M., Khalil, A.M., Melhem, Z.I., Nakad, T.I., and AbuMusa, A.A. 2003. Fetal macrosomia (≥4500 g): perinatal outcome of 231 cases according to the mode of delivery. *J Perinatol* 23:136–41.

34. Hod, M., Bar, J., Peled, Y., et al. 1998. Antepartum management protocol. Timing and mode of delivery in gestational diabetes. *Diabetes Care* 21(Suppl 2):B113–17.

35. Witkop, C.T., Neale, D., Wilson, L.M., Bass, E.B., and Nicholson, W.K. 2009. Active compared with expectant delivery management in women with gestational diabetes: a systematic review. *Obstet Gynecol* 113:206–17.

36. American Diabetes Association. 2004. Gestational diabetes mellitus. *Diabetes Care* 27(Suppl 1):S88–90.

37. Kjos, S.L., Henry, O.A., Montoro, M., Buchanan, T.A., and Mestman, J.H. 1993. Insulin-requiring diabetes in pregnancy: a randomized trial of active induction of labor and expectant management. *Am J Obstet Gynecol* 169:611–15.

38. Lurie, S., Matzkel, A., Weissman, A., Gotlibe, Z., and Friedman, A. 1992. Outcome of pregnancy in class A1 and A2 gestational diabetic patients delivered beyond 40 weeks' gestation. *Am J Perinatol* 9:484–88.

39. Bellamy, L., Casas, J.P., Hingorani, A.D., and Williams, D. 2009. Type 2 diabetes mellitus after gestational diabetes: a systematic review and meta-analysis. *Lancet* 373:1773–79.

40. Vohr, B.R., and Boney, C.M. 2008. Gestational diabetes: the forerunner for the development of maternal and childhood obesity and metabolic syndrome? *J Matern Fetal Neonatal Med* 21:149–57.

41. Vambergue, A., Dognin, C., Boulogne, A., Réjou, M.C., Biausque, S., and Fontaine, P. 2008. Increasing incidence of abnormal glucose tolerance in women with prior abnormal glucose tolerance during pregnancy: DIAGEST 2 study. *Diabet Med* 25:58–64.

42. Noussitou, P., Monbaron, D., Vial, Y., Gaillard, R.C., and Ruiz, J. 2005. Gestational diabetes mellitus and the risk of metabolic syndrome: a population-based study in Lausanne, Switzerland. *Diabetes Metab* 31:361–69.

43. Bo, S., Monge, L., Macchetta, C., et al. 2004. Prior gestational hyperglycemia: a long-term predictor of the metabolic syndrome. *J Endocrinol Invest* 27:629–35.

44. Pallardo, F., Herranz, L., Garcia-Ingelmo, T., et al. 1999. Early postpartum metabolic assessment in women with prior gestational diabetes. *Diabetes Care* 22:1053–58.

45. Heitritter, S., Solomon, C., Mitchell, G., Skali-Ounis, N., and Seely, E. 2005. Subclinical inflammation and vascular dysfunction in women with previous gestational diabetes mellitus. *J Clin Endocrinol Metab* 90:3983–88.

46. Freire, C.M., Nunes Mdo, C., Barbosa, M.M., et al. 2006. Gestational diabetes: a condition of early diastolic abnormalities in young women. *J Am Soc Echocardiogr* 19:1251–56.

47. Bo, S., Valpreda, S., Menato, G., et al. 2007. Should we consider gestational diabetes a vascular risk factor? *Atherosclerosis* 194:e72–79.

48. Anastasiou, E., Lekakis, J.P., Alevizaki, M., et al. 1998. Impaired endothelium dependent vasodilatation in women with previous gestational diabetes. *Diabetes Care* 21:2111–15.

49. Carr, D.B., Utzschneider, K.M., Hull, R.L., et al. 2006. Gestational diabetes mellitus increases the risk of cardiovascular disease in women with a family history of type 2 diabetes. *Diabetes Care* 29:2078–83.

50. Shah, B.R., Retnakaran, R., and Booth, G.L. 2008. Increased risk of cardiovascular disease in young women following gestational diabetes mellitus. *Diabetes Care* 31:1668–69.

51. **Tobias, D.K., Hu, F.B., Forman, J.P., Chavarro, J., and Zhang, C. 2011. Increased risk of hypertension after gestational diabetes mellitus: findings from a large prospective cohort study. *Diabetes Care* 34:1582–84.** *An original paper that highlights the association between GDM and hypertension.*

52. Volpe, L., Cuccuru, I., Lencioni, C., et al. 2008. Early subclinical atherosclerosis in women with previous gestational diabetes mellitus. *Diabetes Care* 31:e32.

53. Schmidt, M.I., Duncan, B.B., Reichelt, A.J., et al. 2001. Gestational diabetes mellitus diagnosed with a 2-h 75-g oral glucose tolerance test and adverse pregnancy outcomes. *Diabetes Care* 24:1151–55.

54. Bradley, R.J., Brudenell, J.M., and Nicolaides, K.H. 1991. Fetal acidosis and hyperlacticaemia diagnosed by cordocentesis in pregnancies complicated by maternal diabetes mellitus. *Diabet Med* 8:464–68.

55. Aberg, A., Westbom, L., and Kallen, B. 2001. Congenital malformations among infants whose mothers had gestational diabetes or preexisting diabetes. *Early Human Dev* 61:85–95.

56. Martínez-Frías, M.L., Bermejo, E., Rodríguez-Pinilla, E., Prieto, L., and Frías, J.L. 1998. Epidemiological analysis of outcomes of pregnancy in gestational diabetic mothers. *Am J Med Genet* 78:140–45.

57. Farrel, T., Cundy, N., and Cundy, T. 2002. Congenital anomalies in the offspring of women with type 1, type 2 and gestational diabetes. *Diabet Med* 19:322–26.

58. Kalter, H. 1998. The non-teratogenicity of gestational diabetes. *Paediatr Perinat Epidemiol* 12:456–58.

59. Waller, D.K., Mills, J.L., Simpson, J.L., et al. 1994. Are obese women at higher risk for producing malformed offspring? *Am J Obstet Gynecol* 170:541–48.

60. Cedergren, MI., and Kallen, B.A. 2003. Maternal obesity and infant heart defects. *Obes Res* 11:1065–71.
61. Watkins, M.L., Rasmussen, S.A., Honeru, M.A., Botto, LD., and Moore, C.A. 2003. Maternal obesity and risk for birth defects. *Pediatrics* 111:1152–58.
62. Pedersen, J., Molstead-Pederson, L., and Pedersen, B. 1974. Assessors of fetal perinatal mortality in pregnancy. Analysis of 1,332 pregnancies in the Copenhagen series, 1946–1972. *Diabetes* 23:302–5.
63. Kitzmiller, J.L., Gavin, L.A., Gin, G.D., Jovanovic-Peterson, L., Main, E.K., and Zigrang, W.D. 1991. Preconception care of diabetes. Glycemic control prevents congenital anomalies. *JAMA* 265:731–36.
64. Roversi, G.D., Gargiulo, M., Nicolini, U., et al. 1979. A new approach to the treatment of diabetic pregnant women. Report of 479 cases seen from 1963 to 1975. *Am J Obstet Gynecol* 135:567–76.
65. Langer, O., and Conway, D.L. 2000. Level of glycemia and perinatal outcome in pregestational diabetes. *J Matern Fetal Med* 9:35–41.
66. Evers, I.M., deValk, H.W., and Visser, G.H. 2004. Risk of complications of pregnancy in women with type 1 diabetes: nationwide prospective study in the Netherlands. *BMJ* 328:915.
67. Atègbo, J.M., Grissa, O., Yessoufou, A., et al. 2006. Modulation of adipokines and cytokines in gestational diabetes and macrosomia. *J Clin Endocrinol Metab* 91:4137–43.
68. Gabbe, S.G., Niebyl, J.R., and Simpson, J.L. 2007. Diabetes mellitus complicating pregnancy. In *Obstetrics, normal and problem pregnancies*, 976–1005. 5th ed. Philadelphia: Churchill Livingstone.
69. Cox, N.J. 1994. Maternal component in NIDDM transmission: how large an effect? *Diabetes* 43:166–68.
70. Jovanovic-Peterson, L., Peterson, C.M., Reed, G.F., et al. 1991. Maternal postprandial glucose levels and infant birth weight: the Diabetes in Early Pregnancy Study. The National Institute of Child Health and Human Development—Diabetes in Early Pregnancy Study. *Am J Obstet Gynecol* 164:103–11.
71. **Ehrenberg, HM., Mercer, BM., and Catalano, P.M. 2004. The influence of obesity and diabetes on the prevalence of macrosomia. *Am J Obstet Gynecol* 191:964–68.** *An original paper showing that with the increasing prevalence and relative frequency of overweight and obese women in pregnancy, abnormal maternal body habitus exhibits the strongest influence on the prevalence of LGA deliveries.*
72. Bhattacharya, S., Campbell, D.M., Liston, W.A., and Bhattacharya, S. 2007. Effect of body mass index on pregnancy outcomes in nulliparous women delivering singleton babies. *BMC Public Health* 7:168.
73. Acker, D.B., Sachs, B.P., and Friedman, E.A. 1985. Risk factors for Erb-Duchenne palsy. *Obstet Gynecol* 66:764.
74. McFarland, M.B., Trylovich, C.G., and Langer, O. 1998. Anthropometric differences in macrosomic infants of diabetic and nondiabetic mothers. *J Matern Fetal Med* 7:292–95.
75. Athukorala, C., Crowther, C.A., and Willson. K. 2007. Women with gestational diabetes mellitus in the ACHOIS trial: risk factors for shoulder dystocia. *Aust N Z J Obstet Gynaecol* 47:37–41.
76. Piper, J.M. 2002. Lung maturation in diabetes in pregnancy: if and when to test. *Semin Perinatol* 26:206–9.
77. Moore, T.R. 2002. A comparison of amniotic fluid fetal pulmonary phospholipids in normal and diabetic pregnancy. *Am J Obstet Gynecol* 186:641–50.
78. Berkowitz, K., Reyes, C., Saadat, P., and Kjos, S.L. 1997. Fetal lung maturation: comparison of biochemical indices in gestational diabetic and nondiabetic pregnancies. *J Reprod Med* 42:793–800.

79. Kjos, S.L., Berkowitz, K.M., and Kung, B. 2002. Prospective delivery of reliably dated term infants of diabetic mothers without determination of fetal lung maturity: comparison to historical control. *J Matern Fetal Neonatal Med* 12:433–37.
80. Kjos, S.L., Walther, F.J., Montoro, M., Paul, R.H., Diaz, F., and Stabler, M. 1990. Prevalence and etiology of respiratory distress in infants of diabetic mothers: predictive value of fetal lung maturation tests. *Am J Obstet Gynecol* 163:898–903.
81. Langer, O. 2002. The controversy surrounding fetal lung maturity in diabetes in pregnancy: a re-evaluation. *J Matern Fetal Neonatal Med* 12:428–32.
82. Metzger, B.E., Persson, B., Lowe, L.P., et al. 2010. Hyperglycemia and adverse pregnancy outcome study: neonatal glycemia. *Pediatrics* 126:e1545–52.
83. Yogev, Y., and Langer, O. 2007. Spontaneous preterm delivery and gestational diabetes: the impact of glycemic control. *Arch Gynecol Obstet* 276:361–65.
84. Smith, G.C.S., Shah, I., Pell, J.P., Crossley, J.A., and Dobbie, R. 2007. Maternal obesity in early pregnancy and risk of spontaneous and elective preterm deliveries: a retrospective cohort study. *Am J Public Health* 97:157–62.
85. **Yessoufou, A., and Moutairou, K. 2011. Maternal diabetes in pregnancy: early and long-term outcomes on the offspring and the concept of "metabolic memory." *Exp Diabetes Res* 2011:218598.** *Summary on the current evidence for alterations in infants of diabetic mothers that persist postnatally into the future life and the concept of metabolic memory.*
86. Hales, C.N., and Barker, D.J.P. 2001. The thrifty phenotype hypothesis. *Br Med Bull* 60:5–20.
87. Palinski, W., and Napoli, C. 2002. The fetal origins of atherosclerosis: maternal hypercholesterolemia, and cholesterol-lowering or antioxidant treatment during pregnancy influence in utero programming and postnatal susceptibility to atherogenesis. *FASEB J* 16:1348–60.
88. Napoli, C., D'Armiento, F.P., Mancini, F.P., et al. 1997. Fatty streak formation occurs in human fetal aortas and is greatly enhanced by maternal hypercholesterolemia. *J Clin Invest* 100:2680–90.
89. Franke, K., Harder, T., Aerts, L., et al. 2005. "Programming" of orexigenic and anorexigenic hypothalamic neurons in offspring of treated and untreated diabetic mother rats. *Brain Res* 1031:276–83.
90. Plagemann, A. 2005. Perinatal programming and functional teratogenesis: impact on body weight regulation and obesity. *Physiol Behav* 86:661–68.
91. Eriksson, J.G., Forsen, T.J., Osmond, C., and Barker, D.J. 2003. Pathways of infant and childhood growth that lead to type 2 diabetes. *Diabetes Care* 26:3006–10.
92. Verma, A., Boney, C.M., Tucker, R., and Vohr, B.R. 2002. Insulin resistance syndrome in women with prior history of gestational diabetes mellitus. *J Clin Endocrinol Metab* 87:3227–35.
93. Hillier, T.A., Pedula, K.L., Schmidt, M.M., Mullen, J.A., Charles, M.A., and Pettitt, D.J. 2007. Childhood obesity and metabolic imprinting: the ongoing effects of maternal hyperglycemia. *Diabetes Care* 30:2287–92.
94. Ludwig, DS., and Currie, J. 2010. The association between pregnancy weight gain and birthweight: a within-family comparison. *Lancet* 376:984–90.
95. Silverman, B.L., Rizzo, T.A., Cho, N.H., and Metzger, B.E. 1998. Long-term effects of the intrauterine environment. The Northwestern University Diabetes in Pregnancy Center. *Diabetes Care* 21(Suppl 2):B142–49.
96. Dabelea, D., Knowler, W.C., and Pettitt, D.J. 2000. Effect of diabetes in pregnancy on offspring: follow-up research in the Pima Indians. *J Matern Fetal Med* 9:83–88.
97. Pettitt, D.J., Bennett, P.H., Saad, M.F., Charles, M.A., Nelson, R.G., and Knowler, W.C. 1991. Abnormal glucose tolerance during pregnancy in Pima Indian women. Long-term effects on offspring. *Diabetes* 40(Suppl 2):126–30.

98. West, N.A., Crume, T.L., Maligie, M.A., and Dabelea, D. 2011. Cardiovascular risk factors in children exposed to maternal diabetes in utero. *Diabetologia* 54:504–7.

99. Beyerlein, A., Nehring, I., Rosario, A.S., and vonKries, R. 2012. Gestational diabetes and cardiovascular risk factors in the offspring: results from a cross-sectional study. *Diabet Med* 29:378–84.

Section IV

Treatments

6 Dietary Therapy for Gestational Diabetes

Colin A. Walsh
Department of Maternal–Fetal Medicine, Royal
North Shore Hospital, Sydney, Australia

Fionnuala M. McAuliffe
Department of Maternal–Fetal Medicine, National
Maternity Hospital, Dublin, Ireland; UCD Obstetrics
and Gynaecology, University College Dublin,
National Maternity Hospital, Dublin, Ireland

CONTENTS

6.1 INTRODUCTION

Recent guidelines from the Royal College of Obstetricians and Gynaecologists in the UK and updated recommendations from the U.S. Institute of Medicine have highlighted the importance of healthy nutrition in pregnant women. Both over- and undernutrition in pregnancy have been associated with adverse short-term and long-term health outcomes for mother and child. Evidence-based dietary guidelines are particularly important for women with gestational diabetes mellitus (GDM), for whom maternal nutritional therapy represents the cornerstone of clinical treatment.

As in diabetes outside pregnancy, some element of carbohydrate control is the foundation of dietary therapy for GDM. While traditionally this has involved restriction of total carbohydrate intake, recent work has focused on the concept of switching to better sources of carbohydrate, i.e., foods with low glycaemic index (GI). To date, only small- to medium-sized randomised controlled trials on low-GI diets in GDM have been performed; although a clear benefit has not yet been demonstrated, the existing trials are small and further studies are ongoing.

Current recommendations for maternal weight gain in GDM pregnancy are based on criteria for pregnant women with normoglycaemia. Recently, several authors have begun to challenge the accepted notion that all women with GDM must achieve gestational weight gain within the recommended limits. There is mounting evidence that obese women (prepregnancy body mass index (BMI) ≥ 30 kg/m^2) may benefit from reduced gestational weight gain (<5 kg) with regards to preeclampsia, caesarean delivery, and large for gestational age infants, although this must be balanced against the increased risk of small for gestational age infants.

6.2 NUTRITIONAL REQUIREMENTS IN UNCOMPLICATED PREGNANCY: LATEST DEVELOPMENTS

Pregnancy represents a unique paradigm, in which the risks of malnutrition in the mother must be balanced against both the woman's increased metabolic demands and the nutritional requirements of the growing foetus. In its 10 key facts on global nutrition, the World Health Organisation (WHO) highlights both the major health challenge brought about by rising rates of obesity and the association between maternal undernutrition and poor foetal development (http://www.who.int/features/factfiles/nutrition/en). Although maternal overnutrition presents a far greater disease burden in Western society, the high rates of immigration from developing to developed countries make knowledge of maternal undernutrition important for all healthcare providers.[1] Both forms of malnutrition represent a threat to a healthy outcome for mother and baby. Furthermore, since the landmark work by Barker and colleagues,[2,3] there has been a growing appreciation of the importance of the transgenerational impact of maternal malnutrition and the resultant "thrifty phenotype" in the foetus.[4]

A comprehensive review of the nutritional requirements of the healthy pregnant woman is beyond the scope of this chapter. Instead, we present a summary of recent evidence for informing women on fundamental nutritional considerations during pregnancy. A 2010 scientific opinion paper from the Royal College of Obstetricians and Gynaecologists (RCOG)[5] in the UK recommends a total daily energy intake of 1,940 kcal in pregnancy, increasing to 2,140 kcal in the third trimester (Table 6.1). The RCOG suggests that the contribution of macronutrients to energy intake in pregnancy remain unchanged from outside pregnancy, namely, 35% derived from fat and 50% from carbohydrate, with an emphasis on healthy eating and the avoidance of potential dietary teratogens.[5]

Certain nutritional recommendations for pregnant women are not novel. The importance of folate in embryonic development has been appreciated for more than half a century. The reduction in foetal neural tube defects through periconceptual intake of folic acid represents one of the major success stories of public health policy in recent decades.[6] Identification of high-risk women, who should be offered an increased daily dose of folate supplementation (4–5 mg), is critical to the success of the folic acid strategy.[7] Maternal folic acid requirements are often linked to the need for adequate iron intake, through strategies such as the WHO Weekly Iron and Folic Acid Supplementation (WIFS) initiative.[8] The current recommendation from the National Institute for Health and Clinical Excellence (NICE) in the UK is that iron supplementation should not be offered routinely to all pregnant women, although screening for anaemia should be undertaken in early pregnancy and again at 28 weeks.[9]

The role of several other micronutrients in pregnancy has been well studied. A recent Cochrane review examined the benefits of calcium supplementation on improving pregnancy and infant outcomes.[10] Data collated from 21 randomised studies demonstrated no effect from calcium supplements in terms of risk of preterm birth or rate of low birth rate infants. However, good quality evidence has previously shown calcium supplementation of ≥1 g daily to halve the risk of preeclampsia, and thus it may be recommended on this basis.[11] In contrast, recent meta-analyses have refuted the long-held hypothesis that rates of preeclampsia are reduced by supplementation of vitamin C and vitamin E in pregnancy.[12,13]

The WHO has declared that iodine deficiency in foetal life and childhood is the single most preventable cause of mental retardation; consequently, a daily iodine intake of 200 μg is recommended during pregnancy and postpartum.[14] Other authors have examined the importance of micronutrient antioxidants, such as selenium, copper, zinc, and manganese, in pregnancy.[15] Micronutrient supplementation in pregnancy has been associated with reduced preeclampsia in women with low-baseline antioxidant status,[16] reduced childhood atopy,[17] and reduced postpartum thyroid dysfunction in women with antithyroid antibodies.[18] Recent work has suggested that multiple micronutrient supplementation may confer advantages over routine iron-folate supplementation in developing countries, with respect to foetal growth and survival.[19–21]

Finally, considerable attention has been paid of late to the role of vitamin D supplementation in pregnancy.[22–24] However, most of the adverse outcomes associated with vitamin D deficiency in pregnancy, including increased risk of caesarean delivery, have not been consistent across all studies.[22,25] There is a suggestion that vitamin D supplementation for pregnant women reduces the incidence of low birth weight

TABLE 6.1
RCOG Recommendations for Nutritional Requirements in Pregnancy

Nutrient/Day	Women (19–50 years)	Pregnancy
Energy (kcal)	1,940	+200[a]
Protein (g)	45	+6
Thiamin (mg)	0.8	+0.1[a]
Riboflavin (mg)	1.1	+0.3
Niacin (mg)	13	[b]
Vitamin B6 (mg)	1.2	[b]
Vitamin B12 (g)	1.5	[b]
Folate (μg)	200	+100
Vitamin C (mg)	40	+10
Vitamin A (μg)	600	+100
Vitamin D (μg)	—	10[c]
Calcium (mg)	700	[b]
Phosphorus (mg)	550	[b]
Magnesium (mg)	270	[b]
Sodium (mg)	1,600	[b]
Potassium (mg)	3,500	[b]
Chloride (mg)	2,500	[b]
Iron (mg)	14.8	[b]
Zinc (mg)	7.0	[b]
Copper (mg)	1.2	[b]
Selenium (μg)	60	[b]
Iodine (μg)	140	[b]

Source: Reproduced from RCOG Scientific Advisory Committee, *Nutrition in Pregnancy*, RCOG Scientific Advisory Committee Opinion Paper 18, Royal College of Obstetricians and Gynaecologists, London, 2010. With permission.

[a] Third trimester only.

[b] No increment.

[c] A 50 μg supplement is required at this level and is not usually achievable through diet. It is especially important for those most at risk of deficiency:

- Women of South Asian, African, Caribbean, or Middle Eastern family origin
- Women who have limited exposure to sunlight, such as women who are predominantly housebound or usually remain covered when outdoors
- Women who eat a diet particularly low in vitamin D, such as women who consume no oily fish, eggs, meat, vitamin D-fortified margarine, or breakfast cereal
- Women with a prepregnancy body mass index above 30 kg/m^2

(<2,500 g) infants, although this requires further study.[26] Many authorities, including the Institute of Medicine (IOM) in the United States[27] and NICE guidelines from the UK[28] now recommend routine supplementation of vitamin D (600 IU/10 µg/day, respectively) for pregnant women, with particular attention paid to obese mothers (Table 6.1).

Despite a wealth of data on nutritional requirements in healthy pregnancy, failure of women to meet recommended daily allowances for several nutrients remains a real concern. The Avon Longitudinal Study of Pregnancy and Childhood published its findings in 1998, and found that although pregnant women reported adequate intake of most nutrients, insufficient levels of iron, magnesium, potassium, and folate were very prevalent.[29] A study of generally well-educated Irish women found that, on average, pregnant women had a suboptimal intake of total carbohydrate, folate, iron, vitamin D, and selenium.[30] A 2012 Australian study of women at high risk for developing GDM reported poor insight on behalf of these women regarding their individual risk of pregnancy complications.[31] Very recent data demonstrated a healthier pregnancy diet in older (>32 years), better-educated women with a normal BMI.[32] It would appear that ongoing education of nutritional requirements in pregnancy is critical for both mothers and health practitioners.

6.3 MATERNAL NUTRITIONAL THERAPY FOR GESTATIONAL DIABETES

It is now well accepted that identification and appropriate management of GDM is associated with reduced infant morbidity and mortality.[33,34] Expert consensus from the Fifth International Workshop on Gestational Diabetes Mellitus dictates that medical nutrition therapy (MNT) is the cornerstone of clinical management of GDM.[35] This is endorsed by guidelines from the National Institute for Health and Clinical Excellence in the UK, which notes that 82–93% of women with GDM will achieve blood glucose targets through diet alone.[36] The goal of GDM management is to optimise outcomes for the mother and foetus without increasing the risk of serious adverse events, such as hypoglycaemia or ketoacidosis, in the mother.[36] Thus, the primary tenet of MNT is to safely optimise maternal glycaemic control. Although MNT is recognised as the first-line management strategy for GDM, the precise nutritional approach for such women, such as nutrient distribution, is less clear.[37] In the landmark ACHOIS study, for example, women in the intervention group received "individualised dietary advice from a qualified dietician," the precise details of which are not made available.[33]

As with diabetes outside of pregnancy, the essential component of nutritional therapy for GDM is some element of carbohydrate control. Indeed, MNT has been described as a "carbohydrate-controlled meal plan that promotes adequate nutrition with appropriate weight gain, normoglycaemia and the absence of ketosis."[37] Individualised MNT programs must also take account of macro- and micronutrient requirements, caloric requirements, and weight gain.[38] In accordance with expert recommendations from the Fifth International Workshop on Gestational Diabetes Mellitus, MNT should be prescribed and supervised by a qualified dietician.[35]

6.3.1 Carbohydrate Control

Because carbohydrate is the principal nutrient affecting postprandial glucose levels, regulation of carbohydrate intake is an essential prerequisite for achieving optimal glycaemic control in GDM. In simple terms, restriction of total carbohydrate intake can be accomplished by either reducing intake of carbohydrates or introducing carbohydrate sources with different glycaemic responses, such as low-GI foods. Worldwide consensus on amount, type, and daily distribution of carbohydrate in GDM does not exist, and controversy still exists over many of these issues.[38]

The Institute of Medicine in the United States has set a minimum carbohydrate intake of 175 g daily for pregnant women, which is higher than the 130 g/day recommended outside of pregnancy.[27] However, there is wide variation in the recommended proportion of carbohydrates for women with GDM. In their advisory paper on nutrition in pregnancy, the RCOG cites the Diabetes UK nutritional advice to patients with diabetes, which recommends 45%–60% total carbohydrates.[5] Other studies of meal plans for diabetics vary in their recommendations for total carbohydrate intake, from 30% to 55%.[39] Reducing carbohydrate intake from 55% to 40% of total energy intake does not appear to reduce the requirement for insulin in GDM.[40] The American Diabetes Association (ADA) recommends that this carbohydrate be divided into three meals and two to four snacks; these recommendations also note that, in general, carbohydrates are less well tolerated at breakfast than at other meals.[41] Several authors have shown benefit to minimising carbohydrate load at breakfast to 30%–40% of the total.[38]

The potential for fibre intake to improve glycaemic control in women with GDM has also been examined. Reece et al. demonstrated no improvement in postprandial glucose levels in women consuming high levels of fibre (70–80 g/day) compared to those consuming no more than 20 g/day.[42] Furthermore, a high intake of fibre is often limited by the difficulty reported by patients in tolerating high levels of fibre. The ADA now recommends the same fibre intake in diabetes as in the general public, which is 14 g/1,000 kcal.[41] Nutrition guidelines from the UK give no quantitative recommendation for fibre intake in GDM, but note that soluble fibre has beneficial effects on glycaemic and lipid metabolism.[5]

In recent years, the focus on carbohydrate control in GDM has evolved from simply restricting total carbohydrate intake toward a greater focus on the different glycaemic effects of different sources of carbohydrate. Recent work has concentrated on the role of carbohydrates of low glycaemic index (GI) in women with GDM. Indeed, the recent NICE guideline on GDM concludes that a diet "high in carbohydrates of low glycaemic index improves overall glucose control."[36] The ADA notes that "the use of glycaemic index ... may provide a modest additional benefit over when total carbohydrate is considered alone."[41] The role of low-GI foods in GDM is discussed in detail later in this chapter.

6.3.2 Macronutrients Other Than Carbohydrates

Given the emphasis on glycaemic control in GDM, other sources of dietary energy have not been studied in as much detail. The ADA recommends that, in the context of normal renal function, there is insufficient evidence to recommend altering the usual protein intake in GDM (15–20% of total energy).[41] The RCOG recommends that protein intake should not be >1 g/kg of body weight in GDM.[5] With regard to fat intake, the RCOG recommends that <35% of total energy intake in GDM be derived from fat, with sources of saturated and trans-unsaturated fat accounting for no more than 10% of total energy.[5] The ADA guidelines are more strict and suggest limiting saturated fat to <7% of total intake while minimising the intake of trans fats in diabetes.[41] Several authors have reported reduced intake of essential fatty acids in women following standardised dietary advice for GDM. Gillen and Tapsell reported higher rates of saturated fat intake in GDM women advised simply to follow a low-fat diet, compared to women given additional targets for dietary sources of unsaturated fats.[43] Ley and colleagues examined the relationship between macronutrient intake distribution in the second trimester and subsequent glucose metabolism. They found that higher intakes of total fat, saturated fat, and trans fat were associated with increased fasting glucose levels at 30 weeks.[44]

A small study from the UK found that while women with GDM had reduced intake of total and saturated fatty acids following dietary advice, their intake of omega-3 fatty acids was below that recommended in pregnancy.[45] This is concerning given the known association between omega-3 polyunsaturated fatty acid intake in pregnancy and subsequent childhood obesity.[46] With this in mind, the ADA recommends two or more servings of fish per week in diabetes, as a source of omega-3 polyunsaturated fatty acids.[41] The RCOG suggests one or two portions, with no more than two portions of oily fish due to the potential for methyl mercury contamination; furthermore, shark, swordfish, and marlin should be avoided in pregnancy.[5]

6.3.3 MICRONUTRIENTS

Vitamin and mineral supplementation is not routinely recommended for women with GDM in the absence of underlying deficiencies.[41] The RCOG recommends encouraging foods that are naturally rich in vitamins and antioxidants.[5] For several decades, researchers have suggested a relationship between low serum levels of chromium and risk of diabetes, including GDM.[47,48] The potential for chromium supplementation as a therapy for improving glycaemic control has shown promising results.[49] However, studies on its association with GDM have been less hopeful. A prospective Australian study of women with abnormal glucose challenge tests in pregnancy found no difference in chromium levels between those with normal and those with abnormal 75 g oral glucose tolerance tests.[50] Another large prospective study of 425 pregnant women demonstrated no difference in serum chromium levels in women with GDM versus those without GDM.[51] Thus, the role of chromium supplementation in treating GDM cannot be recommended. Finally, a recent study found that high dietary glycaemic load predicted poor micronutrient intake in women with GDM, emphasising the need for comprehensive MNT in gestational diabetes.[52]

6.4 NUTRITIONAL PREVENTION OF GESTATIONAL DIABETES

In addition to being the cornerstone of therapy for women with confirmed GDM, several aspects of maternal nutrition have demonstrated benefit in the primary prevention of gestational diabetes.

6.4.1 CALORIE RESTRICTION

Calorimetry studies by Prentice have shown that there is dramatic interpatient variation in the changes in basal metabolic rate between nonpregnancy and pregnancy.[53] Such individual differences render some women "energy-profligate" and others "energy-sparing" in pregnancy,[5] making generalised recommendations on calorie intake for pregnant women fraught with difficulty. Such difficulty is compounded by the high rates of energy intake underreporting amongst pregnant women.[30]

In healthy pregnancy, the U.S. Institute of Medicine suggests no calorie increase in the first trimester, an additional 340 kcal/day in the second trimester, and 452 kcal/day in the third trimester.[27] Women in the UK are recommended 1,940 kcal/day in pregnancy, increasing by 200 kcal/day in the third trimester[5] (Table 6.1). However, it is not entirely clear whether women with GDM should follow these same recommendations for calorie intake.[37] On this issue, most commentators, and most expert consensus documents, draw a distinction between GDM women of normal weight or underweight and those who are overweight or obese.[37,38,41]

Several studies suggest a role for calorie restriction for overweight or obese pregnant women in the prevention of GDM.[36] A randomised crossover trial found that obese pregnant women on a hypocaloric diet lost weight whether the calorie-restricted diet was 40 or 55% carbohydrate. However, the 40% carbohydrate (and thus higher-fat) calorie-restricted diet produced a more favourable effect on triglyceride levels.[54] In an Australian randomised controlled trial (RCT) on the effect of 30% energy restriction in obese pregnant women with GDM, energy restriction did not alter the frequency of insulin therapy, although insulin was commenced later and lower insulin doses were required to achieve glycaemic targets in the energy-restricted group.[55] In contrast, a recent meta-analysis of dietary intervention in pregnancy showed an average 2 kg reduction in gestational weight gain with calorie restriction, although this did not translate into a significant reduction in rates of GDM.[56]

In women who are of normal weight, the recommended calorie intake is 30 kcal/kg/day based on current pregnancy weight.[38] Overweight women with GDM may benefit from calorie restriction as a means of controlling weight gain. However, severe calorie restriction to less than 1,500 kcal/day increases ketonaemia, and a minimum of 1,700–1,800 kcal/day is required to prevent ketoacidosis.[57] This is reflected in expert consensus documents. The 2004 position statement on GDM from the ADA recommends a 30–33% calorie restriction in obese (BMI > 30 kg/m^2) pregnant women with GDM, for a target intake of 25 kcal/kg/day.[58] The NICE guideline on GDM recommends that women with a prepregnancy BMI of >27 kg/m^2 should restrict daily calorie intake to ≤25 kcal/kg.[36]

6.4.2 SPECIFIC NUTRIENT INTAKE IN THE PREVENTION OF GESTATIONAL DIABETES

In addition to larger studies examining the effect of total energy and carbohydrate intake on the development of GDM, several individual studies have explored the association between GDM and individual nutrients. However, for many nutrients the data are conflicting. Several authors have reported a significant association between haeme iron intake in the preconceptual and early pregnancy period and subsequent

GDM.[59,60] The same effect has not been demonstrated with nonhaeme iron[59] or in women receiving iron supplementation in pregnancy.[61]

Several vitamins have also been implicated in the development of GDM. A secondary analysis from the HAPO study cohort reported a significant inverse relationship between mid-gestation 25-hydroxy vitamin D concentrations and fasting glucose levels, among 4,000 normoglycaemic pregnant women.[62] However, a case-control study from the UK did not substantiate the relationship between early pregnancy 25-hydroxy vitamin D and development of GDM.[63] A study of 785 Indian women in pregnancy found that low serum vitamin B_{12} concentrations were associated with a significantly higher risk of GDM, even after controlling for the higher BMI, which was observed among B_{12}-deficient women. Furthermore, B_{12} deficiency in pregnancy was positively and significantly associated with diabetes prevalence at 5-year follow-up.[64]

As discussed earlier, there is increasing evidence of the benefits of antioxidant micronutrients in maternal health. A survey of 500 pregnant women reported significantly lower intakes of selenium and zinc in women with gestational hyperglycaemia.[65] A significant reduction in GDM in women randomised to receive a probiotic-supplemented diet compared to placebo has also been demonstrated.[66] Higher prepregnancy intake of animal fat and cholesterol has also been associated with an increased risk of GDM.[67] Furthermore, higher animal fat intake appears to increase the risk of developing overt post-pregnancy diabetes in women with GDM.[68] A Finnish cluster-randomised controlled trial reported reduced rates of GDM in women who adhered to an early pregnancy intervention package, which included increased intake of *fibre and polyunsaturated fatty acids* and reduced intake of saturated fatty acids.[69] These findings have not been consistent across all studies. Examining first trimester dietary patterns in 1,700 women, Radesky and colleagues did not find any significant predictors of GDM from several dietary components, including saturated and unsaturated fats.[70]

6.5 ROLE OF MATERNAL WEIGHT REGULATION IN GESTATIONAL DIABETES

A wealth of published data has examined the relationship between maternal body weight and gestational diabetes. The association between maternal obesity and GDM has been discussed in detail elsewhere and will not be elaborated on further in this chapter. Here we present a summary of recent findings with regard to gestational weight change in the prevention and treatment of GDM.

6.5.1 RECOMMENDATIONS FOR WEIGHT GAIN IN PREGNANCY

Recent NICE guidelines on weight management during pregnancy advise that women are more likely to achieve and maintain healthy weight by eating a low-fat diet composed of fibre-rich foods, with five portions fruits/vegetables per day and avoiding fried and sugary foods.[28] They also note that weight loss programs:

- Address the reasons why someone finds it difficult to lose weight

TABLE 6.2

Targets for Gestational Weight Gain

Author	Source	Underweight	Normal	Overweight	Obese
Body mass index (kg/m²)		<18.5	18.5–24.9	25–29.9	≥30
Institute of Medicine 1990[75]	United States	28–40 lb 13–18 kg	25–35 lb 11.5–16 kg	15–25 lb 7–11.5 kg	>15 lb >6.8 kg
Institute of Medicine 2009[76]	United States	28–40 lb 13–18 kg	25–35 lb 11.5–16 kg	15–25 lb 7–11.5 kg	11–20 lb 5–9 kg
Cedergren 2007[77]	Sweden	9 – 24–10 kg	5 – 22 lb 2–10 kg	< 20 lb <9 kg	<13 lb <6 kg

[a] All weight ranges relate to singleton pregnancies.

- Are tailored to individual needs and choices and sensitive to the patient's weight concerns
- Are based on a healthy, balanced diet
- Encourage regular physical activity
- Expect weight loss of no more than 1–2 lb (0.5–1 kg) per week

In addition to prepregnancy obesity being a risk factor for development of GDM, there is good evidence that gestational weight gain also increases the risk. A large retrospective study by Gibson et al. found that by 24 weeks gestation, women who ultimately developed GDM had gained more weight in pregnancy (15 lb versus 11 lb) than those with normal glucose tolerance, despite similar prepregnancy BMI.[71] A recent analysis of 2,500 gestational diabetics found that rates of large for gestational age (LGA) infants were doubled in normal and overweight/obese women who gained more than 35 and 15 pounds, respectively, in pregnancy.[72] Although older studies found that the association between gestational weight gain and infant birth weight was higher in women of normal weight,[73] a recent study found that excessive gestational weight gain trebled the risk of LGA infants independent of prepregnancy weight.[74]

It appears that excessive weight gain in pregnancy adversely affects perinatal outcomes; what then is the optimal target range for gestational weight gain? The normal gestational increase in weight varies according to the prepregnancy weight. In 1990 the Institute of Medicine (IOM) in the United States published guidelines for gestational weight gain targets[75]; these were updated in 2009,[76] although the updated targets were identical, save for imposing an upper limit to the recommended weight gain in obese women (Table 6.2). Some commentators have challenged the failure of the IOM guidelines to distinguish between different levels of maternal obesity.[77,78]

There are limited data available on recommended weight gain in pregnancy from other patient populations. A retrospective analysis of 300,000 Swedish pregnancies reported a decreased risk of adverse obstetric and neonatal outcomes associated with gestational weight gain at lower limits than those recommended by the IOM[79] (see Table 6.2). Currently, there are no UK evidence-based guidelines on targets for appropriate gestational weight gain.[28]

6.5.2   THE ROLE OF SUBOPTIMAL WEIGHT GAIN
AND WEIGHT LOSS IN PREGNANCY

Given the established effects of obesity and excessive gestational weight gain on the prevalence of GDM, the logical question arising is whether reduced weight gain, or even weight loss, in pregnancy ameliorates this risk. In view of the proven benefits of weight loss in people with type 2 diabetes[80] and the known overlap between type 2 diabetes and GDM,[81] it could be reasonably hypothesised that weight loss would be beneficial in women with GDM. Indeed, the 2010 NICE guidance states that while prepregnancy weight loss should be encouraged in women with a BMI > 30 kg/m^2, weight loss programs are *not* recommended during pregnancy, as they may harm the health of the foetus, with concerns regarding ketonaemia and foetal growth restriction.[28]

Traditionally, the principal concern with suboptimal weight gain in pregnancy has been the effect on foetal growth. Among women with GDM, Cheng et al. found that those who gained less than the recommended 15–35 lb in pregnancy were more likely to remain on diet control, but 40% more likely to deliver small for gestational age (SGA) infants.[82] Similar studies in nondiabetic pregnancy have demonstrated an association between suboptimal gestational weight gain and SGA infants, both in women with normal prepregnancy BMI[83] and in obese women.[84] However, these same studies showed suboptimal weight gain to significantly reduce the risk of preeclampsia and caesarean delivery across all weight categories.[83,84] Although it must be noted that the 2009 IOM guidelines for gestational weight gain are not specific to diabetic pregnancy, Yee et al. demonstrated higher complication rates in women with type 2 diabetes whose gestational weight gain was excessive by the IOM criteria; they concluded that the 2009 IOM guidelines seem applicable to a diabetic pregnant population.[85]

However, not all experts agree that suboptimal weight gain in pregnancy is invariably deleterious.[78] There is accumulating support for the role of reduced gestational weight gain, particularly in more obese women, in improving overall pregnancy outcomes. Additionally, it is now known that reduced gestational weight gain is protective against future maternal and childhood obesity.[86–88] Analysis on the effect on childhood obesity, however, must factor in the known U-shaped effect, whereby maternal undernutrition in pregnancy has also been linked with higher obesity rates in offspring.[88]

For the first time, the updated guidelines published by the IOM in 2009 took account of outcomes for both mother and child.[76] This was based on several studies that have suggested protective effects to suboptimal gestational weight gain. Among women of normal weight gaining less than the IOM recommended 25 lb, DeVader and colleagues demonstrated significant reductions in preeclampsia (by 44%), LGA (by 60%), and caesarean section (by 18%), but with a doubling of SGA infants.[83] Kiel et al. reported significant protective effects for the same outcome measures across all levels of maternal obesity.[84] Furthermore, in women with BMI ≥ 35 kg/m^2, the rate of SGA in women with gestational weight gain < 15 lb was 5–10%, which is what would be expected for an outcome defined as less than the 10th percentile.[84] Concerns regarding the association between suboptimal weight gain and SGA infants appear to be greater in women with a normal prepregnancy BMI.

Although much has been published on the effects of suboptimal weight gain in pregnancy, less is known about the effect of actual weight loss in pregnant women. Both the Institute of Medicine in the United States[75] and the National Institute for Health and Clinical Excellence in the UK[28] discourage weight loss in pregnant women, based primarily on the dearth of long-term data.[77] Nonetheless, recent work has begun to examine the effects of gestational weight loss on pregnancy outcomes. Blomberg examined pregnancy outcomes in almost 50,000 obese Swedish women, stratified by obesity class and gestational weight change. Compared to women with the recommended 5–9 kg weight gain, women who lost weight during pregnancy had significantly lower caesarean rates (by 25–30%) across all classes of obesity, with no difference in preeclampsia or instrumental delivery rates. Additionally, weight loss during pregnancy was associated with a 27–46% reduction in LGA, with no effect on 5 min Apgar or foetal distress.[88] Compared to women with the recommended gestational weight gain, women with class I or III obesity who lost weight had twice the risk of SGA infants; the rate of SGA across all obesity classes, however, was <5% and was not significantly different from the baseline risk in the same population.[89]

A similar study of 700,000 German women reported outcomes in women with gestational weight loss compared to those with nonexcessive weight gain, stratified by BMI.[90] Rates of preeclampsia, emergency caesarean section, and LGA were reduced in obese women who lost weight. In women with BMI 25–40 kg/m² who lost weight, rates of SGA infants were increased, which was not demonstrated in the most obese (class III) patients. Concerns over the effect on SGA infants were echoed by a recent placental study, which demonstrated significantly lighter placentae, significantly shorter umbilical cords, and significantly lower birth weights in women with gestational weight loss compared to BMI-matched controls.[91]

6.6 GLYCAEMIC INDEX

6.6.1 ABOUT THE GLYCAEMIC INDEX

Different carbohydrate foods have different effects on blood glucose levels. The glycaemic index (GI) of foods was first described more than 30 years ago, as a method of classifying the blood glucose responses generated by different types of carbohydrates.[92] The glycaemic index expresses the rise in blood glucose after a test food against a standard glucose curve, produced after glucose (or white bread) in the same subject.[93] Mathematically, the GI is defined as the incremental area under the blood glucose curve following ingestion of 50 g of a test food, expressed as a percentage of the area under the curve following an equal amount of a reference food (such as glucose) by the same subject on a different occasion[94] (Figure 6.1).

By convention, the GI of glucose is set at 100, with other foods assigned a numerical value relative to this.[93] If white bread is used as the reference, then the GI value must be divided by 1.4 to yield the value relative to glucose.[95] Commonly, foods with a GI less than 55, such as lentils, beans, oats, and green vegetables, are referred to as low GI.[96] In contrast, high-GI foods (GI > 70), such as white bread, breakfast cereals, and potatoes, tend to be more processed and result in more rapid elevations in blood glucose levels.[97,98]

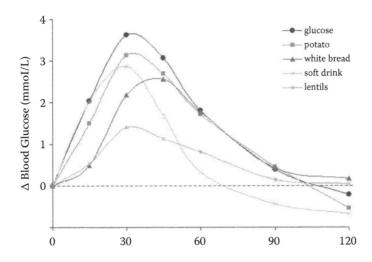

FIGURE 6.1   The glycaemic response to 50 g portions of common foods. (Reproduced from Brand-Miller, J. et al., *J. Am. Coll. Nutr.*, 28(Suppl), 446S–49S, 2009. With permission from the publishers.)

6.6.2   CLINICAL APPLICABILITY OF THE GLYCAEMIC INDEX

Since the earliest descriptions of low-GI foods, patients with diabetes mellitus have been the primary focus of much of the work on the clinical benefits of this dietetic regime.[99] It was hypothesised that since low GI foodstuffs deliver a more gradual supply of glucose, which usually improves insulin sensitivity, a low-GI diet might prove beneficial to diabetic patients. Several small studies in the early 1990s demonstrated improved glucose tolerance in prepregnancy diabetes, both type 1 and type 2 diabetes.[100] A 2003 meta-analysis of RCTs reported a small but clinically useful impact on medium-term glycaemic control in diabetic patients following a low-GI diet.[101] This was confirmed by a 2009 Cochrane review, which found that, on average, low-GI diets reduced glycated haemoglobin levels in diabetics by 0.5% (approximately 6 mmol/mol) and were associated with fewer episodes of hypoglycaemia.[102]

A wealth of literature supporting the role of low-GI diets in the treatment of a variety of other chronic disease states is now emerging.[103,104] Most of this work has concentrated on the treatment and prevention of nondiabetic obesity. A 2007 Cochrane review of six randomised trials reported increased weight loss and improvements in lipid profiles in overweight and obese nonpregnant patients following a low-GI diet, although the average difference in weight loss was only 1 kg.[105] Additionally, both human and animal studies have demonstrated improved lipid and cholesterol profiles associated with low-GI diets.[106,107] Not surprisingly, given the apparent effects on known risk factors, the Nurses' Health Study found that high-GI diets doubled the risk of cardiovascular disease among 82,000 women at 20 years follow-up.[108] Finally, although much work has been done in an attempt to determine the association between GI intake and malignancy, including breast and ovarian cancer, a causal link has thus far proved elusive.[109–111]

6.6.3   Low-GI Diet in Nondiabetic Pregnancy

Although questions over the importance of the glycaemic index in pregnancy were raised as far back as 1988,[112] only in recent years has this issue begun to receive widespread attention.[113,114] It does not appear that the pregnant state per se alters the GI of particular foodstuffs.[110] As such, studies into the role of GI in pregnancy have tended to use published GI values constructed from nonpregnant subjects.[115] Until very recently, studies of the effects of low-GI diets in pregnancy have focused exclusively on low-GI diets in healthy, nondiabetic pregnancies, as a means of preventing GDM, reducing neonatal macrosomia, and controlling maternal weight gain. However, lately preliminary data from low-GI diets in the treatment of established GDM has begun to emerge.[116]

6.6.4   Low-GI Diet for the Prevention of GDM

Several observational studies provide us with useful information regarding the role of the glycaemic index in preventing the development of GDM in pregnant women. Scholl and colleagues recruited 1,082 healthy, nondiabetic pregnant women over a 6-year period in the United States, on whom detailed dietary records were collected and converted to glycaemic indices.[117] They found glycaemic index to be positively and significantly associated with markers of carbohydrate metabolism (blood glucose levels and glycated haemoglobin levels). Although women with formal GDM were excluded from this retrospective analysis, it is notable that both biomarkers increased with every unit increase in GI intake.[117]

Zhang and colleagues examined data from the Nurses' Health Study II, a prospective cohort study of 116,000 female U.S. nurses that was established in 1989.[118] Based on self-reported cases of GDM determined by a follow-up questionnaire, they identified 758 cases of first-time GDM. Prepregnancy consumption of total dietary fibre, cereal, and fruit fibre was inversely associated with GDM risk after adjustment for age and BMI. In contrast, a high dietary glycaemic load more than doubled the risk of GDM on multivariate analysis.[118]

In contrast, Radesky et al. studied 1,700 healthy women with singleton pregnancies, of whom 91 (5%) developed GDM. They found no difference in first trimester glycaemic load, percentage carbohydrate intake, or fibre intake in GDM cases (or indeed in women with impaired glucose tolerance) compared to reference women with normal glucose tolerance.[70] Based on a strong association between prepregnancy BMI and risk of GDM in this study, the authors concluded that nutritional status entering pregnancy was likely a stronger predictor of GDM risk than maternal diet in early pregnancy.

6.6.5   Low-GI Diet for Reducing Neonatal Macrosomia

Several investigators have examined the relationship between maternal GI intake and subsequent neonatal birth weight in nondiabetic pregnancies (Table 6.3). In a

TABLE 6.3
Studies of Low-GI Diet in Healthy, Nondiabetic Pregnancy

Author	Year	n	Study Design	Inclusion Criteria	Maternal Weight Gain (kg)			Neonatal Birth Weight (g)		
					Low GI	Control	p	Low GI	Control	p
Clapp[123]	1997	12	RCT	Healthy gravida	11.8	19.7	<0.01	3,270	4,250	<0.01
Scholl et al.[117]	2004	1,082	Prospective, observational	Healthy gravida	Weight gain by GI quintile		0.28	116 g lighter in the lowest GI quintile		<0.05
Moses et al.[119]	2006	62	Prospective, nonrandomised	Healthy gravida	11.5	10.1	0.16	3,408	3,644	0.051
Deierlein et al.[124]	2008	1,231	Prospective, observational	Healthy gravida	Weight gain by GI quartile		> 0.05	—	—	—
Rhodes et al.[125]	2010	46	RCT	Prepregnancy BMI ≥ 25, < 45	6.4	6.9	0.74	3,507	3,133	0.22
Walsh et al.[122]	2012	720	RCT	Secundigravida with prior < 4 kg	12.2	13.6	0.01	—	—	—

prospective 6-year study of 1,082 healthy nondiabetic pregnant women, Scholl et al. found a nonsignificant reduction in large for gestational age (LGA) infants in the low-GI group, although it was noted that these women were twice as likely to deliver a small for gestational age (SGA) infant.[117] A smaller study by Moses et al., however, provides more compelling evidence regarding the effect of low-GI intake on neonatal macrosomia. They assigned 70 healthy gravidas to either a low-GI or high-GI (high-fibre, low sugar) diet from the second trimester onward.[119] The rates of LGA (defined as > 90th percentile) were 3 and 33% in the low- and high-GI groups, respectively; furthermore, the higher rate of SGA in the low-GI women reported by Scholl was not reproduced. In a follow-up report at a mean of 22 months, infants who were LGA at birth maintained this weight difference up to 2.5 years of age.[120]

More recent data, from both animal and human studies, have confirmed an association between GI intake in nondiabetic pregnancy and birth weight. A study to examine the effect of transient hyperglycaemic intake (as a surrogate for high-GI snacking) in pregnant ewes demonstrated higher birth weights in lambs born to ewes who were fed high-GI meals during the third trimester.[121] Very recently, preliminary results from a novel prospective trial (the ROLO trial) examining the benefits of low-GI diet in preventing recurrence of nondiabetic macrosomia have been published. Secundigravid women, with a previous macrosomic (>4,000 g) infant, were randomised to either a low-GI diet from 14 weeks onward under dietetic supervision or a nonintervention control group.[94] Among 371 women in their second pregnancy, there was no difference in the rate of recurrent macrosomia in the low-GI group (51%) compared to the controls (52%), although maternal weight gain was significantly lower in the interventional group.[122] Larger studies and meta-analyses of existing data will be required to further elucidate the effects of low-GI diets on neonatal birth weight in GDM.

6.6.6   Low-GI Diet for Controlling Maternal Weight Gain

To date, several investigators have examined the correlation between GI intake and maternal weight gain in nondiabetic pregnancy (Table 6.3). Although an early study of 12 women reported increased weight gain in women on the high-GI diet,[123] subsequent larger studies failed to substantiate any direct association.[119,124] Indeed, at 2 years follow-up of the Moses study, no difference was reported in the GI intake of women, irrespective of which regime they had followed in the index pregnancy.[120] Recently, preliminary data from the prospective ROLO trial demonstrated reduced maternal weight gain in women with a prior macrosomic baby, who were randomised to low-GI diet during pregnancy.[122] Finally, a randomised trial from Rhodes et al. was designed to determine the effects of low-GI diets in pregnancy, specifically in obese mothers.[125] Amongst 46 women with a mean BMI > 30 kg/m^2, the low-GI diet was not associated with differences in maternal weight gain, abdominal circumference, or BMI.

6.6.7   Low-GI Diet for Improving Pregnancy Outcomes: The Future

A 2008 Cochrane review on dietary therapy in the prevention of GDM, updated in 2013,[216] noted that while low-GI diet was beneficial for some outcomes, further trials with large numbers and longer follow-up are required before reaching more definite conclusions.[127] Several large trials are currently recruiting, which should help determine the role for dietary therapy in the prevention of GDM and its associated complications.

The Australian Pregnancy and Glycaemic Index Outcomes (PREGGIO) study aims to recruit 700 nondiabetic women with singleton pregnancies before 20 weeks (ACTRN12610000174088). Participants will see a dietician at least twice during the pregnancy and will receive either information on the low-GI diet or general dietary advice. The study aims to determine the effect of low-GI dietary advice on rate of GDM, neonatal birth weight, and childhood obesity at 2 years. The UK Pregnancies Better Eating and Activity (UPBEAT) Trial is currently recruiting nondiabetic women with a BMI $\geq$ 30 kg/m^2 at 10–16 weeks to receive an individualised activity and diet plan, including low-GI advice (ISRCTN89971375). The effect of the dietary intervention on development of GDM and neonatal complications will be determined, with measurement of serum glucose levels at recruitment and again at 32–36 weeks. Finally, the LIMIT study is a randomised trial designed to assess the benefits of dietary and lifestyle advice in reducing neonatal macrosomia among overweight and obese pregnant women (ACTRN12607000161426). It plans to randomise 2,500 women to dietician-led advice with the aim of limiting gestational weight gain to $\leq$5 kg. The results of these studies will tease out the role of maternal nutrition in the prevention of GDM.

6.6.8   Low-GI Diet in the Treatment of GDM

The low-GI diet is the cornerstone of treatment of GDM and is considered the first-line treatment. However, although the association between GI intake and diabetes mellitus has been studied for more than three decades, it is only latterly that level I evidence on the role of low-GI diets in the treatment of GDM has begun to emerge. However, the three randomised trials published to date have incorporated different primary outcomes and have yielded conflicting results[128–130] (Table 6.4).

Moses and colleagues published a randomised Australian trial, designed to assess whether insulin requirements in women with documented GDM would be reduced following the introduction of a low-GI diet.[128] Nonsmoking women with a first-time diagnosis of GDM, seen at 28–32 weeks gestation, were randomised to either a low-GI diet or a high-fibre, low-sugar diet, with no specific mention of the glycaemic index. Dietary intake was scrutinised at four third trimester visits, with insulin therapy commenced for fasting glucose levels $\geq$ 5.5 mmol/L or 1 h postprandial glucose $\geq$ 8.0 mmol/L on more than one occasion per week. Women assigned to the low-GI arm successfully achieved a significantly lower GI intake at all stages of assessment. The need for insulin therapy was significantly lower in the low-GI arm (29%) compared to the high-fibre, low-sugar (high-GI) arm (59%). Furthermore, among women in the high-GI arm who warranted insulin therapy (and who were then changed to a low-GI diet), 50% no longer met criteria for insulin commencement after transition to the low-GI diet.[128] However, no differences in neonatal birth weight or gestational weight gain were observed between arms in this trial.

While the trial by Moses et al. found a reduced need for insulin therapy in GDM women following a low-GI diet,[128] the direct relationship between GI intake and

TABLE 6.4

Studies of Low-GI Diet in the Treatment of GDM

Author	Year	n	Study Design	Inclusion Criteria	Maternal Weight Gain (kg)			Neonatal Birth Weight (g)		
					Low GI	Control	P	Low GI	Control	P
Moses et al.[128]	2009	63	RCT	GDM	No significant differences			No significant differences		
Grant et al.[129]	2011	47	RCT	GDM/IGT	No significant differences			3,124	3,330	>0.05
Louie et al.[130]	2011	92	RCT	GDM	11.9	13.1	0.31	3,300	3,300	0.62

blood glucose levels was not reported. A Canadian randomised trial, by Grant et al., aimed to further assess this relationship, by examining the effect of low-GI diet on maternal glycaemic control (HbA1c and self-monitored blood glucose levels) in 43 pregnant women with GDM or impaired glucose tolerance.[129] However, although blood glucose levels fell in both arms throughout the study, there was no significant difference demonstrated in the low-GI versus control groups. Similarly, women in the low-GI arm had similar rates of macrosomia, SGA infants, HbA1c, maternal weight gain, and need for insulin commencement, despite achieving a significantly lower GI intake[129] (Table 6.4). The only notable finding was a higher proportion of postprandial glucose readings within recommended target ranges in the low-GI arm.

Subsequently, Louie et al. randomised 91 women with confirmed GDM to either a low-GI or a moderate-GI (high-fibre) pregnancy diet, with the primary aim of determining the effect on neonatal birth weight.[130] Proportions of total protein, fat, and carbohydrate were similar for both dietary arms, with a target glycaemic index of ≤50 for the low-GI recruits. The trial demonstrated no difference in birth weight, rate of LGA or SGA infants, ponderal index, maternal weight gain, or rate of emergency caesarean section between the two arms (Table 6.4). Additionally, consistent with the Grant trial,[129] Louie et al. demonstrated no difference in the need for insulin therapy between groups. The authors concluded that the lack of benefit associated with a low-GI diet in women with GDM could be related to the normal BMI range across both arms or to the fact that the GI intake in the high-GI women was also relatively low in this trial (53 at delivery), which minimised the treatment effect of the low-GI intervention.[130]

A fourth RCT, published in 2012, examined the impact of low-GI dietary advice in 107 women at ≤29 weeks.[131] Although the low-GI diet was associated with reduced excessive maternal weight gain, the rate of prematurity was higher in the low-GI subgroup. Furthermore, only approximately 50% of women in the trial had GDM, with pre-gestational type 2 DM comprising the remaining study participants.

6.7 CONCLUSIONS: IDEAL DIET IN GESTATIONAL DIABETES

Gestational diabetes is intrinsically linked to the growing worldwide maternal obesity epidemic. There is general consensus that maternal nutritional therapy is the first-line, and cornerstone, treatment for women who develop GDM. However, unlike other forms of diabetes, any nutritional recommendations must always consider the well-being of both mother and foetus. Furthermore, the evolving appreciation of the long-term effects of maternal nutrition on morbidity in childhood and beyond makes the need for optimising nutrition in pregnancy particularly compelling.

Contemporary expert recommendations suggest that pregnant women require almost 2,000 kcal (30 kcal/kg) per day (Figure 6.2), with increasing energy requirements in the third, and possibly second, trimester. Overall, women with GDM should derive approximately 50% of energy from carbohydrate, 35% from fat, and 15% from protein, with an emphasis on healthy eating, soluble fibre sources, and adequate micronutrient intake, including omega-3 polyunsaturated fatty acids. The effect of micronutrients, such as vitamins D and B_{12}, selenium, and zinc in GDM warrants further study.

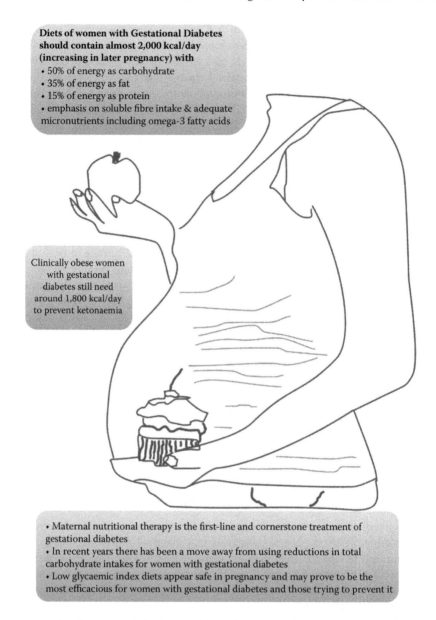

Diets of women with Gestational Diabetes should contain almost 2,000 kcal/day (increasing in later pregnancy) with
- 50% of energy as carbohydrate
- 35% of energy as fat
- 15% of energy as protein
- emphasis on soluble fibre intake & adequate micronutrients including omega-3 fatty acids

Clinically obese women with gestational diabetes still need around 1,800 kcal/day to prevent ketonaemia

- Maternal nutritional therapy is the first-line and cornerstone treatment of gestational diabetes
- In recent years there has been a move away from using reductions in total carbohydrate intakes for women with gestational diabetes
- Low glycaemic index diets appear safe in pregnancy and may prove to be the most efficacious for women with gestational diabetes and those trying to prevent it

FIGURE 6.2 Summary of the basic nutritional recommendations for women with gestational diabetes.

Prepregnancy BMI is central to identifying an ideal diet for women with GDM. A moderate (approximately 30%) calorie restriction in clinically obese (BMI > 30 kg/m^2) women with GDM is appropriate, although 1,800 kcal/day is required to avoid ketonaemia. Consensus statements offer recommendations on target gestational weight gain stratified by BMI. Although weight loss in GDM is not endorsed by expert guidelines, the paradigm is evolving. There is mounting evidence that suboptimal weight gain in obese pregnant women is associated with reductions in preeclampsia, caesarean section, and LGA infants; although the risk of SGA is increased, this appears to be mostly confined to women of normal or low prepregnancy weight.

Women with GDM require a detailed program of carbohydrate control, under the supervision of a qualified dietician. In recent years, there has been a move away from reduction in total carbohydrate intake toward emphasis of low-GI sources as a means of achieving glycaemic control. Although level I evidence of low-GI diet in GDM has not yet shown conclusive benefits in terms of neonatal birth weight or maternal gestational weight gain, the safety of low GI in pregnancy appears to have been established, and further studies of efficacy are ongoing. Reassuringly, women following low-GI dietary advice in pregnancy do not appear to face an increased economic burden.[132] Additionally, low-GI diets may have a valuable role in the primary prevention of GDM.

REFERENCES

Key references are in bold.

1. Lindsay, K., Gibney, E., and McAuliffe, F.M. 2012. Maternal nutrition among women from Sub-Saharan Africa, with a focus on Nigeria, and the potential implications for pregnancy outcomes among immigrant populations in developed countries. *J Hum Nutr Diet* 25:534–46.
2. Barker, D.J. 1992. Fetal growth and adult disease. *Br J Obstet Gynaecol* 99:275–76.
3. Barker, D.J., Osmond, C., Simmonds, S.J., and Wield, G.A. 1993. The relation of small head circumference and thinness at birth to death from cardiovascular disease in adult life. *BMJ* 306:422–26.
4. Ford, S.P., and Long, N.M. 2011. Evidence for similar changes in offspring phenotype following either maternal undernutrition or overnutrition: potential impact on fetal epigenetic mechanisms. *Reprod Fertil Dev* 24:105–11.
5. **RCOG Scientific Advisory Committee. 2010. *Nutrition in pregnancy*. RCOG Scientific Advisory Committee Opinion Paper 18. London: Royal College of Obstetricians and Gynaecologists.** *Recent expert opinion on desired nutrient intakes in pregnancy.*
6. Obican, S.G., Finnell, R.H., Mills, J.L., Shaw, G.M., and Scialli, A.R. 2010. Folic acid in early pregnancy: a public health success story. *FASEB J* 24:4167–74.
7. De-Regil, L.M., Fernández-Gaxiola, A.C., Dowswell, T., and Peña-Rosas, J.P. 2010. Effects and safety of periconceptional folate supplementation for preventing birth defects. *Cochrane Database Syst Rev* CD007950.
8. World Health Organisation. 2009. *Weekly iron–folic acid supplementation (WIFS) in women of reproductive age: its role in promoting optimal maternal and child health. Position statement.* Geneva: World Health Organisation. Available from http://www.who.int/nutrition/publications/micronutrients/weekly_iron_folicacid.pdf (accessed March 2012).
9. National Institute for Health and Clinical Excellence. 2010. *Routine care for the healthy pregnant woman*. Clinical Guideline 62. Available from http://www.nice.org.uk/CG062.
10. Buppasiri, P., Lumbiganon, P., Thinkhamrop, J., Ngamjarus, C., and Laopaiboon, M. 2011. Calcium supplementation (other than for preventing or treating hypertension) for improving pregnancy and infant outcomes. *Cochrane Database Syst Rev* CD007079.

11. Hofmeyr, G.J., Lawrie, T.A., Atallah, A.N., and Duley, L. 2010. Calcium supplementation during pregnancy for preventing hypertensive disorders and related problems. *Cochrane Database Syst Rev* CD001059.

12. Conde-Agudelo, A., Romero, R., Kusanovic, J.P., and Hassan, S.S. 2011. Supplementation with vitamins C and E during pregnancy for the prevention of preeclampsia and other adverse maternal and perinatal outcomes: a systematic review and metaanalysis. *Am J Obstet Gynecol* 204:503.e1–12.

13. Rossi, A.C., and Mullin, P.M. 2011. Prevention of pre-eclampsia with low-dose aspirin or vitamins C and E in women at high or low risk: a systematic review with meta-analysis. *Eur J Obstet Gynecol Reprod Biol* 158:9–16.

14. Perez-Lopez, F.R. 2007. Iodine and thyroid hormones during pregnancy and postpartum. *Gynecol Endocrinol* 23:414–28.

15. Mistry, H.D., and Williams, P.J. 2011. The importance of antioxidant micronutrients in pregnancy. *Oxid Med Cell Longev* 2011:841749.

16. Rumiris, D., Purwosunu, Y., Wibowo, N., Farina, A., and Sekizawa, A. 2006. Lower rate of preeclampsia after antioxidant supplementation in pregnant women with low antioxidant status. *Hypertens Pregnancy* 25:241–53.

17. Patelarou, E., Giourgouli, G., Lykeridou, A., et al. 2011. Association between biomarker-quantified antioxidant status during pregnancy and infancy and allergic disease during early childhood: a systematic review. *Nutr Rev* 69:627–41.

18. Negro, R., Greco, G., Mangieri, T., Pezzarossa, A., Dazzi, D., and Hassan, H. 2007. The influence of selenium supplementation on postpartum thyroid status in pregnant women with thyroid peroxidase autoantibodies. *J Clin Endocrinol Metab* 92:1263–68.

19. Shah, P.S., Ohlsson, A., and Knowledge Synthesis Group on Determinants of Low Birth Weight and Preterm Births. 2009. Effects of prenatal multimicronutrient supplementation on pregnancy outcomes: a meta-analysis. *CMAJ* 180:E99–108.

20. Roberfroid, D., Huybregts, L., Lanou, H., et al. 2012. Prenatal micronutrient supplements cumulatively increase fetal growth. *J Nutr* 142:548–54.

21. Roberfroid, D., Huybregts, L., Lanou, H., et al. 2012. Impact of prenatal multiple micronutrients on survival and growth during infancy: a randomized controlled trial. *Am J Clin Nutr* 95:916–24.

22. Dror, D.K. 2011. Vitamin D status during pregnancy: maternal, fetal, and postnatal outcomes. *Curr Opin Obstet Gynecol* 23:422–26.

23. McGowan, C.A, Byrne, J., Walsh, J., and McAuliffe, F.M. 2011. Insufficient vitamin D intakes among pregnant women. *Eur J Clin Nutr* 65:1076–78.

24. Urrutia, R.P., and Thorp, J.M. 2012. Vitamin D in pregnancy: current concepts. *Curr Opin Obstet Gynecol* 24:57–64.

25. Savvidou, M.D., Makgoba, M., Castro, P.T., Akolekar, R., and Nicolaides, K.H. 2012. First-trimester maternal serum vitamin D and mode of delivery. *Br J Nutr*, 108:1972–75.

26. De-Regil, L.M., Palacios, C., Ansary, A., Kulier, R., and Peña-Rosas, J.P. 2012. Vitamin D supplementation for women during pregnancy. *Cochrane Database Syst Rev* CD008873.

27. Institute of Medicine Food and Nutrition Board. 2002. *U.S. dietary reference intakes: energy, carbohydrates, fiber, fat, fatty acids, cholesterol, protein, and amino acids.* Washington, DC: National Academies Press.

28. **National Institute for Health and Clinical Excellence. 2010. Dietary interventions and physical activity interventions for weight management before, during and after pregnancy. Public Health Guidance 27. Available from http://www.nice. org.uk/guidance/PH27.** *Expert guidance on weight management prior to, during, and immediately after pregnancy.*

29. Rogers, I., and Emmett, P. 1998. Diet during pregnancy in a population of pregnant women in South West England. ALSPAC Study Team. Avon Longitudinal Study of Pregnancy and Childhood. *Eur J Clin Nutr* 52:246–50.
30. McGowan, C.A., and McAuliffe, F.M. 2012. Maternal nutrient intakes and levels of energy underreporting during early pregnancy. *Eur J Clin Nutr* 66:906–13.
31. Harrison, C., Lombard, C., and Teede, H. 2012. Understanding health behaviours in a cohort of pregnant women at risk of gestational diabetes mellitus: an observational study. *BJOG* 119:731–38.
32. McGowan, C.A., and McAuliffe, F.M. 2012. Maternal dietary patterns and associated nutrient intakes during each trimester of pregnancy. *Public Health Nutr* 16:97–107.
33. Crowther, C.A., Hiller, J.E., Moss, J.R., et al. 2005. Effect of treatment of gestational diabetes mellitus on pregnancy outcomes. *N Engl J Med* 352:2477–86.
34. Alwan, N., Tuffnell, D.J., and West, J. 2009. Treatments for gestational diabetes. *Cochrane Database Syst Rev* CD003395.
35. Metzger, B.E., Buchanan, T.A., Coustan, D.R., et al. 2007. Summary and recommendations of the Fifth International Workshop—Conference on Gestational Diabetes Mellitus. *Diabetes Care* 30(Suppl 2):S251–60.
36. National Institute for Health and Clinical Excellence. 2008. *Diabetes in pregnancy*. Clinical Guideline 63. Available from http://www.nice.org.uk/CG063.
37. **Magon, N., and Seshiah, V. 2011. Gestational diabetes mellitus: non-insulin management.** *Indian J Endocrinol Metab* **15:284–93**. *A recent review about the treatment of gestational diabetes with emphasis on the role of nutrition.*
38. Uplinger, N. 2009. The controversy continues: nutritional management of the pregnancy complicated by diabetes. *Curr Diab Rep* 9:291–95.
39. Reader, D.M. 2007. Medical nutrition therapy and lifestyle interventions. *Diabetes Care* 30(Suppl 2):S188–93.
40. Moreno-Castilla, C., Hernandez, M., Bergua, M., et al. 2013. Low-carbohydrate diet for the treatment of gestational diabetes mellitus: A randomized controlled trial. *Diabetes Care* 36:2233–38.
41. American Diabetes Association, Bantle, J.P., Wylie-Rosett, J., et al. 2008. Nutrition recommendations and interventions for diabetes: a position statement of the American Diabetes Association. *Diabetes Care* 31(Suppl 1):S61–78.
42. Reece, E.A., Hagay, Z., Caseria, D., Gay, L.J., and DeGennaro, N. 1993. Do fiber-enriched diabetic diets have glucose-lowering effects in pregnancy? *Am J Perinatol* 10:272–74.
43. Gillen, L.J., and Tapsell, L.C. 2004. Advice that includes food sources of unsaturated fat supports future risk management of gestational diabetes mellitus. *J Am Diet Assoc* 104:1863–67.
44. Ley, S.H., Hanley, A.J., Retnakaran, R., Sermer, M., Zinman, B., and O'Connor, D.L. 2011. Effect of macronutrient intake during the second trimester on glucose metabolism later in pregnancy. *Am J Clin Nutr* 94:1232–40.
45. Thomas, B., Ghebremeskel, K., Lowy, C., Crawford, M., and Offley-Shore, B. 2006. Nutrient intake of women with and without gestational diabetes with a specific focus on fatty acids. *Nutrition* 22:230–236.
46. Donahue, S.M., Rifas-Shiman, S.L., Gold, D.R., Jouni, Z.E., Gillman, M.W., and Oken, E. 2011. Prenatal fatty acid status and child adiposity at age 3 y: results from a US pregnancy cohort. *Am J Clin Nutr* 93:780–88.
47. Mertz, W. 1976. Chromium and its relation to carbohydrate metabolism. *Med Clin North Am* 60:739–44.
48. Anderson, R.A. 2000. Chromium in the prevention and control of diabetes. *Diabetes Metab* 26:22–27.

49. Bartlett, H.E., and Eperjesi, F. 2008. Nutritional supplementation for type 2 diabetes: a systematic review. *Ophthalmic Physiol Opt* 28:503–23.
50. Gunton, J.E., Hams, G., Hitchman, R., and McElduff, A. 2001. Serum chromium does not predict glucose tolerance in late pregnancy. *Am J Clin Nutr* 73:99–104.
51. Woods, S.E., Ghodsi, V., Engel, A., Miller, J., and James, S. 2008. Serum chromium and gestational diabetes. *J Am Board Fam Med* 21:153–57.
52. Louie, J.C., Markovic, T.P., Ross, G.P., Foote, D., and Brand-Miller, J.C. 2013. Higher glycemic load diet is associated with poorer nutrient intake in women with gestational diabetes mellitus. *Nutr Res* 33:259–65.
53. Prentice, A.M., Spaaij, C.J., Goldberg, G.R., et al. 1996. Energy requirements of pregnant and lactating women. *Eur J Clin Nutr* 50(Suppl 1):S82–110; discussion S110–11.
54. Peterson, C.M., and Jovanovic-Peterson, L. 1995. Randomized crossover study of 40% vs. 55% carbohydrate weight loss strategies in women with previous gestational diabetes mellitus and non-diabetic women of 130–200% ideal body weight. *J Am Coll Nutr* 14:369–75.
55. Rae, A., Bond, D., Evans, S., North, F., Roberman, B., and Walters, B. 2000. A randomised controlled trial of dietary energy restriction in the management of obese women with gestational diabetes. *Aust N Z J Obstet Gynaecol* 40:416–22.
56. Tanentsapf, I., Heitmann, B.L., and Adegboye, A.R. 2011. Systematic review of clinical trials on dietary interventions to prevent excessive weight gain during pregnancy among normal weight, overweight and obese women. *BMC Pregnancy Childbirth* 11:81.
57. Reader, D., and Sipe, M. 2001. Key components of care for women with gestational diabetes. *Diabetes Spectrum* 14:188–91.
58. American Diabetes Association. 2004. Gestational diabetes mellitus (position statement). *Diabetes Care* 27(Suppl 1):S88–90.
59. Qiu, C., Zhang, C., Gelaye, B., Enquobahrie, D.A., Frederick, I.O., and Williams, M.A. 2011. Gestational diabetes mellitus in relation to maternal dietary heme iron and non-haeme iron intake. *Diabetes Care* 34:1564–69.
60. Bowers, K., Yeung, E., Williams, M.A., et al. 2011. A prospective study of prepregnancy dietary iron intake and risk for gestational diabetes mellitus. *Diabetes Care* 34:1557–63.
61. Chan, K.K., Chan, B.C., Lam, K.F., Tam, S., and T.T. Lao. 2009. Iron supplement in pregnancy and development of gestational diabetes—a randomised placebo-controlled trial. *BJOG* 116:789–97; discussion 797–98.
62. McLeod, D.S., Warner, J.V., Henman, M., et al. 2012. Associations of serum vitamin D concentrations with obstetric glucose metabolism in a subset of the Hyperglycemia and Adverse Pregnancy Outcome (HAPO) study cohort. *Diabet Med* 29:e199–204.
63. Makgoba, M., Nelson, S.M., Savvidou, M., Messow, C.M., Nicolaides, K., and Sattar, N. 2011. First-trimester circulating 25-hydroxyvitamin D levels and development of gestational diabetes mellitus. *Diabetes Care* 34:1091–93.
64. Krishnaveni, G.V., Hill, J.C., Veena, S.R., et al. 2009. Low plasma vitamin B12 in pregnancy is associated with gestational 'diabesity' and later diabetes. *Diabetologia* 52:2350–58.
65. Bo, S., Lezo, A., Menato, G., et al. 2005. Gestational hyperglycemia, zinc, selenium, and antioxidant vitamins. *Nutrition* 21:186–91.
66. Luoto, R., Laitinen, K., Nermes, M., and Isolauri, E. 2010. Impact of maternal probiotic-supplemented dietary counselling on pregnancy outcome and prenatal and postnatal growth: a double-blind, placebo controlled study. *Br J Nutr* 103:1792–99.
67. Bowers, K., Tobias, D.K., Yeung, E., Hu, F.B., and Zhang, C. 2012. A prospective study of prepregnancy dietary fat intake and risk of gestational diabetes. *Am J Clin Nutr* 95:446–53.
68. Kim, S.H., Kim, M.Y., Yang, J.H., et al. 2011. Nutritional risk factors of early development of postpartum prediabetes and diabetes in women with gestational diabetes mellitus. *Nutrition* 27:782–88.

69. Luoto, R., Kinnunen, T.I., Aittasalo, M., et al. 2011. Primary prevention of gestational diabetes mellitus and large-for-gestational-age newborns by lifestyle counseling: a cluster-randomized controlled trial. *PLoS Med* 8:e1001036.

70. Radesky, J.S., Oken, E., Rifas-Shiman, S.L., Kleinman, K.P., Rich-Edwards, J.W., and Gillman, M.W. 2008. Diet during early pregnancy and development of gestational diabetes. *Paediatr Perinat Epidemiol* 22:47–59.

71. Gibson, K.S., Waters, T.P., and Catalano, P.M. 2012. Maternal weight gain in women who develop gestational diabetes mellitus. *Obstet Gynecol* 119:560–65.

72. Most, O., and Langer, O. 2012. Gestational diabetes: maternal weight gain in relation to fetal growth, treatment modality, BMI and glycemic control. *J Matern Fetal Neonatal Med* 25:2458–63.

73. Abrams, B.F., and Laros, R.K., Jr. 1986. Prepregnancy weight, weight gain, and birth weight. *Am J Obstet Gynecol* 154:503–9.

74. Ferraro, Z.M., Barrowman, N., Prud'homme, D., et al. 2011. Excessive gestational weight gain predicts large for gestational age neonates independent of maternal body mass index. *J Matern Fetal Neonatal Med* 25:538–42.

75. Institute of Medicine. 1990. *Nutrition during pregnancy. Part I. Weight gain.* Available from http:www.iom.edu/Reports/1990/Nutrition-During-Pregnancy-Part-I-Weight-Gain-Part-II-Nutrient-Supplements.aspx.

76. **Institute of Medicine 2009.** *Weight gain during pregnancy: reexamining the guidelines.* **Washington, DC: National Academies. Available from http:www.iom.edu/ Reports/2009/Weight-Gain-During-Pregnancy-Reexamining-the-Guidelines.aspx.** *Expert guidelines concerning weight gain in pregnancy.*

77. Cedergren, M.I. 2007. Optimal gestational weight gain for body mass index categories. *Obstet Gynecol* 110:759–64.

78. Artal, R., Lockwood, C.J., and Brown, H.L. 2010. Weight gain recommendations in pregnancy and the obesity epidemic. *Obstet Gynecol* 115:152–55.

79. Rasmussen, K.M., Abrams, B., Bodnar, L.M., Butte, N.F., Catalano, P.M., and Maria Siega-Riz, A. 2010. Recommendations for weight gain during pregnancy in the context of the obesity epidemic. *Obstet Gynecol* 116:1191–95.

80. Norris, S.L., Zhang, X., Avenell, A., et al. 2004. Long-term effectiveness of lifestyle and behavioral weight loss interventions in adults with type 2 diabetes: a meta-analysis. *Am J Med* 117:762–74.

81. Bellamy, L., Casas, J.P., Hingorani, A.D., and Williams, D. 2009. Type 2 diabetes mellitus after gestational diabetes: a systematic review and meta-analysis. *Lancet* 373:1773–79.

82. Cheng, Y.W., Chung, J.H., Kurbisch-Block, I., Inturrisi, M., Shafer, S., and Caughey, A.B. 2008. Gestational weight gain and gestational diabetes mellitus: perinatal outcomes. *Obstet Gynecol* 112:1015–22.

83. DeVader, S.R., Neeley, H.L., Myles, T.D., and Leet, T.L. 2007. Evaluation of gestational weight gain guidelines for women with normal prepregnancy body mass index. *Obstet Gynecol* 110:745–51.

84. Kiel, D.W., Dodson, E.A., Artal, R., Boehmer, T.K., and Leet, T.L. 2007. Gestational weight gain and pregnancy outcomes in obese women: how much is enough? *Obstet Gynecol* 110:752–58.

85. Yee, L.M., Cheng, Y.W., Inturrisi, M., and Caughey, A.B. 2011. Effect of gestational weight gain on perinatal outcomes in women with type 2 diabetes mellitus using the 2009 Institute of Medicine guidelines. *Am J Obstet Gynecol* 205:257.e251–56.

86. von Kries, R., Ensenauer, R., Beyerlein, A., Amann-Gassner, U., Hauner, H., and Schaffrath Rosario, A. 2011. Gestational weight gain and overweight in children: results from the cross-sectional German KiGGS study. *Int J Pediatr Obes* 6:45–52.

87. Nehring, I., Schmoll, S., Beyerlein, A., Hauner, H., and von Kries, R. 2011. Gestational weight gain and long-term postpartum weight retention: a meta-analysis. *Am J Clin Nutr* 94:1225–31.

88. Herring, S.J., Rose, M.Z., Skouteris, H., and Oken, E. 2012. Optimizing weight gain in pregnancy to prevent obesity in women and children. *Diabetes Obes Metab* 14:195–203.

89. Blomberg, M. 2011. Maternal and neonatal outcomes among obese women with weight gain below the new Institute of Medicine recommendations. *Obstet Gynecol* 117:1065–70.

90. Beyerlein, A., Schiessl, B., Lack, N., and von Kries, R. 2011. Associations of gestational weight loss with birth-related outcome: a retrospective cohort study. *BJOG* 118:55–61.

91. Hasegawa, J., Nakamura, M., Hamada, S., et al. 2012. Gestational weight loss has adverse effects on placental development. *J Matern Fetal Neonatal Med* 25:1909–12.

92. Jenkins, D.J., Wolever, T.M., Taylor, R.H., et al. 1981. Glycemic index of foods: a physiological basis for carbohydrate exchange. *Am J Clin Nutr* 34:362–66.

93. Wolever, T.M., Jenkins, D.J., Jenkins, A.L., and Josse, R.G. 1991. The glycemic index: methodology and clinical implications. *Am J Clin Nutr* 54:846–54.

94. Walsh, J., Mahony, R., Foley, M., and McAuliffe, F. 2010. A randomised control trial of low glycaemic index carbohydrate diet versus no dietary intervention in the prevention of recurrence of macrosomia. *BMC Pregnancy Childbirth* 2010:16.

95. Du, H., Van der A, D.L., and Feskens, E.J. 2006. Dietary glycaemic index: a review of the physiological mechanisms and observed health impacts. *Acta Cardiol* 61:383–97.

96. Standards Australia. 2007. *Glycemic index of foods*. Australia Standards AS4694-2007.

97. Foster-Powell, K., Holt, S.H., and Brand-Miller, J.C. 2002. International table of glycemic index and glycemic load values: 2002. *Am J Clin Nutr* 76:5–56.

98. Levis, S.P., McGowan, C.A., and McAuliffe, F.M. 2011. Methodology for adding and amending glycaemic index values to a nutrition analysis package. *Br J Nutr* 105:1117–32.

99. Jenkins, D.J., Wolever, T.M., Jenkins, A.L., et al. 1983. The glycaemic index of foods tested in diabetic patients: a new basis for carbohydrate exchange favouring the use of legumes. *Diabetologia* 24:257–64.

100. Miller, J.C. 1994. Importance of glycemic index in diabetes. *Am J Clin Nutr* 59(3 Suppl):747S–52S.

101. Brand-Miller, J., Hayne, S., Petocz, P., and Colagiuri, S. 2003. Low-glycemic index diets in the management of diabetes: a meta-analysis of randomized controlled trials. *Diabetes Care* 26:2261–67.

102. Thomas, D., and Elliott, E.J. 2009. Low glycaemic index, or low glycaemic load, diets for diabetes mellitus. *Cochrane Database Syst Rev* CD006296.

103. Ludwig, D.S. 2002. The glycemic index: physiological mechanisms relating to obesity, diabetes, and cardiovascular disease. *JAMA* 287:2414–23.

104. Brand-Miller, J., McMillan-Price, J., Steinbeck, K., and Caterson, I. 2009. Dietary glycemic index: health implications. *J Am Coll Nutr* 28(Suppl):446S–49S.

105. Thomas, D.E., Elliott, E.J., and Baur, L. 2007. Low glycaemic index or low glycaemic load diets for overweight and obesity. *Cochrane Database Syst Rev* CD005105.

106. Pawlak, D.B., Kushner, J.A., and Ludwig, D.S. 2004. Effects of dietary glycaemic index on adiposity, glucose homoeostasis, and plasma lipids in animals. *Lancet* 364:778–85.

107. Ebbeling, C.B., Leidig, M.M., Feldman, H.A., Lovesky, M.M., and Ludwig, D.S. 2007. Effects of a low-glycemic load vs low-fat diet in obese young adults: a randomized trial. *JAMA* 297:2092–102.

108. Halton, T.L., Willett, W.C., Liu, S., et al. 2006. Low-carbohydrate-diet score and the risk of coronary heart disease in women. *N Engl J Med* 355:1991–2002.

109. Mulholland, H.G., Murray, L.J., Cardwell, C.R., and Cantwell, M.M. 2008. Dietary glycaemic index, glycaemic load and breast cancer risk: a systematic review and meta-analysis. *Br J Cancer* 99:1170–75.

110. Mulholland, H.G., Murray, L.J., Cardwell, C.R., and Cantwell, M.M. 2008. Dietary gly-caemic index, glycaemic load and endometrial and ovarian cancer risk: a systematic review and meta-analysis. *Br J Cancer* 99:434–41.

111. Mulholland, H.G., Murray, L.J., Cardwell, C.R., and Cantwell, M.M. 2009. Glycemic index, glycemic load, and risk of digestive tract neoplasms: a systematic review and meta-analysis. *Am J Clin Nutr* 89:568–76.

112. Lock, D.R., Bar-Eyal, A., Voet, H., and Madar, Z. 1988. Glycemic indices of various foods given to pregnant diabetic subjects. *Obstet Gynecol* 71:180–83.

113. Louie, J.C., Brand-Miller, J.C., Markovic, T.P., Ross, G.P., and Moses, R.G. 2010. Glycemic index and pregnancy: a systematic literature review. *J Nutr Metab* 2010:282464.

114. McGowan, C.A., and McAuliffe, F.M. 2010. The influence of maternal glycaemia and dietary glycaemic index on pregnancy outcome in healthy mothers. *Br J Nutr* 104:153–59.

115. Atkinson, F.S., Foster-Powell, K., and Brand-Miller, J.C. 2008. International tables of glycemic index and glycemic load values: 2008. *Diabetes Care* 31:2281–83.

116. Louie, J.C., Brand-Miller, J.C., and Moses, R.G. 2013. Carbohydrates, glycemic index, and pregnancy outcomes in gestational diabetes. *Curr Diab Rep* 13:6–11.

117. **Scholl, T.O., Chen, X., Khoo, C.S., and Lenders, C. 2004. The dietary glycemic index during pregnancy: influence on infant birth weight, fetal growth, and bio-markers of carbohydrate metabolism. *Am J Epidemiol* 159:467–74.** *A study of over 1,000 pregnancies showing the link between dietary glycaemic index and maternal glu-cose concentrations in pregnancy. A low maternal glycaemic index diet was associated with a lower offspring birth weight and a higher risk for the offspring being small for gestational age.*

118. Zhang, C., Liu, S., Solomon, C.G., and Hu, F.B. 2006. Dietary fiber intake, dietary gly-cemic load, and the risk for gestational diabetes mellitus. *Diabetes Care* 29:2223–30.

119. Moses, R.G., Luebcke, M., Davis, W.S., et al. 2006. Effect of a low-glycemic-index diet during pregnancy on obstetric outcomes. *Am J Clin Nutr* 84:807–12.

120. Moses, R.G., Luebke, M., Petocz, P., and Brand-Miller, J.C. 2007. Maternal diet and infant size 2 y after the completion of a study of a low-glycemic-index diet in pregnancy. *Am J Clin Nutr* 86:1806.

121. Smith, N.A., McAuliffe, F.M., Quinn, K., Lonergan, P., and Evans, A.C. 2009. Transient high glycaemic intake in the last trimester of pregnancy increases offspring birthweight and postnatal growth rate in sheep: a randomised control trial. *BJOG* 116:975–83.

122. Walsh, J., McGowan, C.A., Mahony, R., Foley, M.E., and McAuliffe, F.M. 2012. Low glycaemic index diet in pregnancy to prevent macrosomia (ROLO study): randomised control trial. *BMJ* 345:e5605.

123. Clapp, J.F., II. 1997. Diet, exercise, and feto-placental growth. *Grundlagenreferate Arch Gynecol Obstet* 261:101–8.

124. Deierlein, A.L., Siega-Riz, A.M., and Herring, A. 2008. Dietary energy density but not glycemic load is associated with gestational weight gain. *Am J Clin Nutr* 88:693–99.

125. Rhodes, E.T., Pawlak, D.B., Takoudes, T.C., et al. 2010. Effects of a low-glycemic-load diet in overweight and obese pregnant women: a pilot randomized controlled trial. *Am J Clin Nutr* 92:1306–15.

126. Han, S., Crowther, C.A., Middleton, P., and Heatley, E. 2013. Different types of dietary advice for women with gestational diabetes mellitus. *Cochrane Database Syst Rev* 3:CD009275.

127. Tieu, J., Crowther, C.A., and Middleton, P. 2008. Dietary advice in pregnancy for pre-venting gestational diabetes mellitus. *Cochrane Database Syst Rev* 2:CD006674.

128. **Moses, R.G., Barker, M., Winter, M., Petocz, P., and Brand-Miller, J.C. 2009. Can a low-glycemic index diet reduce the need for insulin in gestational diabetes mellitus? A randomized trial. *Diabetes Care* 32:996–1000.** *A randomised trial showing the use of a low-glycaemic index diet can safely reduce the need for insulin to treat GDM.*

129. Grant, S.M., Wolever, T.M., O'Connor, D.L., Nisenbaum, R., and Josse, R.G. 2011. Effect of a low glycaemic index diet on blood glucose in women with gestational hyperglycaemia. *Diabetes Res Clin Pract* 91:15–22.

130. **Louie, J.C., Markovic, T.P., Perera, N., Foote, D., Petocz, P., Ross, G.P., and Brand-Miller, J.C. 2011. A randomized controlled trial investigating the effects of a low-glycemic index diet on pregnancy outcomes in gestational diabetes mellitus. *Diabetes Care* 34:2341–46.** *The largest randomised controlled trial testing the use of low GI diets in non-GDM pregnancy.*

131. Perichart-Perera, O., Balas-Nakash, M., Rodriguez-Cano, A., Legorreta-Legorreta, J., Parra-Covarrubias, A., and Vadillo-Ortega, F. 2012. Low glycemic index carbohydrates versus all types of carbohydrates for treating diabetes in pregnancy: a randomised clinical trial to evaluate the effect of glycemic control. *Int J Endocrinol* 2012:296017.

132. Cleary, J., Casey, S., Hofsteede, C., Moses, R.G., Milosavljevic, M., and Brand-Miller, J. 2012. Does a low glycaemic index (GI) diet cost more during pregnancy? *Nutrients* 4:1759–66.

7 Exercise and Gestational Diabetes

Michel Boulvain
Department of Gynecology and Obstetrics,
Geneva University Hospitals, Faculty of Medicine,
Geneva University, Geneva, Switzerland

CONTENTS

7.1 INTRODUCTION

Reduced physical activity and a sedentary lifestyle are risk factors for both excessive weight gain and reduced insulin sensitivity. These risk factors for gestational diabetes are potentially modifiable. Therefore, promoting exercise during pregnancy could reduce the risk of developing gestational diabetes and may be an intervention to be included in the management of women with gestational diabetes.[1] Pregnancy may also provide an opportunity to improve lifestyle in the longer term, decreasing the risk of obesity and type 2 diabetes for both mother and her child.[2]

7.2 EXERCISE IN NORMAL PREGNANCY

Physical activity had been traditionally discouraged in pregnancy due to theoretical concerns of injury and adverse foetal and maternal outcomes.[3] More recently, observational studies suggested that light to moderate physical activity during a normal pregnancy provides various benefits for the mother and her foetus (Table 7.1).[4,5]

Fourteen randomised trials, including a total of 1,014 women, evaluating the effects of aerobic exercise programs during pregnancy were conducted. A systematic review of these trials concluded that regular aerobic exercise appears to improve (or maintain) physical fitness, but available data are insufficient to exclude important benefits and risks for the mother or infant.[6] A disturbing finding was a nonstatistically significant increase in the risk of preterm delivery in the exercise groups (relative risk 1.82, 95% confidence interval 0.35 to 9.57). This was not accompanied by

TABLE 7.1

Baseline Characteristics of the Study Subjects, the Associated Metabolic Effects, and Delivery Outcomes in an Observational Study of Pregnant Women Grouped According to Their Level of Physical Activity

Characteristic	Active Women ($n = 27$)	Inactive Women ($n = 17$)	p Value
General			
Age (years)	31.5 ± 5.4	30.5 ± 5.8	0.55
Primiparous women (n {%})	19 (70.4)	10 (58.8)	0.52
Height (cm)	167.8 ± 6.4	163.2 ± 5.2	0.01
Prepregnancy weight (kg)	64.3 ± 13.1	60.8 ± 9.9	0.35
Prepregnancy body mass index (kg/m^2)	22.8 ± 4.2	22.8 ± 3.5	0.98
Weight (kg)	79.3 ± 13.4	75.1 ± 11.4	0.88
Body weight gain (kg)	15.9 ± 3.8	15.1 ± 4.3	0.51
Metabolic			
Physical activity level	1.6 ± 0.1	1.4 ± 0.1	0.001
Total energy expenditure (kJ/day)	$12,557 \pm 2,374$	$10,508 \pm 1,751$	0.004
Activity energy expenditure (kJ/day)	$3,478 \pm 1,129$	$1,735 \pm 456$	0.001
Maximal oxygen uptake (ml/min/kg)	34.9 ± 5.6	30.3 ± 6.2	0.01
Maximal oxygen uptake (ml/min)	$2,742 \pm 475$	$2,256 \pm 484$	0.002
Sleeping heart rate (beats/min)	66.7 ± 7.8	74.6 ± 6.4	0.001
Movement (counts/min)	23.5 ± 9.5	13.4 ± 5.6	0.012
Delivery Outcomes			
Birth weight (g)	$3,448 \pm 310$	$3,518 \pm 418$	0.53
First stage of labour (min)	301 (40–770) ($n = 25$)	304 (75–555) ($n = 15$)	0.87
Second stage of labour (min)	88 (9–178) ($n = 24$)	146 (3–212) ($n = 14$)	0.05
Duration of pushing efforts (min)	50 (4–115) ($n = 24$)	83 (1–133) ($n = 14$)	0.14
Apgar score (<7 at 5 min)	1	1	0.74
Meconium	12	6	0.77
Episiotomy/perineal laceration	19 ($n = 25$)	7 ($n = 15$)	0.19
Anaesthesia (spinal/epidural)	20	15	0.45
Postpartum haemorrhage ($\geq$500 ml)	6	7	0.32
Operative delivery (vacuum/forceps/caesarean)	9	11	0.06

Source: Melzer, K. et al., *Am. J. Obstet. Gynecol.*, 202, 266 e1–6, 2010. Copyright © 2010 Mosby, Inc. With permission from Elsevier.

Note: Quantitative data are mean ± standard deviation or mean (range). Active women were those performing ≥30 min of moderate physical activity per day, defined as any activity with an energy expenditure between 3 and 6 metabolic equivalents or multiples of metabolic rate. Inactive women were those doing less than 30 min of this per day.

Study or subgroup	Exercise Mean	SD	Total	Control Mean	SD	Total	Weight	Mean difference IV, Random, 95% CI	Mean difference IV, Random, 95% CI
Barakat, 2009	11.5	3.7	72	12.4	3.4	70	14.1%	−0.90 [−2.07, 0.27]	
Cavalcante, 2009	14.3	2.1	21	15.1	1.6	27	15.5%	−0.80 [−1.88, 0.28]	
Clapp, 2000	15.7	2.2	22	16.3	1.9	24	13.7%	−0.60 [−1.79, 0.59]	
Collings, 1983	15.8	3.6	12	14	3.7	8	2.7%	1.80 [−1.47, 5.07]	
Garshasbi, 2005	14.1	3.8	107	13.8	5.2	105	13.2%	0.30 [−0.93, 1.53]	
Hopkins, 2010	8.2	13.4	47	8	10.3	37	1.2%	0.20 [−4.87, 5.27]	
Marquez-Sterling, 2000	16.2	3.4	9	15.7	4	6	1.9%	0.50 [−3.40, 4.40]	
Ong, 2009	3.7	3.4	6	5.2	1.3	6	3.3%	−1.50 [−4.41, 1.41]	
Prevedel, 2001	14.95	4.2	22	12.5	5.8	19	2.9%	2.45 [−0.69, 5.59]	
Santos, 2005	5.7	8.5	37	6.3	7.7	35	2.1%	−0.60 [−4.34, 3.14]	
Sedaghati, 2007	13.6	1.1	40	15.1	2.1	50	24.2%	−1.50 [−2.17, 0.83]	
Yeo, 2009	15.4	5.9	64	15.9	6.8	60	5.2%	−0.50 [−2.75, 1.75]	
Total (95% CI)			459			447	100.0%	−0.61 [−1.17, −0.06]	

Heterogeneity: Tau² = 0.21; Chi² = 14.76, df = 11 (P = 0.19); I² = 25%
Test for overall effect: Z = 2.17 (P = 0.03)

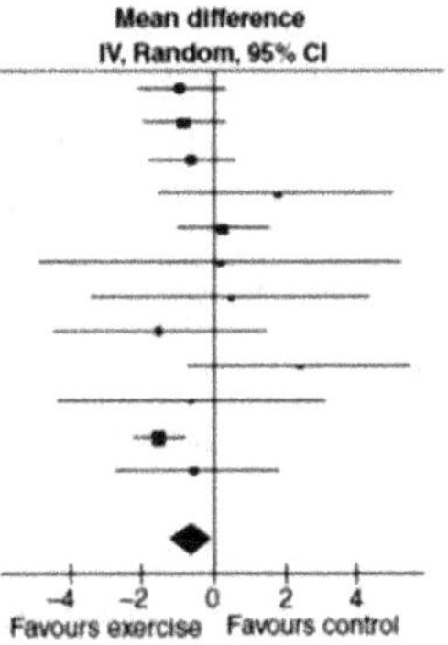

Favours exercise Favours control

FIGURE 7.1 Mean differences in gestational weight gain between exercise and control groups in various related publications, calculated using a random effects model. The squares represent the point estimate for each study included in the meta-analysis; the lines either side of this represent the 95% confidence interval. The diamond represents the overall pooled point estimate of all these studies. (Reproduced from Streuling, I. et al., *BJOG*, 118, 278–84, 2011. Published by John Wiley & Sons, Inc. Copyright © 2010 Streuling, I. et al. With permission.)

a mean reduction of gestational age at birth or a reduction in mean birth weight. Another review, including 12 trials, suggested that exercise programs may reduce pregnancy weight gain (Figure 7.1).[7]

Despite the lack of strong evidence for a clinically significant benefit, recommendations to perform regular physical activity during pregnancy in the absence of medical or obstetric complications have been released based on concensus opinion.[8] Absolute contraindications to aerobic exercise during pregnancy were recommended as haemodynamically significant heart disease, restrictive lung disease, incompetent cervix/cerclage, multiple gestation (at risk of premature labour), persistent second or third trimester bleeding, placenta previa after 26 weeks of gestation, premature labour, ruptured membranes, and preeclampsia/pregnancy-induced hypertension. Relative contraindications were recommended as severe anaemia, unevaluated maternal cardiac arrhythmia, chronic bronchitis, poorly controlled type 1 diabetes/seizure disorder/hyperthyroidism, extreme morbid obesity, extreme underweight (body mass index less than 12 kg/m²), history of extremely sedentary lifestyle, intrauterine growth restriction in current pregnancy, orthopaedic limitations, and being a heavy smoker.

7.3 EXERCISE TO PREVENT GESTATIONAL DIABETES

The prevalence of gestational diabetes is increasing, because of the increasing prevalence of obesity and of sedentary lifestyle. Another factor for this increase is the recently accepted new definition of the condition, which doubles the prevalence in many populations.[9] Because of this high prevalence, it is logical to design interventions to be included in the routine care of the general population of pregnant women to prevent gestational diabetes and eventually other consequences of excessive weight gain during pregnancy. Exercise programs have the potential to reach this goal and to modify lifestyle in the longer term, which might benefit the whole family. But, before introducing such large-scale interventions, it is important to demonstrate that the intervention is feasible, effective, and harmless.

Observational studies have found that physical activity during normal pregnancy decreases insulin resistance, and therefore might help to decrease the risk of gestational diabetes.[10] The largest of these observational studies suggested that the risk of gestational diabetes was decreased by 33% among women in the highest quintile of physical activity, compared to the lowest quintile.[11]

Five randomised trials, including a total of 1,115 women, were conducted to evaluate various exercise programs to prevent gestational diabetes.[12–16] Four of these trials had a small sample size, and only one had sufficient sample size to demonstrate differences in clinically relevant outcomes.[16] The systematic review included in the Cochrane Library found no significant difference in gestational diabetes incidence in women receiving additional exercise interventions, compared with those having routine antenatal care (3 trials, 826 women, relative risk 1.10, 95% confidence interval 0.66 to 1.84).[17]

None of the included studies have reported longer-term outcomes for mothers or their children. A systematic review of randomised and nonrandomised studies evaluating exercise programs in overweight and obese pregnant women found no statistically significant reduction in the incidence of gestational diabetes.[18]

Why is there such a difference between the results of observational studies and those of randomised trials? The first reason may be confounding, as performing exercise may be associated with healthy lifestyle in general, and thus a decreased risk of gestational diabetes. Another reason might be that only a minimal improvement in physical activity has been achieved in the intervention group of the randomised trials, compared to larger differences between active and nonactive women in observational studies. It is difficult to modify lifestyle during the relatively short period of the pregnancy and in the context of a study.

7.4 EXERCISE IN WOMEN DIAGNOSED WITH GESTATIONAL DIABETES

The primary objective of the management of gestational diabetes is to decrease hyperglycaemia, in order to improve pregnancy outcomes. Specific antenatal care for women with gestational diabetes includes glucose monitoring, diet and lifestyle counselling, administration of insulin or oral glucose-lowering agents, and foetal surveillance. This package of interventions was shown effective in improving pregnancy outcomes.[19,20] The package of interventions that was demonstrated effective in randomised trials included dietary and lifestyle advice as initial treatment. In these trials, women were probably encouraged to exercise, but no details on this specific aspect of care were reported. If these interventions alone were not sufficient to achieve glycaemia control, insulin therapy was introduced. Administration of insulin is poorly acceptable to women, because it involves the need for injections, may cause hypoglycaemia, and needs intensive follow-up for adaptation of the dosage. If demonstrated effective in reducing the need for adding insulin to the diet, an exercise program may be an attractive alternative. An additional benefit might be that as women with gestational diabetes are at increased risk of developing type 2 diabetes in later life, long-lasting increase in exercise level may prevent this long-term complication.

Exercise is effective in the prevention and management of type 2 diabetes, by reducing insulin resistance, in men and nonpregnant women.[21,22] Increasing the exercise level has been shown to decrease glycaemia and insulin resistance during pregnancy.[23] The effect was greatest with low-intensity prolonged exercise that uses a large muscle mass in late pregnancy shortly (less than 2 h) after food intake. Regular exercise during pregnancy is associated with decreased circulating tumour necrosis factor (TNF)-alpha levels, and the effect seems to be dose and time dependent.[24] Therefore, exercise programs may be an effective intervention to add in the management of women diagnosed with gestational diabetes.

Several randomised trials were conducted to evaluate the benefit of exercise, in addition to diet, in women with gestational diabetes.[25–30] A systematic review, published in the Cochrane Library, included the trials comparing any type of exercise program with no exercise program or other therapy.[31] Women were recruited during the third trimester of pregnancy, and the intervention was performed for about 6 weeks. All trials included pregnant women with gestational diabetes mellitus, but criteria to define gestational diabetes and strategies for screening varied between studies. Type, frequency, intensity, and duration of the exercise program were also different, but included in general a session of moderate-level exercise during 30 min every other day (Table 7.2). In all the studies, diet was part of the routine care and was not different in the intervention and control groups.

As all trials were of small size, the analysis has low power to detect any clinically significant benefit of the exercise programs. Values of glycaemia were generally lower in women randomised in the exercise groups. The use of insulin was reported in all trials. One trial included women deemed to receive insulin treatment,

TABLE 7.2
Characteristics of Studies Included in the Systematic Review

Author	Experimental Group (n)	Control Group (n)	Intervention
Avery et al. 1997[29]	15	14	Cycle ergometer at 70% VO2 max for 30 min, 3–4 times weekly
Bung et al. 1991[30]	17	17	Cycle ergometer at 50% VO2 max for 45 min, 3 times weekly
Jovanovic-Peterson et al. 1989[27]	10	9	Arm ergometer for 20 min, 3 times weekly
Brankston et al. 2004[25]	16	16	Circuit type resistance training for 30 min, 3 times weekly
de Barros et al. 2010[28]	32	32	Circuit type resistance training for 30 min, 2–3 times weekly, using an elastic band

Source: Ceysens, G. et al., *Cochrane Database Syst. Rev.,* 3, CD004225, 2006.

randomised to insulin or exercise.[30] Therefore, use of insulin should not be considered an outcome in this trial. The meta-analysis of the results of the four other trials[25,27-29] showed promising results from the exercise programs in reducing the need for insulin (relative risk 0.61, 95% confidence interval 0.38 to 0.99). There were no differences between groups in other clinically relevant outcomes. Limited information is available regarding neonatal outcomes.

7.5 SUMMARY

A recommendation to perform regular moderate exercise may be included in routine antenatal care, despite the lack of strong evidence for a benefit in preventing gestational diabetes (Figure 7.2). Exercise programs may be beneficial, in addition to dietary advice, for women with gestational diabetes. In addition to short-term benefits, exercise performed during pregnancy may promote a change in lifestyle persisting after delivery and may help prevent the onset of type 2 diabetes and its long-term complications.

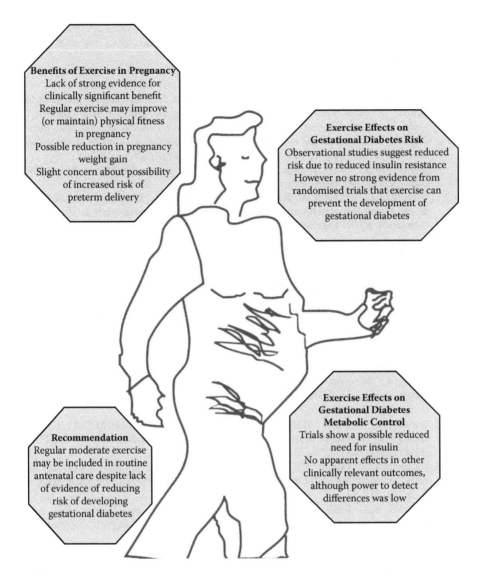

Benefits of Exercise in Pregnancy
Lack of strong evidence for clinically significant benefit
Regular exercise may improve (or maintain) physical fitness in pregnancy
Possible reduction in pregnancy weight gain
Slight concern about possibility of increased risk of preterm delivery

Exercise Effects on Gestational Diabetes Risk
Observational studies suggest reduced risk due to reduced insulin resistance
However no strong evidence from randomised trials that exercise can prevent the development of gestational diabetes

Recommendation
Regular moderate exercise may be included in routine antenatal care despite lack of evidence of reducing risk of developing gestational diabetes

Exercise Effects on Gestational Diabetes Metabolic Control
Trials show a possible reduced need for insulin
No apparent effects in other clinically relevant outcomes, although power to detect differences was low

FIGURE 7.2 Summary diagram showing current knowledge about the effects of moderate exercise on pregnancy, including effects on gestational diabetes risk and as a treatment adjunct for it.

REFERENCES

Key references are in bold.

1. Petry, C.J. 2010. Gestational diabetes: risk factors and recent advances in its genetics and treatment. *Br J Nutr* 104:775–87.
2. Ratner, R.E., Christophi, C.A., Metzger, B.E., et al. 2008. Prevention of diabetes in women with a history of gestational diabetes: effects of metformin and lifestyle interventions. *J Clin Endocrinol Metab* 93:4774–79.

3. Melzer, K., Schutz, Y., Boulvain, M., and Kayser, B. 2010. Physical activity and pregnancy: cardiovascular adaptations, recommendations and pregnancy outcomes. *Sports Med* 40:493–507.

4. Melzer, K., Schutz, Y., Soehnchen, N., et al. 2010. Effects of recommended levels of physical activity on pregnancy outcomes. *Am J Obstet Gynecol* 202:266 e1–6.

5. **Kalisiak, B., and Spitznagle, T. 2009. What effect does an exercise program for healthy pregnant women have on the mother, fetus, and child? *P M R* 1:261–66.** *A review assessing the effects of moderate exercising on the mother and her offspring, in both the foetal period and childhood, and a recommendation based on a comparison with American College of Obstetrics and Gynecologists (ACOG) guidelines.*

6. Kramer, M.S., and McDonald, S.W. 2006. Aerobic exercise for women during pregnancy. *Cochrane Database Syst Rev* 3:CD000180.

7. **Streuling, I., Beyerlein, A., Rosenfeld, E., Hofmann, H., Schulz, T., and von Kries, R. 2011. Physical activity and gestational weight gain: a meta-analysis of intervention trials. *BJOG* 118:278–84.** *A contemporary meta-analysis of studies assessing the effects of increasing physical activity on gestational weight gain in pregnant, obese women.*

8. ACOG Committee Opinion. 2002. Exercise during pregnancy and the postpartum period. Number 267, January 2002. American College of Obstetricians and Gynecologists. *Int J Gynaecol Obstet* 77:79–81.

9. Metzger, B.E., Gabbe, S.G., Persson, B., et al. 2010. International Association of Diabetes and Pregnancy Study Groups recommendations on the diagnosis and classification of hyperglycemia in pregnancy. *Diabetes Care* 33:676–82.

10. Reece, E.A., Leguizamon, G., and Wiznitzer, A. 2009. Gestational diabetes: the need for a common ground. *Lancet* 373:1789–97.

11. Zhang, C., Solomon, C.G., Manson, J.E., and Hu, F.B. 2006. A prospective study of pregravid physical activity and sedentary behaviors in relation to the risk for gestational diabetes mellitus. *Arch Intern Med* 166:543–48.

12. Barakat, R., Pelaez, M., Montejo, R., Luaces, M., and Zakynthinaki, M. 2011. Exercise during pregnancy improves maternal health perception: a randomized controlled trial. *Am J Obstet Gynecol* 204:402 e1–7.

13. Callaway, L.K., Colditz, P.B., Byrne, N.M., et al. 2010. Prevention of gestational diabetes: feasibility issues for an exercise intervention in obese pregnant women. *Diabetes Care* 33:1457–59.

14. Hopkins, S.A., Baldi, J.C., Cutfield, W.S., McCowan, L., and Hofman, P.L. 2010. Exercise training in pregnancy reduces offspring size without changes in maternal insulin sensitivity. *J Clin Endocrinol Metab* 95:2080–88.

15. Ong, M.J., Guelfi, K.J., Hunter, T., Wallman, K.E., Fournier, P.A., and Newnham, J.P. 2009. Supervised home-based exercise may attenuate the decline of glucose tolerance in obese pregnant women. *Diabetes Metab* 35:418–21.

16. **Stafne, S.N., Salvesen, K.A., Romundstad, P.R., Eggebo, T.M., Carlsen, S.M., and Morkved, S. 2012. Regular exercise during pregnancy to prevent gestational diabetes: a randomized controlled trial. *Obstet Gynecol* 119:29–36.** *A randomised controlled trial assessing the effect of a 12-week exercise program on insulin sensitivity and the development of gestational diabetes.*

17. **Han, S., Middleton, P., and Crowther, C.A. 2012. Exercise for pregnant women for preventing gestational diabetes mellitus. *Cochrane Database Syst Rev* 7:CD009021.** *A contemproary meta-analysis of studies assessing the effect of exercise on the development of gestational diabetes or impaired glucose tolerance in pregnancy.*

18. **Oteng-Ntim, E., Varma, R., Croker, H., Poston, L., and Doyle, P. 2012. Lifestyle interventions for overweight and obese pregnant women to improve pregnancy outcome: systematic review and meta-analysis. *BMC Med* 10:47.** *A contemporary*

systematic review and meta-analysis of the effects of antenatal dietary, activity, behaviour, or lifestyle interventions in overweight and obese women on pregnancy outcomes such as gestational weight gains and the development of gestational diabetes.

19. Crowther, C.A., Hiller, J.E., Moss, J.R., McPhee, A.J., Jeffries, W.S., and Robinson, J.S. 2005. Effect of treatment of gestational diabetes mellitus on pregnancy outcomes. *N Engl J Med* 352:2477–86.

20. Landon, M.B., Spong, C.Y., Thom, E., et al. 2009. A multicenter, randomized trial of treatment for mild gestational diabetes. *N Engl J Med* 361:1339–48.

21. Dunkley, A.J., Charles, K., Gray, L.J., Camosso-Stefinovic, J., Davies, M.J., and Khunti, K. 2012. Effectiveness of interventions for reducing diabetes and cardiovascular disease risk in people with metabolic syndrome: systematic review and mixed treatment comparison meta-analysis. *Diabetes Obes Metab* 14:616–25.

22. Tuomilehto, J., Lindstrom, J., Eriksson, J.G., et al. 2001. Prevention of type 2 diabetes mellitus by changes in lifestyle among subjects with impaired glucose tolerance. *N Engl J Med* 344:1343–50.

23. Clapp, J.F. 2006. Effects of diet and exercise on insulin resistance during pregnancy. *Metab Syndr Relat Disord* 4:84–90.

24. Clapp, J.F., 3rd. 2000. Exercise during pregnancy. A clinical update. *Clin Sports Med* 19:273–86.

25. Brankston, G.N., Mitchell, B.F., Ryan, E.A., and Okun, N.B. 2004. Resistance exercise decreases the need for insulin in overweight women with gestational diabetes mellitus. *Am J Obstet Gynecol* 190:188–93.

26. Bung, P., Artal, R., and Khodiguian, N. 1993. Regular exercise therapy in disorders of carbohydrate metabolism in pregnancy—results of a prospective, randomized longitudinal study. *Geburtshilfe Frauenheilkd* 53:188–93.

27. Jovanovic-Peterson, L., Durak, E.P., and Peterson, C.M. 1989. Randomized trial of diet versus diet plus cardiovascular conditioning on glucose levels in gestational diabetes. *Am J Obstet Gynecol* 161:415–19.

28. de Barros, M.C., Lopes, M.A., Francisco, R.P., Sapienza, A.D., and Zugaib, M. 2010. Resistance exercise and glycemic control in women with gestational diabetes mellitus. *Am J Obstet Gynecol* 203:556 e1–6.

29. Avery, M.D., Leon, A.S., and Kopher, R.A. 1997. Effects of a partially home-based exercise program for women with gestational diabetes. *Obstet Gynecol* 89:10–15.

30. Bung, P., Artal, R., Khodiguian, N., and Kjos, S. 1991. Exercise in gestational diabetes. An optional therapeutic approach? *Diabetes* 40(Suppl 2):182–85.

31. **Ceysens, G., Rouiller, D., and Boulvain, M. 2006. Exercise for diabetic pregnant women. *Cochrane Database Syst Rev* 3:CD004225.** *A meta-analysis of clinical trials testing the effectiveness of exercise on perinatal and maternal morbidity in pregnant women with diabetes.*

8 Pharmacological Treatment of Gestational Diabetes

David Simmons
Wolfson Diabetes and Endocrinology Clinic, Institute of
Metabolic Science, Cambridge University Hospitals NHS
Foundation Trust, Addenbrooke's Hospital, Cambridge,
United Kingdom; Department of Rural Health, University
of Melbourne, Shepparton, Victoria, Australia

CONTENTS

8.1   BACKGROUND

Hyperglycaemia in the antenatal period can have a major impact on foetal beta cell and adipocyte development[1] and can lead to neonatal hypoglycaemia, macrosomia, polycythaemia, hyperbilirubinaemia, and hypomagnesaemia.[2] There is growing evidence that exposure to hyperglycaemia in utero may increase the risk of future obesity and diabetes in the offspring.[3-5] The relationship between maternal hyperglycaemia and adverse maternal/neonatal adverse outcomes is continuous with no threshold.[6]

Managing hyperglycaemia in the antenatal period is associated with a reduction in perinatal and maternal pregnancy-related complications,[7] although there remains debate over the optimal glycaemic criteria for both diagnosis and initiating/intensifying pharmacological therapy. As gestational diabetes mellitus (GDM) is diagnosed when "hyperglycaemia is detected for the first time during pregnancy,"[8] there may have been preexisting dysglycaemia (diabetes, impaired glucose tolerance, impaired fasting glucose) as well as newly developed hyperglycaemia, and this will clearly influence likelihood of pharmacological therapy. Generally, GDM is detected after organogenesis (i.e., after the first 8 weeks), and this chapter will focus on the impact of pharmacological agents after this time, although comment on malformations will be made where relevant.

8.2   WHICH OUTCOMES SHOULD BE CONSIDERED WHEN TESTING THE EFFICACY OF A PHARMACEUTICAL AGENT IN GDM?

There are a growing number of randomised controlled trials that demonstrate that identification and management of GDM improves maternal and neonatal outcomes.[9,10] Obstetric management is a major component in the multifaceted approach to improving pregnancy outcomes in GDM. Earlier delivery, through induction and, where necessary, caesarean section, can prevent the occurrence of the major adverse obstetric outcomes in GDM: stillbirth, birth trauma, and severe perineal trauma. Technically, obstetric care that is able to predict 100% of such adverse events would result in randomised controlled trials where the only possible differences in the efficacy of antihyperglycaemic agents able to be shown would be through caesarean section rates (with perhaps a different mix of indications), neonatal intensive care unit admissions, neonatal hypoglycaemia rates, neonatal breathing problems, and long-term outcomes in the offspring and mother. As obstetric intervention and neonatal intensive care unit admission rates are dependent on many other factors (e.g., local policies), criteria for neonatal hypoglycaemia vary and can be dependent on local neonatal feeding policies, breathing difficulties and shoulder dystocia are variably diagnosed, and long-term outcomes require long-term studies, it is not surprising that there has been much debate over the usefulness of managing maternal hyperglycaemia. However, trials of more vs. less tight glycaemic control, such as twice a day insulin therapy vs. four times a day therapy,[11] and a focus on preprandial vs. postprandial glycaemic targets[12] have also shown the benefits of tighter glycaemic control.

Using birth weight as an outcome is particularly fraught, as both small and large for gestational age babies are seen as undesirable, and higher birth weight itself is not a "harm"; it is the associates that are important. However, as macrosomia/large for gestational age (LGA) infants and maternal hypertension are indications for earlier obstetric intervention, these, and birth weight itself, should be seen as intermediate outcomes. With the recognition that induction even as late as 38 weeks might be associated with adverse outcomes,[13] there is a need to delay obstetric intervention to as near term as possible. In this setting, management of hyperglycaemia is likely to become more, rather than less, important as the ability to wait an additional 3–7 days could be beneficial. There is also evidence that macrosomia in association with GDM predicts metabolic syndrome in those offspring 11 years downstream, compared with other offspring from mothers with and without GDM.[14] An increased long-term risk of diabetes in the offspring has been shown to be associated with higher levels of maternal glycaemia at diagnosis of GDM,[15] and adiposity in the offspring is less when mothers have insulin-treated GDM compared with those treated with diet alone.[16]

With the evidence that pregnancy-related outcomes, and potentially the incidence of long-term diabetes-related complications, can be optimised through the achievement of better glycaemic control comes the necessity to use the available management strategies to control the blood glucose. The standard approach to managing hyperglycaemia, after lifestyle therapy (i.e., nutrition and physical activity), has been insulin therapy. However, insulin therapy has its problems. Balancing medication dosage, food, and activity with the frequency of hypoglycaemic episodes, overall glycaemia, weight management, and life, in general, remains a constant struggle for many pregnant women. When medication is used, approaches to mimicking postprandial insulin release, tailoring insulin action in special circumstances (e.g., exertion, intercurrent illness), improving insulin sensitivity, and providing adequate background insulin remain imperfect. The utility of the new insulins and the use of oral antihyperglycaemic agents therefore need to be viewed in the light of the known benefits of near normoglycaemia and the potential difficulties in achieving tighter glucose control.

8.3   GLYCAEMIC TARGETS FOR PREGNANCY

The importance of achieving tight postprandial glycaemia was shown by De Veciana's randomised controlled trial comparing preprandial and postprandial targets,[12] and most studies[17] have used a 2 h target of 6.7 mmol/L. The two major trials of the efficacy of the management of GDM, the Australian Carbohydrate Intolerance Study in

Pregnant Women (ACHOIS) and Maternal–Fetal Medicine Unit Network Randomized Clinical Trial (MFMN),[9,10] focused their diagnostic criteria on the postprandial glucose, with entry fasting thresholds of 7.0 and 5.3 mmol/L, respectively. However, the Hyperglycemia and Adverse Pregnancy Outcome (HAPO) study[6] showed that fasting hyperglycaemia is associated with adverse outcomes at much lower levels than previously used and led to a recommendation that the fasting glucose criterion for the diagnosis of GDM be lowered to 5.1 mmol/L.[18] Of course, increasing the proportion with lower overall risk may mean benefits are less. On the other hand, the mean fasting and 2 h glucose concentrations on OGTT in ACHOIS/MFMN were 4.8/4.8 and 8.6/9.6 mmol/L respectively, with no lower threshold for benefit from intervention shown.

Most clinical guidelines for GDM recommend targeting preprandial levels between 3.9 and 5.3 mmol/L and 1 and 2 h postprandial levels of <7.8 and 6.7 mmol/L, respectively. These targets need to be maintained until the end of pregnancy, even though demand for insulin is increasing, and the glucose trend will be upwards. Naturally, the dose of medication and potential for women using oral antihyperglycaemic agents to require insulin supplementation depend upon the targets set. There is evidence to suggest that use of therapy could be guided by the presence of an increased abdominal circumference on ultrasound.[19] However, in a randomised controlled trial (RCT), Schaefer-Graf et al.[20] subsequently compared introducing insulin when the preprandial glucose was 5.0 mmol/L or 2 h postprandial glucose was 6.7 mmol/L with introducing insulin when the foetal abdominal circumference on ultrasound was > 75th percentile or pre-/postprandial glucose was 6.7 or 11.1 mmol/L, respectively. Insulin treatment was in place for approximately 8 weeks, and there were no significant differences in proportion using insulin, caesarean section, LGA, small for gestational age (SGA), neonatal hypoglycaemia, or admission.

As obesity is associated with an independent risk of macrosomia and adverse outcomes,[21] there may also be a case for earlier (i.e., using a lower glycaemic threshold) for the introduction of medication among obese pregnant women with GDM, but this has not been tested.

So which medications are available?

8.4 PHARMACEUTICAL AGENTS IN GDM

Traditionally, insulin has been used as the recommended agent when lifestyle change is insufficient to control hyperglycaemia in GDM, although some countries have used oral agents for many years.[22] However, early studies suggested potential foetal harm from agents such as the first-generation sulphonylureas.[22,23] More recently, large trials of metformin[24] and glibenclamide[25] have suggested noninferiority compared with insulin, and some advantages, when using such oral agents. Safety and benefits have also needed to be shown with the insulin analogues.

8.4.1 RAPID-ACTING INSULIN ANALOGUES

There are three rapid-acting insulin analogues: lispro/Humalog, aspart/Novorapid, and glulisine/Apidra. All exist as hexamers in storage but dissociate into monomer upon subcutaneous injection, leading to their rapid action. Glulisine, the third rapid-acting insulin analogue introduced, has not been the subject of studies in pregnancy, and no case reports could be found on Medline, so it has not been described in any further detail. No reports were found in a literature review in 2009.[26]

The rapid-acting insulin analogues are not known to cross the placenta, with no reports of antibody-insulin complexes crossing the placenta. It is not known whether they are excreted into human milk.

8.4.1.1 Lispro/Humalog

Insulin lispro (Humalog, Eli Lilly, LysB28, ProB29—human insulin) was approved for clinical use in 1996 and was the first insulin analogue to enter clinical practice. Action is immediate, reaches a peak after 1 h, and lasts 4 h. In comparison with regular insulin, use of insulin lispro is associated with a 1.5–2.5 mmol/L lower postprandial glucose rise, a consistent reduction in HbA1c of 0.3–0.5%, 20–30% less severe hypoglycaemia (especially nocturnal), and less need for snacks.[27,28]

8.4.1.2 Insulin Aspart/Novorapid

Insulin aspart (Novorapid, Novo Nordisk, AspB28—human insulin) was approved for use in 1999. Insulin aspart also acts immediately, with peak action approximately 31–70 min after subcutaneous injection and lasts a similar length of time as insulin lispro. In comparison with regular insulin, use of insulin aspart is associated with 1.5 mmol/L lower postprandial glucose, 0.12% lower HbA1c, and less hypoglycaemic episodes needing third-party assistance.[29,30]

8.4.2 Long-Acting Insulin Analogues

There are currently two long-acting insulin analogues: insulin glargine and insulin levemir. A new insulin analogue, insulin degludec, entered use in 2013; there are no reports on use in pregnancy.

8.4.2.1 Insulin Glargine

Insulin glargine (Lantus, Aventis Pharma, 21A-Gly-30Ba-L-Arg-30Bb-L-Arg—human insulin) was the first new long-acting insulin analogue, having been approved for use in 2000. Two modifications of human insulin have been made: the addition of two arginine molecules to the C-terminal of the B-chain and the replacement of A21 asparagine by glycine. These result in the shifting of the isoelectric point from pH 5.4 to 6.7 (thereby decreasing solubility in subcutaneous tissue) and greater stability (by preventing dimerisation and deamidation), respectively.

Insulin glargine acts from approximately 90 min after subcutaneous injection and lasts 24 h and is considered "peakless." When compared with neutral protamine Hagedorn (NPH) insulin, use of insulin glargine has been associated with less nocturnal hypoglycaemia, reduced fasting glucose, reduced postdinner glucose concentrations, less weight gain, and reduced insulin dose with an impact similar to that of HbA1c.[31–33]

Insulin glargine is not known to cross the placenta, nor are there reports of antibody-insulin complexes crossing the placenta. It is not known whether insulin glargine is excreted into human milk.

No randomised controlled trials of insulin glargine have taken place in GDM, but there have been a number of prospective, retrospective, and case studies of insulin glargine use among women with GDM, and no evidence of harm has been shown.[34,35]

8.4.2.2 Insulin Detemir

Insulin detemir (Levemir, Novo-Nordisk) was originally approved by the U.S. Food and Drug Administration (USFDA) for use among adults with diabetes in 2005. At that time it was a category C drug in pregnancy. Following recent trials, it has now been recategorised as a category B drug. Unlike human insulin, insulin detemir has no amino acid threonine in position B30, and the amino acid B29 has a C14 fatty acid chain attached (Levemir online data sheet, http://www.accessdata.fda.gov/drugsatfda_docs/label/2012/021536s037lbl.pdf (accessed April 15, 2012)). This is associated with slowed systemic absorption through self-association at the injection site and 98% binding to albumin. With insulin detemir doses of between 0.2 and 0.4 units/kg, more than 50% of its maximum effect occurs between 3–4 and 14 h after injection. The effect can last up to 24 h and has no peak. Compared with NPH and insulin glargine, insulin detemir has lower variability in action.[36] As with insulin glargine, insulin detemir use is associated with comparable glycaemic control as NPH insulin, with lower rates of hypoglycaemia and less weight gain.[37–39]

Insulin detemir is not known to cross the placenta, nor are there reports of antibody-insulin complexes crossing the placenta. It is not known whether insulin detemir is excreted into human milk.

No randomised controlled trials of insulin detemir have taken place in GDM. There has been one randomised trial of insulin detemir vs. NPH in type 1 diabetes in pregnancy,[40] with no significant difference in obstetric outcomes.

8.4.3   Continuous Subcutaneous Insulin Infusion in GDM

Where women with GDM need large amounts of insulin to overcome their insulin resistance, a basal bolus regimen can become increasingly ineffective in maintaining euglycaemia. The addition of metformin can reduce insulin needs.[24] U500 insulin can also be considered.

Another strategy is to introduce continuous subcutaneous insulin infusion (CSII) through an insulin pump. A retrospective case control study has been undertaken in South Auckland, New Zealand,[41] where there is a multiethnic population with a high proportion of Polynesian women (indigenous Maori and those from Pacific Islands), many of whom require large amounts of insulin. The diabetes in pregnancy service introduced CSII for women where a single dose of insulin at a given time point exceeded 100 units, where three premeal and one prebed injection failed to provide adequate glycaemic control, or where foetal growth remained accelerated, despite optimal conventional insulin therapy. Over time, it became clear that continuing hyperglycaemia in women requiring over 200 units per day was best controlled using insulin pump therapy.

The subsequent retrospective nested case control study of 30 women on CSII (20 GDM, 10 type 2 diabetes in pregnancy) was compared with a multiple dose insulin (MDI) regimen among 60 non-pump-using age-ethnicity matched controls

(45 GDM/15 type 2 diabetes). The controls had a later gestation at booking (15 ± 7 vs. 19 ± 8 weeks; $p = 0.009$) and nonsignificantly lower diagnostic fasting glucose (7.6 ± 1.6 vs. 6.8 ± 1.6 mmol/L; $p = 0.105$). Weight at booking was similar (99.4 ± 18.6 vs. 95.9 ± 15.8 kg, respectively) as was gestation at delivery (39 ± 2 weeks). The maximum insulin used was higher in the CSII group (258 ± 99 vs. 157 ± 108 IU; $p < 0.001$). In spite of the greater insulin need and relatively higher fasting glucose, the rates of induction, foetal 1 h glucose, and birth weight were similar. More babies from CSII-treated mothers were admitted to the special care baby unit. Of the women who had a postnatal OGTT, 29% ($n = 7$) of those on CSII had abnormal glucose tolerance postpartum vs. 8% ($n = 12$) on MDI.

CSII would appear to be a safe and reasonable intervention among women with GDM requiring more than 200 units of insulin or where increasing insulin appears to be increasingly ineffective.

8.4.4 Continuous Glucose Monitoring Systems in GDM

There have been no randomised controlled trials of the impact of continuous glucose monitoring on the maternal or perinatal outcomes of GDM. One RCT in GDM among 73 women found that antihyperglycaemic therapy was more likely to be introduced using CGMS than conventional five times/day self blood glucose monitoring (31 vs. 8%; $p = 0.0149$).[42] Medication was commenced if the fasting plasma glucose was twice >5.5 mmol/L or once >5.5 mmol/L and the postprandial glucose was >7.8 mmol/L once, or the postprandial glucose was >7.8 mmol/L on at least two occasions. The study was too small to show any difference in maternal or foetal/neonatal outcomes.

8.4.5 Oral Antihyperglycaemic Agents

8.4.5.1 Metformin

The structural formula of metformin or metformin hydrochloride (*N,N*-dimethylimidodicarbonimidic diamide hydrochloride) is shown in Figure 8.1. The other biguanides, phenformin and buformin, were withdrawn following deaths from lactic acidosis. Metformin has been very rarely associated with lactic acidosis (0.03 cases/1,000 patients—same as background[43]), and even then only in those with significant hepatic, renal, or cardiac dysfunction. Metformin was introduced to the United Kingdom in 1958, to Canada in 1972, but was not used in the United States

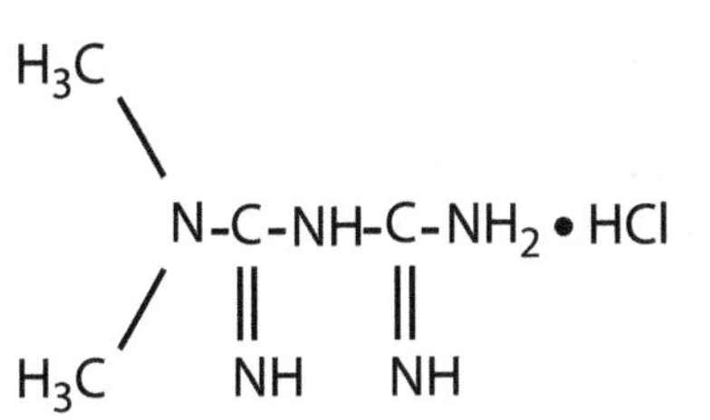

FIGURE 8.1   The structural formula of metformin.

until 1995. It is not chemically or pharmacologically related to any other classes of oral antihyperglycaemic agents.

How metformin acts remains unclear but it reduces hyperglycaemia through suppression of hepatic glucose output (hepatic gluconeogenesis), increasing hepatic insulin sensitivity and enhancing peripheral glucose uptake.[44] As pregnancy is associated with deterioration in glucose control due to changes in both preprandial and postprandial glucose metabolism and insulin resistance, metformin has been seen as a logical choice of oral antihyperglycaemia agent for the management of GDM. It has been suggested that postprandial glucose spikes could lead to a higher concentration of glucose in the amniotic fluid and its subsequent reabsorption/recirculation,[45] and that, as a result, control of postprandial hyperglycaemia is of particular importance during pregnancy. A randomised controlled trial targeting postprandial rather than preprandial glucose[12] did improve pregnancy outcomes, although a high proportion of women probably had overt diabetes in pregnancy (likely undiagnosed type 2 diabetes in pregnancy). Metformin affects background as well as postprandial glycaemia, and hence the importance of the Metformin in Gestational Diabetes (MiG) study, testing the efficacy and safety of metformin relative to insulin therapy in pregnancy.[24]

Metformin has altered pharmacokinetics during pregnancy, through enhanced renal elimination, varying food absorption, and different gastrointestinal transit times. This may mean that a greater dose of metformin is required during pregnancy, by up to 20%.[46] It is not known whether the sustained and immediate release preparations of metformin in GDM have different effects, although it has been suggested that the sustained release version is less useful than the immediate release preparation in reducing postprandial hyperglycaemia among women with polycystic ovary syndrome (PCOS) and type 2 diabetes.[47,48]

As there is transplacental passage of metformin,[49–51] there is a genuine potential for both risk and benefit to the offspring from the use of metformin during and after pregnancy. Such effects could be discovered many years after birth, and many clinicians remain cautious with their use.

Very little metformin is transferred into human milk (<0.4% of the maternal concentration).[52,53] As a result, metformin is thought to be safe to use during breastfeeding.[54]

One aspect of metformin therapy that may need consideration during pregnancy is vitamin B12 deficiency.[55,56] In older people, there may be a dose-dependent relationship, with 1 g/day of metformin being associated with a 2.88-fold (95% confidence interval (CI) 2.15–3.87) risk of developing vitamin B12 deficiency. However, in GDM the exposure is likely to be short, and it is unclear whether any significant reduction occurs. In pregnant women with polycystic ovary syndrome, homocysteine levels (which increase with worsening vitamin B12 deficiency) are not in altered with metformin therapy.[57] It is therefore unlikely that metformin initiated during pregnancy leads to meaningful vitamin B12 deficiency, but measurement of vitamin B12 levels prior to commencing metformin may be prudent in those at risk (e.g., vegetarians).

8.4.5.2 Sulphonylureas

Sulphonylureas act very differently from metformin, acting as insulin secretagogues rather than insulin sensitisers. Increased insulin secretion occurs following sulphonylurea blinding to the ATP-dependent K^+ (K_{ATP}) channel on the pancreatic beta cell

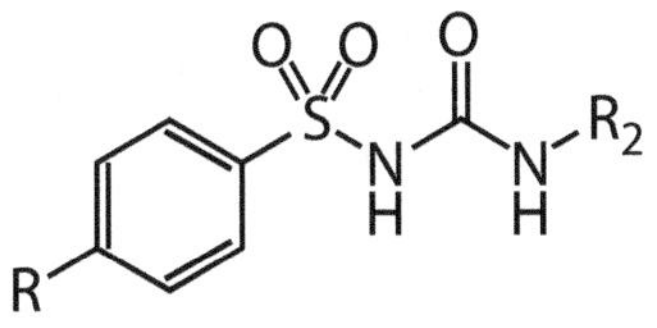

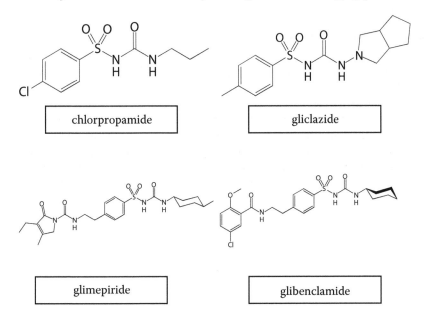

FIGURE 8.2   The core structure of sulphonylureas.

membrane, with subsequent inhibition of potassium efflux, depolarisation, and the opening of voltage-gated Ca^{2+} channels. The rise in intracellular calcium concentration increases fusion of insulin granulae with the cell membrane, and insulin secretion.

The first wave (generation) of sulphonylureas included acetohexamide, chlorpropamide, and tolbutamide. The second generation includes the more current sulphonylureas gliclazide, glipizide, glimepiride, and glibenclamide. The core structure for the sulphonylureas is shown in Figure 8.2, and the structural formula of various sulphonylureas in Figure 8.3.

Neither chlorpropamide nor tolbutamide is used in the management of GDM, as both cross the placenta[51] and are known to be associated with neonatal hypoglycaemia, which can be severe.[58] Both are also excreted into breast milk.[59]

Gliclazide has not undergone trials in GDM, although two case reports showed normal pregnancy outcomes following its use in women with type 2 diabetes in early pregnancy.[60,61] Glimepiride has neither case studies nor trials in pregnancy. In animal studies, pregnant or lactating rats and rabbits exposed to glimepiride experienced an increase in stillbirths, reduced growth, skeletal deformations, and miscarriages. It did not cause any birth defects. Foetotoxicity is thought to be due to hypoglycaemia.[62]

FIGURE 8.3   The structural formula of various sulphonylureas.

It is not known if gliclazide or glimepiride crosses the placenta or enters human breast milk. Both are category C medications. Glipizide does not cross the placenta in clinically significant amounts in in vitro studies,[51] and in one study was not found in breast milk.[63]

Glibenclamide (glyburide, 5-chloro-N-(4-[N-(cyclohexylcarbamoyl)sulphamoyl] phenethyl)-2-methoxybenzamide) is currently in use during pregnancy, and there are a growing number of studies describing its use.[64] Indeed, in a recent international diabetes in pregnancy meeting, 67.4% of participants reported using glibenclamide in GDM, particularly obstetricians (88.6 vs. 45.9% (other doctors)) and in the United States (76.1 vs. 35.5% (outside the United States)).[65] As with all sulphonylureas, the major side effects are weight gain and hypoglycaemia. It does not cross the placenta in clinically significant amounts in vitro,[66] and in two early studies among women with GDM, glibenclamide was not found in cord blood.[67,68] Plasma levels in pregnant women with GDM in the third trimester are approximately 50% lower than those in nonpregnant women.[69]

In one study among eight women, glibenclamide was not detected in breast milk and no hypoglycaemia occurred in the infants who were wholly breastfed when the glibenclamide was at steady state.[63]

8.4.5.3   Meglitinides

There are two meglitinides approved in adults, repaglinide (Prandin/Novonorm—in use since 1997) and nateglinide (Starlix), but neither is approved for use in pregnancy. They are insulin secretagogues working through a different binding site to sulphonylureas. Side effects are hypoglycaemia and weight gain. There are few reports of their use in pregnancy. One report covers use up to 7 weeks gestation resulting in a normal pregnancy.[70] Meglitinides are not recommended in the management of GDM.

8.4.5.4   Thiazolidinediones

Thiazolidenediones (TZDs) were introduced in the late 1990s, initially with troglitazone (Rezulin), and then with rosiglitazone (Avandia) and pioglitazone (Actos). The chemical structure is shown in Figure 8.4.

Thiazolidenediones act by binding to, and activating, the peroxisome proliferation activator receptor gamma (PPAR gamma), which decreases peripheral insulin resistance.[71] They seem to play a role in placental maturation and endometrial attachment by the embryo.[72,73] Inactivation of PPAR gamma results in the death of the embryo in animals. PPAR gamma is expressed in human placental cytotrophoblast and syncytiotrophoblast, and is associated with trophoblast differentiation.[74]

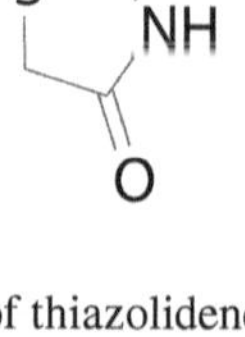

FIGURE 8.4   The chemical structure of thiazolidenediones.

In humans, placental PPAR gamma activation is associated with an increase in placental hormone secretion, including human placental growth hormone and leptin.[75]

Severe hepatic side effects (drug-induced hepatitis) led to the withdrawal of troglitazone, and an increased risk of cardiovascular disease led to the withdrawal of rosiglitazone. Pioglitazone is not recommended for use where there is a risk of heart failure or past bladder cancer. They are associated with weight gain (especially when compared with metformin[76]) but not hypoglycaemia.

TZDs do cross the placenta,[77] and pioglitazone is a category C drug. Animal studies suggest that TZDs are not teratogenic[78]; however, their use has been associated with foetal death and growth retardation. It is not known if TZDs cross into human breast milk.

TZDs have been used in polycystic ovary syndrome, with similar improvements in ovulation, pregnancy rate, and menstrual patterns.[79,80] Metformin was associated with a greater reduction in body mass index, but more nausea, diarrhoea, and abdominal cramping. No differences in adverse foetal outcome were reported, but there remains concern over its safety. High rates of miscarriage have been shown in PCOS-associated infertility, but this would be expected in this group of patients.

No studies using TZDs in GDM have been reported, although there are two case reports associated with normal pregnancies in women with type 2 diabetes.[62,81] Use is not recommended in GDM.

8.4.5.5 Alpha-Glucosidase Inhibitors

Alpha-glucosidase inhibitors reduce breakdown of starch into simpler carbohydrates in the small intestine through inhibition of alpha-glucosidase and pancreatic alpha-amylase. Acarbose (Glucobay) is the major alpha-glucosidase in use outside of pregnancy. Figure 8.5 shows its chemical structure.

It is weight neutral and does not cause hypoglycaemia in monotherapy. Use is associated with gastrointestinal side effects. Very little acarbose (2%) is absorbed as active drug, although 34% of the metabolites are found in the systemic circulation. High doses are not teratogenic in animals. There has been a suggestion that the greater carbohydrate breakdown by gut flora could increase butyrate production, which could increase prostaglandin E secretion and induce labour. One Mexican study of acarbose given three times a day before meals among six women was

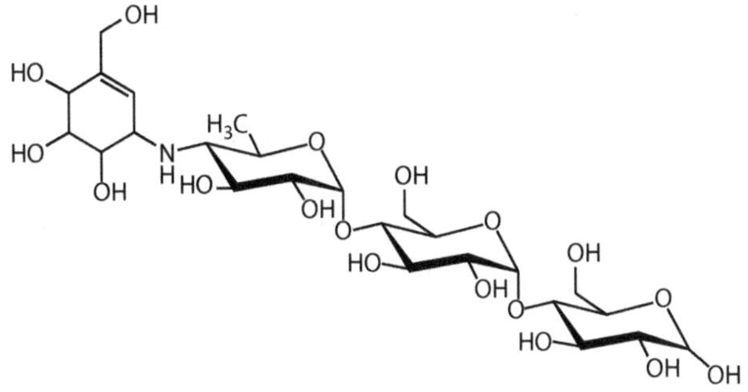

FIGURE 8.5 The chemical structure of acarbose.

associated with improved fasting and postprandial glucose levels and uneventful pregnancies. Intestinal discomfort was present throughout pregnancy.[82] An RCT among 91 women with GDM needing medication reported in an abstract a low need for insulin (6%), but very little other information was provided.[83]

Acarbose is not recommended for the management of GDM.

8.4.5.6   DPP IV Inhibitors

The dipeptidyl peptidase 4 (DPP IV) gene encodes for an enzyme expressed on the surface of many cells associated with immune regulation, signal transduction, and apoptosis. Two of the peptides that are metabolised by DPP IV are the incretins glucagon-like peptide 1 (GLP-1) and gastric inhibitory polypeptide (GIP). The incretins are released from the small intestine in association with meals and stimulate insulin biosynthesis, inhibit glucagon secretion, slow gastric emptying, reduce appetite, and stimulate regeneration of islet beta cells. These incretins are inactivated very quickly by DPP IV, and DPP IV inhibitors prolong the incretin effects.

There are a growing number of DPP IV inhibitors or "gliptins." The first to obtain approval from the USFDA for use in diabetes was sitagliptin in October 2006. Since then, other gliptins have emerged, including saxagliptin,[84] vildagliptin, and linagliptin. Alogliptin is awaiting FDA approval. Gliptins are weight neutral and do not cause hypoglycaemia on their own. They are associated with increased nasopharyngeal infections.

None of the gliptins are approved for use in pregnancy. Sitagliptin, vildagliptin, linagliptin, and saxagliptin are pregnancy category B antidiabetic agents that cross the placenta in animal studies and are known to be excreted into milk. Passage through placenta and to milk in humans is unknown.

8.4.5.7   GLP-1 Analogues

While gliptins inhibit the breakdown of the incretins GLP-1 and GIP by DPP IV, the GLP-1 analogues are largely resistant to DPP IV action, thereby prolonging the incretin effect. There are two GLP-1 agonists currently available, exenatide and liraglutide. Lixisenatide has just been approved for use. All are injected. Exenatide also has an extended release version. Side effects are nausea, vomiting, diarrhoea, and rarely pancreatitis. Hypoglycaemia is rare unless used with other antidiabetes drugs, and they are associated with weight loss. Exenatide, the first GLP-1 analogue, was approved in 2005, and the extended release form (Bydureon) was approved in 2012. It is not known if exenatide or liraglutide crosses the placenta or enters human milk. An ex vivo human placental perfusion study detected low levels on the foetal side (a foetal:maternal ratio of 0.017).[85]

There is a case report of exenatide use in early pregnancy up to 16 weeks with no evidence of harm.[86] It is not known whether exenatide or liraglutide[87] crosses the placenta or enters breast milk in vivo in humans. Both are pregnancy category C. Neither is recommended in pregnancy.

8.4.6   Bariatric Surgery

Bariatric surgery during GDM is not recommended. However, a growing number of women have had bariatric surgery, and some of these do become pregnant.

TABLE 8.1

Association between Weight Gain and Adverse Pregnancy Outcomes among 481 Obese Danish Women with a Normal Glucose Tolerance Test

Adverse Outcome	Weight Gain		
	5–9.9 kg	10–14.9 kg	15.0+ kg
Hypertension	2.1	3.6	4.8
Caesarean section	2.4	3.0	3.6
Induction of labour	2.7	2.8	3.7
Large for gestational age baby	2.4	2.1	2.7

Note: Numbers shown are odds ratios in comparison with women who gained <5 kg in weight.

Gestational diabetes occurs less frequently after bariatric surgery (in one study, 8 vs. 27%, odds ratio (OR) 0.23, 95% CI 0.15–0.36), and when it does, there is less likelihood of the need for caesarean section (28 vs. 43%, OR 0.53, 95% CI 0.39–0.72).[88–91] Other obstetric complications are comparable. Rapid weight loss and nutritional deficiency postsurgery are a concern for at least 1–2 years after surgery, and some recommend that pregnancy be avoided during this time.

8.5 IMPORTANCE OF WEIGHT, WEIGHT GAIN, AND WEIGHT LOSS IN PREGNANCY

Obesity is independently associated with adverse pregnancy outcomes that are additive to those from GDM.[21,92] Weight loss is associated with improved outcomes overall.[93] A range of studies have also shown that antenatal weight gain is associated with adverse pregnancy outcomes among women who are obese.[94–100] As insulin and sulphonylureas (e.g., glibeclamide) are associated with weight gain (unlike metformin and lifestyle change alone), benefits from improved glycaemia might not accrue to the extent required, and this has to be taken into account in any management plan. Furthermore, weight gain during pregnancy often remains postnatally.[101] Table 8.1 shows the weight gain and associated pregnancy complications in one study from Denmark among obese women (prepregnancy body mass index greater than 30 kg/m^2) with a normal antenatal oral glucose tolerance test as an example.[102]

8.6 USE OF MEDICATIONS IN THE DIFFERENT TRIMESTERS

8.6.1 USE OF MEDICATIONS DURING THE FIRST TRIMESTER

GDM can be diagnosed in the first trimester, including the first 8 weeks of pregnancy. This may indicate preexisting diabetes, usually undiagnosed type 2 diabetes, with its associated risk of foetal malformation and spontaneous abortion.[103] Hyperglycaemia, less than overt diabetes in pregnancy (i.e., fasting glucose < 7.0

mmol/L, HbA1c < 6.5% (48 mmol/mol), random glucose < 11.1 mmol/L[18]), might also reflect undiagnosed preexisting diabetes, but could also indicate preexisting impaired fasting glucose or impaired glucose tolerance. Medication is likely to be needed at this point, along with the self glucose monitoring, weight management, physical activity, and dietary management. There is no evidence that targets should differ from those later in pregnancy.

The traditional clinical approach has been to avoid oral hypoglycaemic agents during organogenesis, although animal studies suggest that exposure of the human foetus to metformin and glibenclamide is likely to be safe.

Evidence for use of oral hypoglycaemic agents in pregnant humans has been confounded by three major problems:

1. The legacy of any preexisting diabetes
2. The need to match unexposed and exposed women for baseline metabolic state
3. The need to differentiate between different drugs when more than one is being used.

A good example is the study by Piacquadio et al.[104] This observational study among women with type 2 diabetes reported a major association between oral diabetes agents and congenital defects. However, metformin was grouped with other agents (e.g., older sulphonylureas) and compared women with different degrees of hyperglycaemia in the periconceptual period. Metformin appears to be safe in the first trimester.[105] A number of reviews of metformin have been undertaken across humans and animals, adjusting for hyperglycaemia, and do not suggest an increased risk of malformations.[106] In one meta-analysis,[107] first trimester use in either PCOS or type 2 diabetes was associated with a reduced risk of major malformations, with an odds ratio of 0.57 for malformations with metformin compared with control (1.7% (3/172) vs. 7.2% (17/235)). A subsequent study in PCOS suggested that periconceptual metformin use was associated with less early foetal loss (11.6 vs. 36.3%).[108]

As yet, there has been no evidence of long-term harm among the offspring of women who have taken metformin alone during pregnancy, although such studies so far have been for less than 10 years.

If first trimester exposure to metformin is not associated with foetal anomalies, studies using other hypoglycaemic agents on their own or in combination with metformin warrant a more critical view of the additional agent(s): usually a sulphonylurea. Early reports did implicate first-generation sulphonylureas in foetal loss after exposure in the first trimester. Since then, reports have largely included second- and third-generation sulphonylureas, and results are mixed. In Denmark, higher perinatal mortality rates were found among women with type 2 diabetes compared with women with type 1 diabetes (6.7 vs. 1.7%),[109] in spite of less hyperglycaemia. A range of medications had been used periconceptually. In New Zealand, comparable rates of foetal anomalies were found between women with type 1 and type 2 diabetes, with the latter again on a range of oral glycaemic agents.[110]

Early glibenclamide use is not above suspicion, with evidence coming from a 10-year retrospective analysis of outcomes in 379 pregnancies in South Africa[105] among women with pregestational type 2 diabetes. In this study, when glycaemic targets (fasting glucose < 5.5 mmol/L, 2 h glucose < 6.7 mmol/L) were not met within 1 week, women commenced on metformin for 1 week if obese or glibenclamide for 1 week if nonobese. If hyperglycaemia continued, both agents were used for 1 week, before conversion to insulin therapy if needed. Insulin therapy was commenced immediately where the fasting glucose was 8.0 mmol/L or higher after dietary therapy alone. Overall, 93 women used oral glycaemic agents alone, 249 were transferred from the agent to insulin, and 37 went straight onto insulin. Glycaemic control was best in the group using oral glycaemic agents alone. There was no difference in ethnicity or initial body mass index, but the gestational age at presentation booking differed significantly (21.6 ± 0.9 vs. 18.1 ± 0.5 vs. 13.4 ± 1.4 weeks, respectively; $p < 0.001$). The foetal anomaly rates were 5.7, 2.0, and 0% respectively ($p = 0.175$). The perinatal morality rates were significantly higher on oral agents alone (12.5%) than when switched to insulin (2.8%) or commenced on insulin immediately (3.3%) ($p = 0.003$), and stillbirth rates were 9.1, 2.0, and 3.3%, respectively ($p = 0.010$). No perinatal mortality was seen in women on metformin alone. The authors concluded that early exposure to metformin or glibenclamide did not increase foetal anomalies, but were concerned over the association between perinatal mortality and continuation of gliclazide, glibenclamide, or glibenclamide and metformin. No significant differences in caesarean section (58–63%), neonatal hypoglycaemia (19–24%), macrosomia (17–23%), preeclampsia (0–3%), or neonatal jaundice (9–19%) were found. First trimester exposure to ACE inhibitors and poor glucose control confounded the comparison. The authors wondered if early insulin use was protective.

There have been no major concerns over the rapid-acting insulin analogues or insulin detemir in the first trimester.[34,111] However, insulin glargine remains under closer scrutiny because of its greater in vitro affinity to the IGF-1 receptor than other insulin analogues.[112] These studies have not been undertaken among pregnant women with diabetes, but in nonpregnant subjects; while insulin detemir had a mean ± standard error insulin receptor affinity relative to human insulin of 18 ± 2%, an IGF-1 receptor affinity of 16 ± 1%, and a mitogenic potency of ~11%, the values for insulin glargine were 86 ± 3, 641 ± 51, and 783 ± 132%, respectively. Affinities were also similar to human insulin with insulin aspart, 92 ± 6, 81 ± 9, and 58 ± 22%, and for insulin lispro, 84 ± 6, 156 ± 16, and 66 ± 10%, respectively. Insulin glargine has been used in pregnancy with no evidence of foetal anomalies, but no major trials have yet been undertaken to confirm this conclusively.

8.6.2 USE OF INSULIN DURING THE SECOND AND THIRD TRIMESTERS

There have been two major randomised controlled trials comparing usual care and contemporary management (including insulin therapy where lifestyle alone was inadequate to control hyperglycaemia) of GDM: the ACHOIS and MFN studies.[9,10] A systematic review and meta-analysis in 2010 identified and included three other RCTs from between 1966 and 2005.[113] The meta-analysis included the studies by Bonomo et al. (2005) that did not use pharmacological agents and included women with a raised 50 g glucose challenge test but excluded women with GDM,[114] by O'Sullivan (1966) that did not have access to, e.g., self blood glucose monitoring,[115] and by Langer (1989) that was small ($n = 63$ in each group) and which had issues with randomisation and blinding.[116]

Both ACHOIS and MFN used a two-step screening approach (50 g glucose challenge, then OGTT), with ACHOIS using WHO criteria and MFN using Carpenter and Coustan criteria. ACHOIS excluded women with a fasting glucose of greater than 7.8 mmol/L, and MFN excluded women with a fasting glucose of greater than 5.3 mmol/L. Table 8.2 compares the interventions in the two major studies, and Table 8.3 shows the results, including the meta-analysis that included the other studies. Relatively few women received insulin in the studies, particularly in MFN, which had lower targets, more obese and non-European women, and excluded women with a fasting glucose above 5.3 mmol/L. Even so, it is clear that a clinical strategy including insulin therapy for those above target is associated with reductions in shoulder dystocia, caesarean section (not significant in the meta-analysis), macrosomia/large for dates, and preeclampsia. There are several areas of heterogeneity, including

TABLE 8.2
Major RCTs of the Management of GDM Using Insulin vs. Usual Care

	ACHOIS: Rx vs. control	MFN: Rx vs. control
N	1,000	958
BMI	26.8 vs. 26.0	30.1±5.0 vs. 30.2±5.1
Ethnicity (Europid/Asian/ Hispanic)	73 vs. 78%/19 vs. 14 vs. 0%	25.4 vs. 25.2%/4.5 vs. 5.9%/57.9 vs. 56.0%
Primigravida	43 vs. 49%	21.4 vs. 26.0%
Gestational age at entry (years)	29.1 vs. 29.2	28.8 ± 1.6 vs. 28.9 ± 1.5
Fasting/2 h glucose on OGTT (mmol/L)	4.8 ± 0.7/8.6 vs. 4.8 ± 0.6/8.5	4.8 ± 0.3/9.7 ± 1.2 vs. 4.8 ± 0.3/9.6 ± 1.1 (100 g glucose load)
Intervention	Individualised dietary advice Self blood glucose monitoring 4×/day—fasting and 2 h postprandial	Individualised dietary advice Self blood glucose monitoring 4×/day—asting and 2 h postprandial
Targets	Fasting 3.5–5.5 mmol/L Preprandial 5.5 mmol/L 2 h postprandial 7.0 mmol/L	Fasting 5.3 mmol/L 2 h postprandial 6.7 mmol/L
Insulin therapy if (−35/40; >35/40)	2× Fasting 5.5+; 5.5+ mmol/L Postprandial > 7.0; >8.0 1× 9.0 mmol/L anytime	Majority above target Fasting 5.3+ mmol/L Random blood glucose > 8.9 mmol/L
Insulin Rx	20 vs. 3%	7.7 vs. 0.4%
Weight gain ACHOIS—from first to last visit MFN—from enrollment to birth	8.1 ± 0.3 vs. 9.8 ± 0.4 kg	1.2 vs. 2.1 kg/m² 2.8 ± 4.5 vs. 5.0 ± 3.3 kg
Gestational age at birth (weeks)	39.0 vs. 39.3	39.0 ± 1.8 vs. 38.9 ± 1.8

Note: RCT, randomised controlled trial; Rx, treatment; N, number; BMI, body mass index; OGTT, oral glucose tolerance test.

TABLE 8.3
Outcomes of Major RCTs of the Management of GDM Using Insulin vs. Usual Care and Meta-Analysis Including Other Studies

	ACHOIS Intensive vs. Control	MFN Intensive vs. Control	Meta-Analysis
Composite[a]	—	32.4 vs. 37.0%	—
Any serious perinatal complication	1 vs. 4% 0.33 (0.14–0.75)	—	—
Death	0 vs. 1% 0.19 (0.04–0.96)	0	H
Shoulder dystocia	1 vs. 3% 0.46 (0.19–1.10)	0.36 (0.15–0.88)	0.40 (0.21–0.75)
Bone fracture/nerve palsy	0 vs. 1%	0.6 vs. 1.3%	0.39 (0.13–1.15)
Admission to NICU	71 vs. 61% 1.13 (1.03–1.23)	9.0 vs. 11.6% 0.77 (0.51–1.18)	0.73 (0.50–1.06)
Induction if labour	39 vs. 29% 1.36 (1.15–1.62)	27.3 vs. 26.8% 1.02 (0.81–1.29)	—
Caesarean delivery	31 vs.32% 0.97 (0.91–1.16)	26.9 vs. 33.8% 0.79 (0.64–0.99)	0.86 (0.72–1.02)
Birth weight > 4 kg	10 vs. 21% 0.47 (0.34–0.64)	5.9 vs. 14.3% 0.41 (0.26–0.66)	0.38 (0.30–0.49)
Large for gestational age	13 vs. 22% 0.62 (0.47–0.81)	7.1 vs. 14.5% 0.49 (0.32–0.76)	0.48 (0.38–0.62)
Hypoglycaemia	7 vs. 5%—needing i.v. glucose 1.42 (0.87–2.32)	16.3 vs. 15.4%—any 5.3 vs. 6.8%—i.v. glucose 0.77 (0.44–1.36)	H
Hyperbilirubinaemia	9 vs. 9%—0.93 (0.63–1.37)	9.6 vs. 12.9%	—
Elevated C-peptide	—	17.7 vs. 22.8%	—
Respiratory distress syndrome	5 vs. 4%—1.52 (0.86–2.71)	1.9 vs. 2.9%—0.66 (0.26–1.67)	—
Antenatal preeclampsia	12 vs. 18% 0.70 (0.51–0.95)	2.5 vs. 5.5% 0.46 (0.22–0.97)	—

[a] Composite = stillbirth, neonatal death, hypoglycaemia, hyperbilirubinaemia, elevated cord blood C-peptide level, and birth trauma. H = heterogeneous.

hypoglycaemia requiring intravenous glucose—as controls required a clinical indication, these data would be expected to be weak.

8.6.2.1 Use of Metformin during the Second and Third Trimesters

One Danish study suggesting excess adverse outcomes with metformin therapy[117] was seriously confounded by the greater prepregnancy body mass index (31.2 vs. 22.8–24.8 kg/m^2) and maternal age (32 vs. 28–29 years) in the metformin-treated group. While there was a greater risk of preeclampsia and stillbirth with metformin, this could all be explained by their higher preexisting risk from the greater maternal age, obesity, and proportion with preexisting type 2 diabetes. Indeed, in New Zealand, those who are prescribed metformin during type 2 diabetes in pregnancy have a greater body mass index, more chronic hypertension, and worse glucose control at baseline.[118] In that study, there were no differences in birth weight, proportion of large for gestational age births, prematurity (<37 weeks), neonatal unit admissions, respiratory support, or intravenous dextrose required, or perinatal loss between controls and women using metformin either throughout the pregnancy or in whom metformin was stopped beyond the first trimester.

The Metformin in Gestational Diabetes (MiG) study, with 751 participants, has provided substantial data about the safety, acceptability, and efficacy of metformin treatment in the second and third trimesters.[24] Women were randomised to either metformin or insulin therapy at 20–33 weeks. The characteristics at baseline intervention are described in Table 8.3, and outcomes in Table 8.4, alongside the major RCT with glibenclamide[25] for comparison. The insulin- and metformin-based strategies had comparable perinatal and obstetric outcomes. Among those on metformin, 27 (7.4%) had the metformin stopped (7 of whom 1.9% overall stopped due to gastrointestinal side effects). Overall, 46.3% required additional insulin therapy. The MiG study showed that in this group of women, when compared with an insulin-based regimen, the metformin protocol was associated with the following:

- Better 2 h postprandial glycaemic control from randomisation until delivery and at 1 week
- Comparable fasting glucose and HbA1c
- Better weight management, i.e.:
  - Less weight gain to 37/40 from enrollment—0.4 vs. 2.0 kg
  - More weight loss postpartum from enrollment—8.1 vs. 6.9 kg
- Better patient reports:
  - Women were more likely to choose metformin initially and onward in a subsequent pregnancy (81% metformin vs. 54% of insulin-treated women would choose insulin therapy).
  - 59% of women said that taking metformin was the easiest part of their management plan.

Women randomised to metformin therapy who required supplementary insulin therapy to manage their hyperglycaemia were found to require less insulin. No adverse effects were reported with this combination therapy.

A case control study comparing women with GDM treated with metformin (n = 100) with those treated with insulin therapy (n = 100, without reporting the proportion with diabetes afterward) showed comparable results to the MiG study.[119] Metformin needed to be stopped in 14%. Outcomes were better on metformin than insulin-alone therapy, with less preeclampsia (2 vs. 9%), less preterm delivery (0 vs. 10%), a lower birth weight percentile, less jaundice (8 vs. 30%), less special care baby unit (SCBU) admissions (6 vs. 19%), and similar caesarean section rates. There was less weight gain to 37 weeks gestation with metformin (0.94 vs. 2.72 kg). Obviously,

TABLE 8.4

Major RCTs of the Management of GDM Using Metformin and Glibenclamide

	MiG—Metformin	Langer—Glibenclamide
N	Metformin-363 Insulin-370	Glibenclamide-201 Insulin-203
BMI in early enrolment	32.2 ± 5.82 vs. 31.9 ± 7.6	Obese 70 vs. 65%
Previous GDM	25.9 vs. 21.9%	12 vs. 11%
Ethnicity (Europid/Asian/ Hispanic/Polynesian)	48.2/24.0/0/20.1 vs. 45.4/24.9/0/22.4	12/0/83/0
Primigravida	31.7 vs. 31.9%	28 vs. 29%
Gestational age at entry (weeks)	30 vs. 30	24 vs. 25
Fasting/2 h glucose on OGTT (100 g Langer)	5.7 vs. 5.7 mmol/L 9.7 vs. 9.4 mmol/L	5.4 vs. 5.4 mmol/L 9.7 vs. 9.7 mmol/L
Intervention	Clinic visits every 1–2 weeks, diet treatment, 7-point glucose monitoring; standard protocols (labour, delivery) 500 mg o.d. or b.d. increased over 1–2 weeks to maximum 2,500 mg/day to achieve targets Insulin local guidelines	Weekly clinic visits, diet treatment, 7-point blood glucose monitoring; standard protocols (labour, delivery) Insulin 0.7 U/kg—given t.d.s. and increased weekly Glibenclamide 2.5 mg increased to 20 mg max, then insulin
Targets—above which insulin started	FBG < 5.5 mmol/L	Mean 5.0–5.9 mmol/L
	2 h postprandial < 7.0 mmol/L Some sites had lower levels	FBG 3.4–5.0 mmol/L Preprandial 4.5–5.3 mmol/L Postprandial < 6.7 mmol/L
Insulin Rx in oral agent group	46.3%	4% switched to insulin
Oral agent stopped	7.4%	No information
Maternal hypoglycaemia	Not reported	2.0% vs. 20.2%
Weight gain from enrollment to birth	0.4 vs. 2.0	21 vs. 21 lb
Gestational age at birth (weeks)	38.3 vs. 38.5	38.7 vs. 38.5

Note: BMI, body mass index; FGB, fasting blood glucose; lb, pounds; Rx, treatment.

there could be confounding with the differential selection of who was to be treated with either insulin or metformin therapy.

8.6.2.2   Use of Glibenclamide during the Second and Third Trimesters

The major randomised controlled trial comparing glibenclamide with insulin therapy in GDM involved 404 women using open-label insulin therapy.[25] The study was powered to detect a 4.8% absolute difference (80% power) in adverse outcomes and used no composite score. GDM diagnosis involved a 50 g glucose challenge test with a 1 h postload glucose of greater than 7.3 mmol/L, followed by a 100 g OGTT using

TABLE 8.5

Outcomes of Major RCTs of the Management of GDM Using Insulin vs. Usual Care and Meta-Analysis Including Other Studies

	MiG—Metformin vs. Insulin	Langer—Glibenclamide vs. Insulin
Composite[a]	32.0 vs. 32.2%	NR
Death	0 (0%) vs. 1 (0.3%)	1 vs. 1%
Shoulder dystocia	1.7 vs. 3.0%	NR
Bone fracture/nerve palsy	4.4 vs. 4.6%	NR
Admission to NICU	18.7 vs. 21.1%	6 vs. 7%
Induction if labour	54.0 vs. 56.2%	NR
Caesarean delivery	36.1 vs. 38.4%	23 vs. 24%
Birth weight > 4 kg	NR	7 vs. 4%
Large for gestational age	19.3 vs. 18.6%	12 vs. 13%
Hypoglycaemia	15.2 vs. 18.6%	9 vs. 6%
	(IVG 6.9 vs. 5.9%)	(IVG 14 vs. 11%)
Hyperbilirubinaemia	8.0 vs. 8.4% (phototherapy)	6 vs. 4%
Respiratory distress	3.3 vs. 4.3%	8 vs. 6%
Antenatal preeclampsia	5.5 vs. 7.0%	6 vs. 6%

Note: IVG = intravenous glucose; NR = not reported.

[a] Composite = neonatal hypoglycaemia, phototherapy, respiratory distress, birth trauma, 5 min APGAR < 7, premature birth < 37 weeks.

Carpenter-Coustan criteria. Only women with a fasting glucose of 5.3–7.7 mmol/L were included. Women were randomised if the fasting glucose was greater than 5.3 mmol/L or the 2 h postprandial glucose was greater than 6.7 mmol/L following dietary therapy. Pregnancies were between 11 and 33 weeks gestation upon entry.

Table 8.4 describes the study and cohort in more detail. Table 8.5 describes the pregnancy outcomes. No glibenclamide was detected in cord blood. There has been no follow-up of the offspring. Generally, outcomes were similar, although hypoglycaemia was nonsignificantly higher. There was very little need for insulin, and there was comparable weight gain (unlike with metformin). Since this time, there have been a number of other trials and cohort studies among women with GDM. A meta-analysis in 2008 comparing the use of glibencamide with insulin therapy in GDM included 745 glibenclamide-exposed pregnancies and 637 insulin-treated pregnancies across nine studies. The use of glibenclamide was not associated with increased macrosomia, large for gestational age birth, intensive care admission, or neonatal hypoglycaemia.[120]

In spite of this experience, there remains doubt over whether glibenclamide should be used in GDM or not. A review of the evidence in 2007 described a higher failure rate than in the Langer trial (approximately 20%), particularly if the fasting glucose was above 6.4 mmol/L.[121] The review also queried whether neonatal hypoglycaemia and hyperbilirubinaemia occurred more frequently with glibenclamide than with

insulin. The most recent study[122] supports these concerns over the use of glibenclamide. Among 10,682 women with GDM needing pharmacological intervention,
2,073 (19.4%) received glibenclamide and the remainder used insulin. Glibenclamide
use was associated with 29% (3–64%) more babies with a birth weight greater than
4,000 g and 46% (7–100%) more admissions to the intensive care nursery.

8.7   COMPARISONS BETWEEN ORAL AGENTS AND INSULIN

Beyond the varying clinician preferences for insulin, metformin, and glibenclamide,
a number of meta-analyses have now been undertaken comparing insulin and oral
therapy. The meta-analysis by Dhulkotia et al.[17] shows the dominance of the Langer
and MiG studies, with no significant difference between insulin and oral agents
on large for gestational age babies or birth weight (56 (43–155) g heavier with oral
agents) (Figures 8.6 and 8.7).

There is a suggestion of greater neonatal hypoglycaemia with oral agents, but there is
heterogeneity (Figure 8.8). Similarly, there is a suggestion of greater caesarean section
rates with insulin (Figure 8.9). Neither of these differences is statistically significant.

The meta-analyses found no significant difference in fasting or postprandial glycaemic control.

Table 8.6 compares the benefits and disadvantages for insulin, metformin, and
glibenclamide. As metformin is the only treatment with no effect on weight, it is

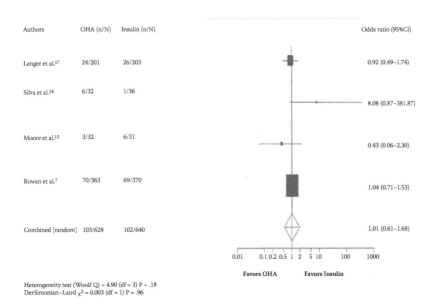

Authors	OHA (n/N)	Insulin (n/N)		Odds ratio (95%CI)
Langer et al.[17]	24/201	26/203		0.92 (0.49–1.74)
Silva et al.[14]	6/32	1/36		8.08 (0.87–381.87)
Moore et al.[13]	3/32	6/31		0.43 (0.06–2.30)
Rowan et al.[7]	70/363	69/370		1.04 (0.71–1.53)
Combined [random]	103/628	102/640		1.01 (0.61–1.68)

0.01   0.1 0.2 0.5 1 2   5 10   100   1000

Favors OHA   Favors Insulin

Heterogeneity test (Woolf Q) = 4.90 (df = 3) P = .18
DerSimonian–Laird χ^2 = 0.003 (df = 1) P = .96

CI, confidence interval; LGA, large-for-gestational-age; OHA, oral hypoglycemic agent

Dhulkotia. Oral hypoglycemic agents vs. insulin in gestational diabetes. *Am J Obstet Gynecol* 2010.

FIGURE 8.6   Effects of oral hypoglycaemic agents (OHAs) vs. insulin on large for gestational age babies. (Reprinted from Dhulkotia, J.S. et al., *Am. J. Obstet. Gynecol.*, 203, 457.
e1–9, 2010. Copyright © 2010 Mosby. With permission from Elsevier.)

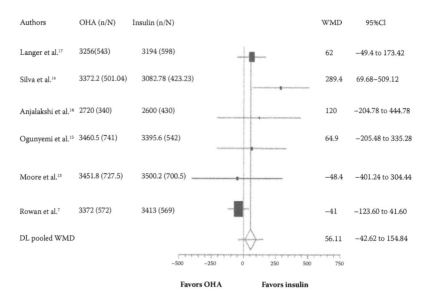

Authors	OHA (n/N)	Insulin (n/N)	WMD	95%CI
Langer et al.[17]	3256(543)	3194 (598)	62	−49.4 to 173.42
Silva et al.[14]	3372.2 (501.04)	3082.78 (423.23)	289.4	69.68–509.12
Anjalakshi et al.[16]	2720 (340)	2600 (430)	120	−204.78 to 444.78
Ogunyemi et al.[15]	3460.5 (741)	3395.6 (542)	64.9	−205.48 to 335.28
Moore et al.[13]	3451.8 (727.5)	3500.2 (700.5)	−48.4	−401.24 to 304.44
Rowan et al.[7]	3372 (572)	3413 (569)	−41	−123.60 to 41.60
DL pooled WMD			56.11	−42.62 to 154.84

Favors OHA   Favors insulin

X^2(for wmd+) = 0.59 (df = 1) P = .44

Q ("combinability" for wmd+) = 8.93 (df = 5) P = .11

DerSimonian–Laird X^2 = 1.24 (df = 1) P = .27

CI, confidence interval; DL, DerSimonian-Laird; OHA, oral hypoglycemic agent; WMD, weighted mean difference.

Dhulkotia. Oral hypoglycemic agents vs. insulin in gestational diabetes. *Am J Obstet Gynecol* 2010.

FIGURE 8.7 Effects of oral hypoglycaemic agents (OHAs) vs. insulin on birth weight. (Reprinted from Dhulkotia, J.S. et al., *Am. J. Obstet. Gynecol.*, 203, 457.e1–9, 2010. Copyright © 2010 Mosby. With permission from Elsevier.)

described within the context of for and against metformin. There have been two head-to-head comparisons between metformin and glibenclamide.[124] The key finding was that in one study, babies from mothers treated with glibenclamide were 200 g heavier than those from metformin-treated mothers.

8.8 INTENSITY OF TREATMENT

The paper by Horvath et al. also included a second series of meta-analyses, comparing the outcomes among women with GDM, using less and more intensive management.[113] There were 13 studies accepted, but only one[11] had a low probability of bias, included a comparison of insulin regimens, and had sufficient numbers. Overall, the only significant difference in outcomes was a reduction in shoulder dystocia (0.31 (0.14–0.70)). Table 8.7 summarises the 13 studies in the meta-analysis.

A key, but small, study by De Veciana et al.,[12] comparing pre- and postprandial targets (unclear as to whether 1 or 2 h after a meal), was omitted from the meta-analysis and included a high proportion of women with likely undiagnosed diabetes—all women used insulin (77 vs. 100 U, respectively, or 0.9 vs. 1.1 U/kg). Compared with monitoring and a preprandial target of 3.3–5.9 mmol/L, women

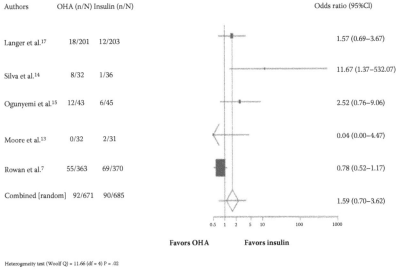

Authors	OHA (n/N)	Insulin (n/N)		Odds ratio (95%CI)
Langer et al.[17]	18/201	12/203		1.57 (0.69–3.67)
Silva et al.[14]	8/32	1/36		11.67 (1.37–532.07)
Ogunyemi et al.[15]	12/43	6/45		2.52 (0.76–9.06)
Moore et al.[13]	0/32	2/31		0.04 (0.00–4.47)
Rowan et al.[7]	55/363	69/370		0.78 (0.52–1.17)
Combined [random]	92/671	90/685		1.59 (0.70–3.62)

Favors OHA   Favors insulin

Heterogeneity test (Woolf Q) = 11.66 (df = 4) P = .02
DerSimonian–Laird X² = 1.24 (df = 1) P = .27

OHA, oral hypoglycemic agent.

Dhulkotia. Oral hypoglycemic agents vs. insulin in gestational diabetes. *Am J Obstet Gynecol* 2010.

FIGURE 8.8 Effects of oral hypoglycaemic agents (OHAs) vs. insulin on neonatal hypogly-caemia. (Reprinted from Dhulkotia, J.S. et al., *Am. J. Obstet. Gynecol.*, 203, 457.e1–9, 2010. Copyright © 2010 Mosby. With permission from Elsevier.)

monitoring with a postprandial target of 7.8 mmol/L had fewer large for gestational age babies (42 vs. 12%), fewer babies > 4 kg (36 vs. 9%), fewer babies with neonatal hypoglycaemia (21 vs. 3%), and the three stillbirths were in the preprandial moni-toring group. Mean birth weight was approximately 400 g lower (3,848 ± 434 g vs. 3,469 ± 668 g) at the same mean gestation. HbA1c dropped from 8.6 ± 2.3 to 8.1 ± 2.2% in the preprandial group, but from 8.9 ± 3.2 to 6.5 ± 1.4% in the postprandial group. There was also a nonsignificant reduction in caesarean sections (39 vs. 24%) and perineal lacerations (24 vs. 9%).

8.9 POTENTIAL LONG-TERM BENEFITS AND RISKS OF METFORMIN AND GLIBENCLAMIDE USE AMONG THE OFFSPRING

There are no follow-up studies among the offspring of women treated with gliben-clamide in pregnancy. Theoretically, as glibenclamide does not generally cross the placenta, there should be no sequelae.

As metformin reduces insulin resistance, it could potentially help protect beta cell function in the offspring and reduce intergenerational transmission of obesity and type 2 diabetes.[137] One possible mechanism for foetal harm from metformin could be in the production of foetal lactic acidosis, for example, during labour. However, this would be more likely to manifest as stillbirth or foetal distress, rather than long-term complications, and this has not been found in studies to date.

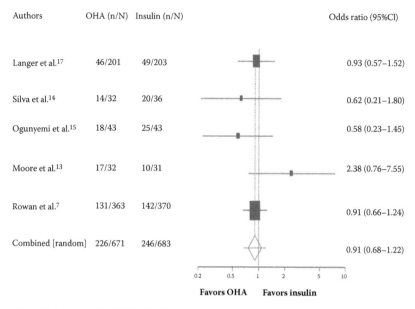

Authors	OHA (n/N)	Insulin (n/N)	Odds ratio (95%CI)
Langer et al.[17]	46/201	49/203	0.93 (0.57–1.52)
Silva et al.[14]	14/32	20/36	0.62 (0.21–1.80)
Ogunyemi et al.[15]	18/43	25/43	0.58 (0.23–1.45)
Moore et al.[13]	17/32	10/31	2.38 (0.76–7.55)
Rowan et al.[7]	131/363	142/370	0.91 (0.66–1.24)
Combined [random]	226/671	246/683	0.91 (0.68–1.22)

Favors OHA   Favors insulin

Heterogeneity test (Cochran Q) = 5.12 (df = 4) P = .28
DerSimonian–Laird X^2 = 0.43 (df = 1) P = .51

CI, confidence interval; OHA, oral hypoglycemic agent.

Dhulkotia. Oral hypoglycemic agents vs. insulin in gestational diabetes. *Am J Obstet Gynecol* 2010.

FIGURE 8.9   Effects of oral hypoglycaemic agents (OHAs) vs. insulin on caesarean section rates. (Reprinted from Dhulkotia, J.S. et al., *Am. J. Obstet. Gynecol.*, 203, 457.e1–9, 2010. Copyright © 2010 Mosby, with permission from Elsevier.)

Long-term carcinogenicity studies performed in rats (dosing duration of 104 weeks) and mice (dosing duration of 91 weeks) at doses < 900 mg/kg/day and 1,500 mg/kg/day, respectively, with four times the maximum recommended human daily dose have shown no evidence of carcinogenicity with metformin in either male or female mice. No tumorigenic potential has been observed with metformin in male rats, although there was an increased incidence of benign stromal uterine polyps in female rats treated with 900 mg/kg/day. There has been no evidence of a mutagenic potential of metformin in several in vitro tests (Ames test (*Salmonella typhimurium*), a gene mutation test (mouse lymphoma cells), a chromosomal aberrations test (human lymphocytes), and an in vivo mouse micronucleus test. There has also been no effect shown on the fertility of male or female rats.[138]

Follow-up in humans with GDM treated with metformin has been limited. In polycystic ovary syndrome, preconceptual and antenatal use of metformin has been common, and an 18-month follow-up study showed no difference (when compared with controls) in motor-social development, growth, or length.[139] The offspring from the MiG study are being followed up,[140] and at 2 years, the offspring from mothers treated with metformin (vs. those from insulin-treated mothers) had larger subscapular and biceps skinfolds, larger mid-upper arm circumferences, but no difference in

TABLE 8.6

Reasons for and against Choosing Metformin Therapy over Glibenclamide and Insulin Therapy in the Management of Type 2 Diabetes in Pregnancy

	Insulin	Metformin	Glibenclamide
For Metformin			
Weight control	Weight gain associated with adverse foetal outcomes	No weight gain	Weight gain associated with adverse foetal outcomes
Hypoglycaemia	Significant risk	No risk unless due to other agents in use	Risk
Complexity of regimen	Complex—needs subcutaneous delivery equipment	Simple—up to three times a day oral treatment	Very simple—once a day oral treatment
Injection site issues	Injection site infection, bruising	Not an issue	Not an issue
Inconvenience of the regimen	Very inconvenient	Easy	Easy
Psychological insulin resistance, needle phobia	In some women	Not an issue	Not an issue
Cost	More expensive	Less expensive	Less expensive
Against Metformin			
Known intrauterine effects	Generally known, but some uncertainty over some analogues	Probably OK—some uncertainty (see below)	Probably OK—some uncertainty
Known long-term effect on offspring	Generally known, but some uncertainty over some analogues	Not known (see below)	Not known
Efficacy	High	Some need insulin as well	May need insulin instead
Do not want to take tablets	Not an issue	In some women	In some women
Gastrointestinal side effects	Not an issue	Can be significant—sustained release version available; no studies in pregnancy	Not usually an issue
All Medications			
Adherence	Can be an issue	Can be an issue	Can be an issue

Source: Simmons, D., *Best Pract. Res. Clin. Endocrinol. Metab.,* 24, 625–34, 2010.

TABLE 8.7
Studies Included in the Horvath et al.[113] Meta-Analysis of Intensive vs. Less Intensive Treatment

Study		Risk of Bias—Patient Flow Transparency
Bancroft et al. 2000[125]	32 vs. 36; D/I vs. D	High—not transparent
Bevier et al. 1999[126]	35 vs. 48; I and sbgm vs. bgm at visits	High—not transparent
Bung et al. 1991[127]	20 vs. 21; D/I vs. D/PA	High—not transparent
Elnour et al. 2008[128]	99 vs. 66; I and intensive monitoring vs. usual care	High
Garner et al. 1997[129]	149 vs. 150—intensive vs. routine: lower vs. higher glucose targets, unrestricted vs. calorie-reduced diet	High—pilot study
Homko et al. 2002[130]	31 vs. 27; D/I and sbgm vs. bgm at visits	High–not transparent
Homko et al. 2007[131]	34 vs. 29; D/G-I and sbgm vs. bgm at visits	High–not transparent
Kestila et al. 2007[132]	36 vs. 37; D/M-I/cgms vs. sbgm	High—not transparent
Nachum et al. 1999[11]	138 vs. 136; qid vs. bd insulin	Low
Persson et al. 1985[133]	97 vs. 105; D/I-higher vs. lower targets	High
Rae et al. 2000[134]	67 vs. 58; I/diet rct	Low—not transparent
Rey 1997[135]	172 vs. 170; D/I sbgm vs. bgm at visits	High—not transparent
Rossi et al. 2000[136]	73 vs. 68; ultrasound-guided treatment	High—not transparent

Note: bd, 2 times/day; bgm, blood glucose monitoring; cgms, continuous glucose monitoring system; D, diet; G-I, glibenclamide or insulin; I, insulin; M-I, metformin or insulin; PA, physical activity; Qid, 4 times/day; sbgm, self blood glucose monitoring.

total fat mass or percentage body fat. The implications of these finds are unclear, but follow-up of this cohort remains very important.

8.10 THE WAY AHEAD

Figure 8.10 collates the trial and meta-analysis data to date. The foundation of management remains patient education, diet, physical activity, and glucose monitoring. If medication is needed to achieve glycaemic targets, then insulin therapy remains the default. Oral agents have substantial advantages from a practical point of view and are now considered safe. The UK National Institute for Health and Clinical Excellence (NICE) guidelines for the management of GDM already include the use of metformin and glibenclamide during pregnancy.[141] Obviously, women need to be advised that metformin crosses the placenta, and that while there has been no harm found, there remains uncertainty over the very long term. Many clinics use an information sheet to form the basis of these discussions. The weight gain with glibenclamide is also a concern, and hence many sites use it sparingly, if at all. Generally, if insulin is needed, clinics use a quick-acting insulin analogue to cover meals, or an isophane insulin overnight (sometimes twice a day). Insulin detemir is also safe in pregnancy but is more expensive. Women on large amounts of insulin

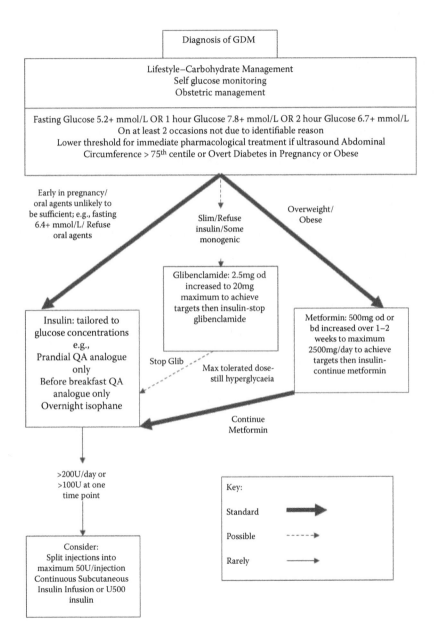

FIGURE 8.10 Summary of the pharmacological treatment of GDM: the way ahead.

have the options of several strategies. Combining oral therapies (metformin and glibenclamide) is not recommended, and some support for this approach comes from the South African 10-year review, which was suggestive of greater problems with combined therapy (than metformin alone or switching to insulin).[105]

REFERENCES

Key references are in bold.

1. Metzger, B.E. 1991. Biphasic effects of maternal metabolism on fetal growth: quintessential expression of fuel-mediated teratogenesis. *Diabetes* 40(Suppl. 2):99–105.
2. Hay, W.W. 1986. Fetal metabolic consequences of maternal diabetes. In *Diabetes and pregnancy*, ed. L. Jovanovic. 1st ed. New York: Praeger.
3. Reece, E.A., Coustan, D.R., Sherwin, R.S., et al. 1991. Does intensive glycaemic control in diabetic pregnancies result in normalization of other metabolic fuels? *Am J Obstet Gynecol* 165:126–30.
4. Nolan, C.J., Walstab, J.E., Riley, S.F., Sheedy, M.T., and Beischer, N.A. 1995. Maternal serum triglyceride, glucose tolerance and neonatal birth weight ratio in pregnancy. *Diabetes Care* 18:1550–56.
5. Plagemann, A., Harder, T., Kohlhoff, R., Rohde, W., and Dorner, G. 1997. Glucose tolerance and insulin secretion in children of mothers with pregestational IDDM or gestational diabetes. *Diabetologia* 40:1094–100.
6. The HAPO Study Cooperative Research Group. 2008. Hyperglycemia and adverse pregnancy outcomes. *N Engl J Med* 358:1999–2002.
7. Simmons D. 2010. Epidemiology of diabetes in pregnancy. In *Practical management of diabetes in pregnancy*, ed. D. McCance and M. Maresh. London: Blackwell Publishing.
8. Metzger, B.E., and Coustan, D.R. 1998. Summary and recommendations of the Fourth International Workshop Conference on Gestational Diabetes Mellitus. *Diabetes Care* 21(Suppl. 2):B161–67.
9. Crowther, C.A., Hiller, J.E., Moss, J.R., McPhee, A.J., Jeffries, W.S., Robinson, J.S., and Australian Carbohydrate Intolerance Study in Pregnant Women (ACHOIS) Trial Group. 2005. Effect of treatment of gestational diabetes mellitus on pregnancy outcomes. *N Engl J Med* 352:2477–86.
10. **Landon, M., Spong, C.Y., Thom, E., et al. 2009. A multicenter, randomized trial of treatment for mild gestational diabetes.** *N Engl J Med* **361:11–20.** *A recent trial showing that incidences of some adverse pregnancy outcomes are reduced by treatment in women with mild gestational diabetes.*
11. Nachum, Z., Ben-Shlomo, I., Weiner, E., and Shalev, E. 1999. Twice daily versus four times daily insulin dose regimens for diabetes in pregnancy: randomised controlled trial. *BMJ* 319:1223–27.
12. De Veciana, M., Major, C.A., Morgan, M.A., et al. 1995. Postprandial versus prepran-dial blood glucose monitoring in women with gestational diabetes mellitus requiring insulin therapy. *N Engl J Med* 333:1237–41.
13. Stock, S.J., Ferguson, E., Duffy, A., Ford, I., Chalmers, J., and Norman, J.E. 2012. Outcomes of elective induction of labour compared with expectant management: population based study. *BMJ* 344:e2838.
14. Boney, C.M., Verma, A., Tucker, R., and Vohr, B.R. 2005. Metabolic syndrome in childhood: association with birth weight, maternal obesity, and gestational diabetes mellitus. *Pediatrics* 115:e290.
15. Franks, P.W., Looker, H.C., Kobes, S., et al. Gestational glucose tolerance and risk of type 2 diabetes in young Pima Indian offspring. *Diabetes* 55:460–65.

16. Simmons, D., and Robertson, S. 1997. Influence of maternal insulin treatment on the infants of women with gestational diabetes. *Diabet Med* 14:762–65.

17. **Dhulkotia, J.S., Ola, B., Fraser, R., and Farrell, T. 2010. Oral hypoglycemic agents vs insulin in management of gestational diabetes: a systematic review and meta-analysis. *Am J Obstet Gynecol* 203:457.e1–9.** *A recent review and meta-analysis showing that in gestational diabetes there was no difference in glycaemic control or incidences of adverse pregnancy outcomes when comparing treatments with oral hypoglycaemic agents vs. insulin.*

18. IADPSG Consensus Panel, International Association of Diabetes and Pregnancy Study Groups (IADPSG). 2010. Recommendations on the diagnosis and classification of hyperglycemia in pregnancy. *Diabetes Care* 33:676–82.

19. Buchanan, T.A., Kjos, S.L., Montoro, M.N, et al. 1994. Use of fetal ultrasound to select metabolic therapy for pregnancies complicated by mild gestational diabetes. *Diabetes Care* 17:275–83.

20. Schaefer-Graf, U.M., Kjos, S.L., Fauzan, O.H., et al. 2004. A randomized trial evaluating a predominantly fetal growth–based strategy to guide management of gestational diabetes in Caucasian women. *Diabetes Care* 27:297–302.

21. Simmons, D. 2011. Diabetes and obesity in pregnancy. *Best Pract Res Clin Obstet Gynaecol* 25:25–36.

22. Jackson, W.P.U., Campbell, G.D., Notelovitz, M., and Blumsohn, D. 1962. Tolbutamide and chlorpropamide during pregnancy in human diabetics. *Diabetes* 11(Suppl.):98–103.

23. Malins, J.M., Cooke, A.M., Pyke, D.A., and Fitzgerald, M.G. 1964. Sulphonylurea drugs in pregnancy. *Br Med J* 2:187.

24. **Rowan, J.A., Hague, W.M., Gao, W., Battin, M.R., and Moore, M.P., MiG Trial Investigators. 2008. Metformin vs insulin for the treatment of gestational diabetes. *N Eng J Med* 358:2003–15.** *A trial showing that treatment of GDM using metformin is not associated with a higher incidence of adverse pregnancy outcomes (in the short term) when compared to treating with insulin alone.*

25. Langer, O., Conway, D.L., Berkus, M.D., Xenakis, E.M., and Gonzales, O. 2000. A comparison of glyburide and insulin in women with gestational diabetes mellitus. *N Engl J Med* 343:1134–38.

26. Torlone, E., Di Cianni, G., Mannino, D., and Lapolla, A. 2009. Insulin analogs and pregnancy: an update. *Acta Diabetologia* 46:163–72.

27. Bolli, G.B., Di Marchi, R.D., Park, G.D., Pramming, S., and Koivisto, V.A. 1999. Insulin analogues and their potential in the management of diabetes mellitus. *Diabetologia* 42:1151–67.

28. Rönnemaa, T., and Viikari, J. 1998. Reducing snacks when switching from conventional soluble to lispro insulin treatment: effects on glycaemic control and hypogylycaemia. *Diabet Med* 15:602–7.

29. Home, P.D., Lindholm, A., Hylleberg, A., Round, P., and UK Insulin Aspart Group. 1998. Improved glycemic control with insulin aspart. *Diabetes Care* 21:1904–9.

30. Home, P.D., Lindholm, A., Riist, A., and European Insulin Aspart Study Group. 2000. Insulin aspart vs human insulin in the management of long term blood glucose control in type 1 diabetes mellitus: a randomized controlled trial. *Diabet Med* 17:762–70.

31. Heinemann, L., Linkeschova, R., Rave, K., Hompesch, B., Sedlak, M., and Heise, T. 2000. Time action profile of the long acting insulin analogue insulin glargine (HOE901) in comparison with those of NPH insulin and placebo. *Diabetes Care* 23:6440–49.

32. Ratner, R.E., Mecca, T.E., Hirsch, I.B., Wilson, C.A., Neifing, J.L., and Garg, S.K. 2000. Less hypoglycaemia with insulin glargine in intensive insulin therapy for type 1 diabetes. *Diabetes Care* 23:639–43.

33. Rosenstock, J., Donley, D.W., Schwartz, S.L., Edwards, M.B., Clark, C.M., and Park, G.D. 2001. Basal insulin therapy in type 2 diabetes. *Diabetes Care* 24:631–36.

34. Mathiesen, E.R., Damm, P., Jovanovic, L., et al. 2011. Basal insulin analogues in diabetic pregnancy: a literature review and baseline results of a randomised, controlled trial in type 1 diabetes. *Diabetes Metab Res Rev* 27:543–51.

35. Pollex, E.K., Feig, D.S., Lubetsky, A., Yip, P.M., and Koren, G. 2010. Insulin glargine safety in pregnancy. *Diabetes Care* 33:29–33.

36. Heise, T., Nosek, L., Rønn, B.B., et al. 2004. Lower within-subject variability of insulin detemir in comparison to NPH insulin and insulin glargine in people with type 1 diabetes. *Diabetes* 53:1614–20.

37. Hermansen, K., Fontaine, P., Kukolja, K.K., Peterkova, V., Leth, G., and Gall, M.A. 2004. Insulin analogues (insulin detemir and insulin aspart) versus traditional human insulins (NPH insulin and regular human insulin) in basal-bolus therapy for patients with type 1 diabetes. *Diabetologia* 47:622–29.

38. Russell-Jones, D., Simpson, R., Hylleberg, B., Draeger, E., and Bolinder, J. 2004. Effects of QD insulin detemir or neutral protamine Hagedorn on blood glucose control in patients with type I diabetes mellitus using a basal-bolus regimen. *Clin Ther* 26:724–36.

39. Bartley, P.C., Bogoev, M., Larsen, J., and Philotheou, A. 2008. Long-term efficacy and safety of insulin detemir compared to neutral protamine Hagedorn insulin in patients with type 1 diabetes using a treat-to-target basal-bolus regimen with insulin aspart at meals: a 2-year, randomized, controlled trial. *Diabet Med* 25:442–49.

40. Hod, M., McCance, D.R., Ivanisevic, M., et al. 2011. Perinatal outcomes in a randomised trial comparing insulin detemir with NPH insulin in 310 pregnant women with type 1 diabetes. In *ADA Annual Scientific Conference*, San Diego, 2011, abstract 62-LB.

41. Simmons, D., Thompson, C.F., Conroy, C., and Scott, D.J. 2001. Use of insulin pumps in pregnancies complicated by type 2 diabetes and gestational diabetes in a multiethnic community. *Diabetes Care* 24:2078–82.

42. **Kestilä, K.K., Ekblad, U.U., and Rönnemaa, T. 2007. Continuous glucose monitoring versus self-monitoring of blood glucose in the treatment of gestational diabetes mellitus. *Diabetes Res Clin Pract* 77:174–79.** *A recent study showing that hyperglycaemia of sufficient magnitude to require drug therapy is detected more frequently in women with gestational diabetes who used continuous glucose monitoring systems than in those who self-monitored using glucose sticks.*

43. Scale, T., and Harvey, J.N. 2011. Diabetes, metformin and lactic acidosis. *Clin Endocrinol* 74:191–96.

44. Andújar-Plat, P., Pi-Sunyer, X., and Laferrère, B. 2012. Metformin effects revisited. *Diabetes Res Clin Pract* 95:1–9.

45. Jovanovic, L. 2007. Point: oral hypoglycaemic agents should not be used to treat diabetic women. *Diabetes Care* 30:2976–79.

46. Hughes, R.C.S., Gardiner, S.J., Begg, E.J., and Zhang, M. 2006. Effect of pregnancy on the pharmacokinetics of metformin. *Diabet Med* 23:323–26.

47. Fujioka, K., Pans, M., and Joyal, S. 2003. Glycemic control in patients with type 2 diabetes mellitus switched from twice-daily immediate release metformin to a once-daily extended-release formulation. *Clin Ther* 25:515–29.

48. Gao, H., Xiao, W., Wang, C., et al. 2008. The metabolic effects of once daily extended-release metformin in patients with type 2 diabetes: a multicentre study. *Int J Clin Pract* 62:695–700.

49. Vanky, E., Zahlsen, K., Sprigset, O., and Carlsen, S.M. 2005. Placental passage of metformin in women with polycystic ovary syndrome. *Fertil Steril* 83:1575–78.

50. Hague, W.M., Davoran, P.H., McIntyre, D., Norris, R., Xiaonian, X., and Charles, B. 2003. Metformin crosses the placenta: a modulator for fetal insulin resistance. *BMJ* 327:880–81.

51. Elliott, B.D., Schenker, S., Langer, O., Johnson, R., and Prihoda, T. 1994. Comparative placental transport of oral hypoglycaemic agents in humans: a model of human placental drug transfer. *Am J Obstet Gynecol* 171:653–60.
52. Hale, T.W., Kristensen, J.H., Hackett, L.P., Kohan, R., and Ilett, K.F. 2002. Transfer of metformin into human milk. *Diabetologia* 45:1509–14.
53. Gardiner, S.J., Kirkpatrick, C.M., Begg, E.J., Zhang, M., Moore, M.P., and Saville, D.J. 2003. Transfer of metformin into human milk. *Clin Pharmacol Ther* 73:71–77.
54. International Diabetes Federation. 2009. *Global guideline: pregnancy and diabetes.* Brussels: International Diabetes Federation.
55. Tomkin, G.H., Hadden, D.R., Weaver, J.A., and Montgomery, D.A.D. 1971. Vitamin-B_{12} status of patients on long-term metformin therapy. *Br Med J* 2:685–87.
56. Ting, R.Z.W., Szeto, C.C., Ho-Ming Chan, M., Ma, K.K., and Chow, K.M. 2006. Risk factors of vitamin B12 deficiency in patients receiving metformin. *Arch Intern Med* 166:1975–79.
57. Carlsen, S.M., Kjotrod, S., Vanky, E., and Romundstad, P. 2007. Homocysteine levels are unaffected by metformin treatment in both nonpregnant and pregnant women with polycystic ovary syndrome. *Acta Obstet Gynecol* 86:145–50.
58. Fanelli, C.G., and Bolli, G.B. 1998. Sulphonylureas and pregnancy. *Eur J Endocrinol* 138:615–16.
59 Benz, J. 1992. Antidiabetic agents and lactation. *J Hum Lact* 8:27.
60. Yaris, F., Yaris, E., Kadioglu, M., Ulku, C., Kesim, M., and Kalyoncu, N.I. 2004. Normal pregnancy outcome following inadvertent exposure to rosiglitazone, gliclazide, atorvastatin in a diabetic and hypertensive woman. *Reprod Toxicol* 18:619–21.
61. Kolagasi, O., Sari, F., Akar, M. and Ramazan, S. 2009. Normal pregnancy and healthy child after continued exposure to gliclazide and ramipril during pregnancy. *Ann Pharmacother* 43:147–49.
62. Amaryl product monograph. 2009. Available from http://products.sanofi.ca/en/amaryl.pdf (accessed April 8, 2012).
63. Feig, D.S., Briggs, G.G., Kraemer, J.M., et al. 2005. Transfer of glyburide and glipizide into breast milk. *Diabetes Care* 28:1851–55.
64. Holt, R.I.G., Clarke, P., Parry, E.C., and Coleman, M.A.G. 2008. The effectiveness of glibenclamide in women with gestational diabetes. *Diabetes Obes Metab* 10:906–911.
65. Ogunyemi, D.A., Fong, A., Rad, S., Fong, S., and Kjos, S.L. 2011. Attitudes and practices of healthcare providers regarding gestational diabetes: results of a survey conducted at the 2010 meeting of the International Association of Diabetes in Pregnancy Study Group (IADPSG). *Diabet Med* 28:976–86.
66. Elliott, B.D., Langer, O., Schenker, S., and Johnston, R.F. 1991. Insignificant transfer of glyburide occurs across the human placenta. *Am J Obstet Gynecol* 165:807–12.
67. Langer, O., Conway, D.L., Berkus, M.D., Xenakis, E.M., and Gonzales, O. 2000. A comparison of glyburide and insulin in women with gestational diabetes mellitus. *N Engl J Med* 343:1134–38.
68. Koren, G. 2001. Glyburide and fetal safety: transplacental pharmacokinetic considerations. *Reprod Toxicol* 15:227–29.
69. Hebert, M.F., Ma, X., Naraharisetti, S.B., et al. 2009. Are we optimizing gestational diabetes treatment with glyburide? The pharmacologic basis for better clinical practice. *Clin Pharmacol Ther* 85:607–14.
70. Mollar-Puchades, M.A., Martin-Cortes, A., Perez-Calvo, A., and Diaz-Garcia, C. 2007. Use of repaglinide on a pregnant woman during embryogenesis. *Diabetes Obes Metab* 9:146–47.
71. Spiegelman, B.M. 1998. PPAR-gamma: adipogenic regulator and thiazolidinedione receptor. *Diabetes* 47:507–14.

72. Froment, P., Gizard, F., Staels, B., Dupont, J., and Monget, P. 2005. A role of PPAR gamma in reproduction? *Med Sci* 21:507–11.

73. Barak, Y., Nelson, M.C., Ong, E.S., et al. 1999. PPAR gamma is required for placental, cardiac, and adipose tissue development. *Mol Cell* 4:585–95.

74. Schaiff, W., Carlson, M.G., Smith, S.D., Levy, R., Nelson, D.M., and Sadovsky, Y. 2000. Peroxisome proliferator-activated receptor-gamma modulates differentiation of human trophoblast in a ligand-specific manner. *J Clin Endocrinol Metab* 85:3874–81.

75. Tarrade, A., Schoonjans, K., Guibourdenche, J., et al. 2001. PPAR gamma/RXR alpha heterodimers are involved in human CG beta synthesis and human trophoblast differentiation. *Endocrinology* 142:4504–14.

76. Ceriello, A., Johns, D., Widel, M., Eckland, D.J., Gilmorfe, K.J., and Tan, M.H. 2005. Comparison of effect of pioglitazone with metformin or sulfonylurea (monotherapy and combination therapy) on postload glycemia and composite insulin sensitivity index during an oral glucose tolerance test in patients with type 2 diabetes. *Diabetes Care* 28:266–72.

77. Chan, L., Yeung, J.H., and Lau, T.K. 2005. Placental transfer of rosiglitazone in the first trimester of human pregnancy. *Fertil Steril* 83:955–58.

78. Briggs, C., Freeman, R.K., and Yaffe, S.J. 2002. *Drugs in pregnancy and lactation.* 6th ed. Baltimore: Williams & Wilkins Co.

79. Li, X.J., Yu, Y.X., Liu, C.Q., et al. 2011. Metformin vs thiazolidinediones for treatment of clinical, hormonal and metabolic characteristics of polycystic ovary syndrome: a meta-analysis. *Clin Endocrinol* 74:332–39.

80. Ota, H., Goto, T., Yoshioka, T., and Ohyama, N. 2008. Successful pregnancies treated with pioglitazone in infertile patients with polycystic ovary syndrome. *Fertil Steril* 90:709–13.

81. Demissie, Y., Fiad, T.M., Klemm, K., et al. 2006. Spontaneous singleton and twin pregnancy in two patients with polycystic ovary syndrome and type 2 diabetes following treatment with metformin combined with rosiglitazone. *Ann Saudi Med* 26:296–99.

82. Zarate, A., Ochoa, R., Hernadez, M., and Basurto, L. 2000. Efficacy of acarbose to control deterioration of glucose tolerance during gestation. *Ginecol Obstet Mex* 68:42–45.

83. de Veciana, M., Trail, P.A., Lau, T.K., and Dulaney, K. 2002. A comparison of oral acarbose and insulin in women with gestational diabetes mellitus. *Obstet Gynecol* 99(Suppl. 4):S5.

84. Lam, S., and Saad, M. 2010. Saxagliptin: a new dipeptidyl peptidase-4 inhibitor for type 2 diabetes. *Cardiol Rev* 18:213–17.

85. Hiles, R.A., Bawdon, R.E., and Petrella, E.M. 2003. Ex vivo human placental transfer of the peptides pramlintide and exenatide. *Hum Exp Toxicol* 22:623–28.

86. Williams, J., Pomeroy, N.E., Pop-Busui, R., et al. 2009. Case Report: exenatide use during pregnancy. *Endocrinologist* 19:119–21.

87. Liraglutide information sheet. Available from http://www.accessdata.fda.gov/drugsatfda_docs/label/2010/022341lbl.pdf (accessed 26 May 2012).

88. Patel, J.A., Colella, J.J., Esaka, E., Patel, N.A., and Thomas, R.L. 2007. Improvement in infertility and pregnancy outcomes after weight loss surgery. *Med Clin North Am* 91:515–28, xiii.

89. Sheiner, E., Menes, T.S., Silverberg, D., et al. 2006. Pregnancy outcome of patients with gestational diabetes mellitus following bariatric surgery. *Obstet Gynecol* 194:431–35.

90. Sheiner, E., Levy, A., Silverberg, D., et al. 2004. Pregnancy after bariatric surgery is not associated with adverse perinatal outcome. *Obstet Gynecol* 190:1335–40.

91. **Burke, A.E., Bennett, W.L., Jamshidi, R.M., et al. 2010. Reduced incidence of gestational diabetes with bariatric surgery. *J Am Coll Surg* 211:169–75.** *A recent study showing that in high-risk women there is a reduced incidence of gestational diabetes after bariatric surgery.*

92. Catalano, P.M., McIntyre, H.D., Cruickshank, J.K., et al. 2012. The Hyperglycemia and Adverse Pregnancy Outcome study: associations of GDM and obesity with pregnancy outcomes. *Diabetes Care* 35:780–86.
93. Thangaratinam, S., Rogozińska, E., Jolly, K., et al. 2012. Effects of interventions in pregnancy on maternal weight and obstetric outcomes: meta-analysis of randomised evidence. *Br Med J* 344:e2088.
94. Ludwig, D.S., and Currie, J. 2010. The association between pregnancy weight gain and birthweight: a within-family comparison. *Lancet* 376:937–38.
95. Schack-Nielsen, L., Michaelsen, K.F., Gamborg, M., Mortensen, E.L., and Sørensen, T.I. 2010. Gestational weight gain in relation to offspring body mass index and obesity from infancy through adulthood. *Int J Obes* 34:67–74.
96. Olson, C.M., Strawderman, M.S., and Dennison, B.A. 2009. Maternal weight gain during pregnancy and child weight at age 3 years. *Matern Child Health J* 13:839–46.
97. Wrotniak, B.H., Shults, J., Butts, S., and Stettler, N. 2008. Gestational weight gain and risk of overweight in the offspring at age 7 y in a multicenter, multiethnic cohort study. *Am J Clin Nutr* 87:1818–24.
98. Oken, E., Rifas-Shiman, S.L., Field, A.E., Franzier, A.L., and Gillman, M.W. 2008. Maternal gestational weight gain and offspring weight in adolescence. *Obstet Gynecol* 112:999–1006.
99. Mamun, A.A., O'Callaghan, M., Callaway, L., Williams, G., Najman, J., and Lawlor, D.A. 2009. Associations of gestational weight gain with offspring body mass index and blood pressure at 21 years of age: evidence from a birth cohort study. *Circulation* 119:1720–27.
100. Laitinen, J., Jääskeläinen, A., Hartikainen, A., et al. 2012. Maternal weight gain during the first half of pregnancy and offspring obesity at 16 years: a prospective cohort study. *BJOG* 119:716–23.
101. Herring, S.J., Rose, M.Z., Skouteris, H., and Oken, E. 2012. Optimizing weight gain in pregnancy to prevent obesity in women and children. *Diabetes Obes Metab* 14:195–203.
102. Jensen, D.M., Oversen, P., Beck-Nielsen, H., et al. 2005. Gestational weight gain and pregnancy outcomes in 481 obese glucose-tolerant women. *Diabetes Care* 28:2118–22.
103. Feig, D.S., and Palda, V.A. 2002. Type 2 diabetes in pregnancy: a growing concern. *Lancet* 359:1690–92.
104. Piacquadio, K., Hollingsworth, D.R., and Murphy, H. 1991. Effects of in-utero exposure to oral hypoglycaemic drugs. *Lancet* 338:866–69.
105. Ekpebegh, C.O., Coetzee, E.J., van der Merwe, L., and Levitt, N.S. 2007. A 10 year retrospective analysis of pregnancy outcome in pregestational type 2 diabetes: comparison of insulin and oral glucose lowering agents. *Diabet Med* 24:253–58.
106. Simmons, D., Walters, B.N.J., Rowan, J.A., and McIntyre, H.D. 2004. Metformin therapy and diabetes in pregnancy. *Med J Aust* 180:462–64.
107. Gilbert, C., Valois, M., and Koren, G. 2006. Pregnancy outcome after first trimester exposure to metformin: a meta analysis. *Fertil Steril* 86:658–63.
108. Khattab, S., Mohsen, I.A., Foutouh, I.A., Ramadan, A., Moaz, M., and Al-Inany, H. 2006. Metformin reduces abortion in pregnant women with polycystic ovary syndrome. *Gynecol Endocrinol* 22:680–84.
109. Clausen, T.D., Mathiesen, E., Ekbom, P., Hellmuth, E., Mandrup-Poulsen, T., and Damm, P. 2005. Poor pregnancy outcome in women with type 2 diabetes. *Diabetes Care* 28:323–28.
110. Hughes, R.C.E., and Rowan, J.A. 2006. Pregnancy in women with type 2 diabetes: who takes metformin and what is the outcome? *Diabet Med* 23:318–22.
111. Simmons, D. 2002. The utility and efficacy of the new insulins in the management of diabetes and pregnancy. *Curr Diab Rep* 2:331–36.

112. Kurtzhals, P., Schäffer, L., Sørensen, A., et al. 2000. Correlations of receptor binding and metabolic and mitogenic potencies of insulin analogs designed for clinical use. *Diabetes* 49:999–1005.

113. **Horvath, K., Koch, K., Jeitler, K., et al. 2010. Effects of treatment in women with gestational diabetes mellitus: systematic review and meta-analysis.** *Br Med J* **340:c1395.** *A recent review and meta-analysis of the benefits associated with treating gestational diabetes.*

114. Bonomo, M., Corica, D., Mion, E., et al. 2005. Evaluating the therapeutic approach in pregnancies complicated by borderline glucose intolerance: a randomized clinical trial. *Diabet Med* 22:1536–41.

115. Langer, O., Levy, J., Brustman, L., Anyaegbunam, A., Merkatz, R., and Divon, M. 1989. Glycemic control in gestational diabetes mellitus: how tight is tight enough; small for gestational age versus large for gestational age? *Am J Obstet Gynecol* 161:646–53.

116. O'Sullivan, J.B., Gellis, S.S., Dandrow, R.V., Tenney, and B.O. 1966. The potential diabetic and her treatment in pregnancy. *Obstet Gynecol* 27:683–89.

117. Hellmuth, E., Damm, P., and Molsted-Pedersen, L. 2000. Oral hypoglycaemic agents in 118 diabetic pregnancies. *Diabet Med* 17:507–11.

118. Hughes, R.C.E., and Rowan, J.A. 2006. Pregnancy in women with type 2 diabetes: who takes metformin and what is the outcome? *Diabet Med* 23:318–22.

119. Balani, J., Hyer, S.L., Rodin, D.A., and Shehata, H. 2009. Pregnancy outcomes in women with gestational diabetes treated with metformin or insulin: case control study. *Diabet Med* 2009; 26:798–802.

120. Moretti, M.E., Rezvani, M., and Koren, G. 2008. Safety of glyburide for gestational diabetes: a meta-analysis of pregnancy outcomes. *Ann Pharmacother* 42:483–90.

121. Moore, T.R. 2007. Glyburide for the treatment of gestational diabetes. A critical appraisal. *Diabetes Care* 30(Suppl. 2):S209–13.

122. Cheng, Y.W., Chung, J.H., Block-Kurbisch, I., Inturrisi, M., and Caughey, A.B. 2012. Treatment of gestational diabetes mellitus: glyburide compared to subcutaneous insulin therapy and associated perinatal outcomes. *J Mat Fetal Neonat Med* 25:379–84.

123. **Simmons, D. 2010. Metformin treatment for type 2 diabetes in pregnancy?** *Best Pract Res Clin Endocrinol Metab* **24:625–34.** *A recent review about the benefits and problems associated with the use of metformin in pregnancy.*

124. **Nicholson, W., and Baptiste-Roberts, K. 2011. Oral hypoglycaemic agents during pregnancy: the evidence for effectiveness and safety.** *Best Pract Res Clin Obstet Gynae* **25:51–63.** *A recent review about the benefits and problems associated with the use of a range of different oral hypoglycaemic agents in pregnancy.*

125. Bancroft, K., Tuffnell, D.J., Mason, G.C., Rogerson, L.J., and Mansfield, M.A. 2000. Randomised controlled pilot study of the management of gestational impaired glucose tolerance. *BJOG* 107:959–63.

126. Bevier, W.C., Fischer, R., and Jovanovic, L. 1999. Treatment of women with an abnormal glucose challenge test (but a normal oral glucose tolerance test) decreases the prevalence of macrosomia. *Am J Perinatol* 16:269–75.

127. Bung, P., Artal, R., Khodiguian, N., and Kjos, S. 1991. Exercise in gestational diabetes: an optional therapeutic approach? *Diabetes* 40(Suppl. 2):S182–85.

128. Elnour, A.A., El Mugammar, I., Jaber, T., Revel, T., and McElnay, J.C. 2008. Pharmaceutical care of patients with gestational diabetes mellitus. *J Eval Clin Pract* 14:131–40.

129. Garner, P., Okun, N., Keely, E., et al. 1997. A randomized controlled trial of strict glycemic control and tertiary level obstetric care versus routine obstetric care in the management of gestational diabetes: a pilot study. *Am J Obstet Gynecol* 177:190–95.

130. Homko, C.J., Sivan, E., and Reece, E.A. 2002. The impact of self-monitoring of blood glucose on self-efficacy and pregnancy outcomes in women with diet-controlled gestational diabetes. *Diabetes Educ* 28:435–43.

131. Homko, C.J., Santamore, W.P., Whiteman, V., et al. 2007. Use of an Internet-based telemedicine system to manage underserved women with gestational diabetes mellitus. *Diabetes Technol Ther* 9:297–306.

132. Kestila, K.K., Ekblad, U.U., and Ronnemaa, T. 2007. Continuous glucose monitoring versus self-monitoring of blood glucose in the treatment of gestational diabetes mellitus. *Diabetes Res Clin Pract* 77:174–79.

133. Persson, B., Stangenberg, M., Hansson, U., and Nordlander, E. 1985. Gestational diabetes mellitus (GDM): comparative evaluation of two treatment regimens, diet versus insulin and diet. *Diabetes* 34(Suppl. 2):S101–5.

134. Rae, A., Bond, D., Evans, S., North, F., Roberman, B., and Walters, B. 2000. A randomised controlled trial of dietary energy restriction in the management of obese women with gestational diabetes. *Aust N Z J Obstet Gyanecol* 40:416–22.

135. Rey, E. 1997. Usefulness of a breakfast test in the management of women with gestational diabetes. *Obstet Gynecol* 89:981–88.

136. Rossi, G., Somigliana, E., Moschetta, M., Bottani, B., Barbieri, M., and Vignali, M. 2000. Adequate timing of fetal ultrasound to guide metabolic therapy in mild gestational diabetes mellitus: results from a randomized study. *Acta Obstet Gynecol Scand* 79:649–54.

137. Sobngwi, E., Boudou, P., Mauvais-Jarvis, F., et al. 2003. Effect of a diabetic environment in utero on predisposition to type 2 diabetes. *Lancet* 361:1862–65.

138. Medsafe. Datasheet: Metformin. Available from http://www.medsafe.govt.nz/Profs/datasheet/a/ArrowMetformintab.htm (accessed March 31, 2010).

139. Glueck, C.J., Goldenberg, N., Pranikoff, J., Loftspring, M., Sieve, L., and Wang, P. 2004. Height, weight, and motor-social development during the first 18 months of life in 126 infants born to 109 mothers with polycystic ovary syndrome who conceived on and continued metformin through pregnancy. *Hum Reprod* 19:1323–30.

140. Rowan, J.A., Rush, E.C., Obolonkin, V., Battin, M., Wouldes, T., and Hague, W.M. 2011. Metformin in gestational diabetes: the offspring follow-up (MiG TOFU): body composition at 2 years of age. *Diabetes Care* 34:2279–84.

141. **National Institute for Health and Clinical Excellence. 2008. NICE clinical guideline 63. Diabetes in pregnancy: management of diabetes and its complications from pre-conception to the postnatal period. London: National Institute for Health and Clinical Excellence.** *Recommendations for current practice for treating gestational diabetes in the United Kingdom.*

Section V

Future Prospects

9 Future Prospects for Gestational Diabetes

Clive J. Petry
Department of Paediatrics, University of Cambridge,
Addenbrooke's Hospital, Cambridge, United Kingdom

CONTENTS

9.1 INTRODUCTION

Intense research effort has greatly increased the understanding of gestational diabetes mellitus (GDM), along with other forms of diabetes, in recent years. Despite this, due to the transgenerational transmission of diabetes risk associated with GDM, more effective treatments and ideally preventive measures are urgently required before GDM in pregnancy and type 2 diabetes thereafter become closer to the norm rather than just being the exception. In the UK the total cost associated with treating all types of diabetes currently stands at around £23.7 billion (approximately US$38.3 billion), and a recently published report predicts that this will rise to £39.8 billion (approximately US$64.3; around 17% of the total UK National Health Service budget based on current spending levels) by 2035–2036, as the number of people with diabetes rises from the current 3.8 million to a projected 6.25 million.[1] Even the chief executive of Diabetes UK, one of the foremost diabetes charities in the UK, described the projected costs of treating all forms of diabetes by 2035 as "unsustainable."[2] Globally diabetes healthcare costs were estimated to be US$376 billion in 2010 and are predicted to be as high as US$490 billion by 2030,[3] which are clearly unsupportable. As GDM increases the future of risk of developing type 2 diabetes (and even type 1 diabetes) in certain women and their offspring (reviewed in

Petry[4]), its potential prevention through modifiable risk factors such as reductions in maternal prepregnancy weight and weight gain during pregnancy could make a big contribution toward reducing these burdensome costs in both the short and the long terms. Indeed, pregnancy may be a time when women are more amenable to altering lifestyles to more healthy ones than at other stages of their lives. Intervention studies aimed at reducing the incidence of GDM will therefore form a vital part of future GDM research.

Two of the main findings from the Hyperglycemia and Adverse Pregnancy Outcome (HAPO) study were that raised maternal glucose concentrations in pregnancy are associated with adverse pregnancy outcomes, and that there is no threshold under which these effects are not apparent.[5] These findings are potentially as important for the understanding of GDM as the Diabetes Control and Complications Trial[6] and the UK Prospective Diabetes Study,[7,8] which found conclusive links between raised glucose concentrations and increased incidence of complications, were for type 1 and 2 diabetes, respectively.

In the remainder of this chapter I present a rather personal view of where I see the future prospects of various aspects related to GDM, including highlighting current knowledge gaps that need to be filled. By necessity many important points have been omitted. Others have been included but not given the depth of insight they deserve. Where possible in these cases, the reader is referred to one or more recent reviews to help fill in the gaps.

9.2   DIAGNOSING AND SCREENING FOR GESTATIONAL DIABETES

As outlined in Chapter 2, it is crucial that the issue of what is defined as GDM is resolved, or even whether it should be considered a disease in its own right or instead a risk factor for adverse pregnancy outcomes. The issue of its definition seems to have been the case ever since John O'Sullivan coined the term *gestational diabetes* to describe the form of diabetes that first presents in pregnancy, in his landmark paper published in the *New England Journal of Medicine*.[9] O'Sullivan wrote, "There is disagreement about the diagnostic criteria. The answer to this situation is complicated by problems of definition, confused by spontaneous remissions and hindered by lack of well documented longitudinal studies with the available diagnostic tools, which are, unfortunately, far from ideal." Unfortunately, rather than defining a threshold of glucose concentrations above which there was a progressive increase in the incidence of adverse pregnancy outcomes and which could be used in the diagnostic criteria for GDM, results from the multinational HAPO study suggested a linear relationship between maternal glucose concentrations and the risk of adverse pregnancy outcomes even in the subdiabetes range.[5] This leaves the criteria for the diagnosis of GDM to be defined by expert consensus opinion. Indeed, this led the International Association of Diabetes in Pregnancy Study Groups (IADPSG) to suggest diagnostic criteria[10] with lower glucose concentrations than those suggested by the National Diabetes Data Group in the United States[11] and the World Health Organisation,[12] both of which were based on circulating glucose concentrations outside of pregnancy. The glucose concentrations that were suggested by the IADPSG as thresholds for diagnosis were the glucose concentrations at which the odds for adverse birth outcomes (greater than the 90th percentile for birth weight, percentage body fat, and cord blood serum C-peptide concentrations) reached 1.75 times the estimated odds for these outcomes at mean glucose concentrations in the HAPO study. This criterion was published in order to stimulate debate, and therefore ultimately gain further consensus. The increased number of women that are classified as having GDM and the resulting increased healthcare costs have led some to criticise the implementation of the criteria,[13–15] although others have accepted them.[16,17] A recent meta-analysis of studies using WHO criteria and IADPSG criteria for diagnosing GDM found that although both were able to highlight those women at minimal increased risk of adverse pregnancy outcomes, the relative risks for these when using the IADPSG were heterogeneous and reduced if the HAPO data were removed.[18]

One difficulty with the use of a uniform criterion for diagnosing GDM was highlighted in a recent study of a multiethnic population from Norway. When comparing IADPSG and WHO criteria for diagnosing GDM, it was found that whilst use of the IADPSG criteria was associated with a raised prevalence of GDM in general, this increase was significantly more evident in those of South Asian origin, many of whom had a relatively mild increase in fasting plasma glucose concentrations.[19] In a further study, this time of a multiethnic population in California, it was found that the risk of GDM at different body mass indices (BMIs) was disparate in different ethnicities. In particular, the risk for women of South Asian or Filipino origin occurred at lower BMIs than equivalent risks for women of other ethnicities.[20] Further studies are therefore necessary in populations of Asian women, in particular to see if those who would be diagnosed with GDM using the IADPSG criteria but not WHO (or even National Diabetes Data Group) criteria have an increased risk of adverse pregnancy outcomes.

The IADPSG criteria for the diagnosis of GDM are based on glucose concentrations from a single 2 h 75 g oral glucose tolerance test (OGTT).[10] Others, mainly in the United States, still prefer the use of a 100 g OGTT following a 50 g glucose challenge test.[21] However, as an alternative to all the diagnostic criteria based on OGTT results, due to technical difficulties in performing OGTTs and the lack of reproducibility inherent in the test, it has been suggested that the diagnosis be based on glycated haemoglobin (HbA_{1c}) concentrations.[22,23] In comparison to OGTT-based techniques, HbA_{1c} has the advantage of being a single measurement (that reflects average glucose concentrations over the lifetime of red blood cells) that does not require the person being tested to fast. As a test it is also far more reproducible than OGTTs and reflects real glucose concentrations rather than those resulting from a high-glycaemic index drink of glucose dissolved in water. However, questions have been raised over the sensitivity of using HbA_{1c} as a diagnostic test, and unless serial measurements are made (which loses one of the advantages of using the test in the first place), there can be problems when testing women with haemoglobin variants or anaemia. As an alternative to the use of HbA_{1c}, using a fasting plasma glucose of greater than 5.1 mmol/L has the advantages of being more reproducible than the OGTT and not being affected by haemoglobin variants. However, again it has relatively low sensitivity for detecting GDM, which may be particularly problematic for certain populations (such as South Asians) in comparison to others whose postload glucoses tend to rise earlier than fasting concentrations in the development of gestational diabetes.[24] These considerations probably make sticking with OGTT for the diagnosis of GDM the preferred option, albeit with its limitations. Whilst use of a mixed meal rather than a glucose load would give a more representative meal glycaemic index, the lack of agreement of the constituents that should make up a mixed meal and the greater complexity of formulating it in comparison to a standard weight of glucose dissolved in a standard amount of water in a global sense again argue for glucose's continued use, even with its inherent limitations. The IADPSG criteria have recently been shown to be cost-effective, but only when postpartum care reduces the incidence of progression to type 2 diabetes.[15]

Further need for expert consensus opinion regarding the diagnosis of GDM led the U.S. National Institutes of Health to hold a Consensus Development Conference in Bethesda, Maryland, in early 2013 (http://prevention.nih.gov/cdp/conferences/2012/gdm/default.aspx). The final statement from this conference highlighted a number of research needs, including the need to develop an approach to the diagnosis of GDM in the United States that is more consistent with international approaches and the need to assess whether women who would be considered free from GDM using current methods but have the condition using IADPSG criteria actually benefit from treatment or not.[25] This is important, as a recent study of 186 women in Canada who were considered to have GDM by IADPSG criteria but who were not considered to have it using current Canadian Diabetes Association criteria, when compared to pregnancy outcomes from 372 women without GDM, were found to have similar (and *not* raised) prevalences of large for gestational age newborns, delivery complications, preeclampsia, prematurity, neonatal complications at delivery, and metabolic complications.[26] Whether current IADPSG, NDDG, WHO, or even other new recommendations (such as using the glucose thresholds from HAPO that are associated with a doubling of risk of adverse pregnancy outcomes, rather than the 1.75-fold increased risk currently suggested by the IADPSG) are adopted, it is hoped that an international standard will emerge that is cost-effective and, most importantly, highlights those women with an increased risk for adverse pregnancy outcomes associated with GDM in both the short and long terms, whatever their ethnicities.

A related question to how should you diagnose GDM is, which women should you screen for this condition, if you even accept that it is worth such screening. An executive summary produced for the Institute for Quality and Efficiency in Health Care in Germany in 2009[27] concluded that at least at that time, there was no direct proof or indications that showed benefit or harm from GDM screening since the authors had not identified any suitable screening studies. Despite this, the authors found that an indication could be indirectly deduced that screening for GDM leads to a reduction in perinatal complications. Since that time, large prospective trials have confirmed the benefit of treating the condition (outlined in Chapter 8). A recent modestly sized retrospective study of 249 women with GDM diagnosed either by screening or by symptoms found that those identified through screening were diagnosed an average of 4 weeks earlier than those identified symptomatically, and their offspring had reduced rates of abdominal circumferences above the 90th percentile at maternal diagnosis, and a reduced proportion that were born large for their gestational age.[28]

Thus, this study suggests that it is worth screening for GDM, although confirmatory studies in larger populations and with different ethnicities are required.

Even amongst those that favour screening pregnant women for GDM, like with its actual diagnosis, different considerations of exactly which women to screen (relating to such factors as cost, sensitivity, specificity, and practicality) have led to a wide range of different national and international criteria.[29] The IADPSG favour a universal screening approach (with a single 75 g OGTT at 24–28 weeks gestation),[10] adoption of which has obvious cost and practicality consequences both in terms of managing the OGTTs themselves and in relation to treating the increased number of women who will be diagnosed with GDM. The alternative to universal screening is selective screening of women who have one or more major risk factors for GDM (such as having had GDM in previous pregnancies, being obese, or being aged over 40 years). A number of studies have been published over the past 15 years comparing the merits of the two screening strategies (Table 9.1).[30–41] Of these, the majority favour universal screening (due to the relatively low specificity of selective screening, the fact that selective screening does not reduce the amount of screening necessary by very much, and the difficulties in successfully implementing it, such as the need for somebody to judge whether the pregnant woman in question has a major risk factor or not). In fact, one study[33] usefully states that universal screening should be used everywhere unless resources are very scarce and its implementation is unfeasible. With the increased incidence of GDM worldwide, it seems likely therefore that unless resources specifically preclude it, universal screening will ultimately become commonplace.

9.3   PREVENTION OF GESTATIONAL DIABETES

As well as diagnosing GDM, another area where there are important gaps in our understanding is how to prevent the development of GDM in the first place.

9.3.1   Maternal Obesity and Gestational Diabetes

The HAPO study showed that the risk of adverse pregnancy outcomes increased with obesity, independently from the increased risk associated with GDM.[42] Indeed, when obesity and GDM were both present, the associated effect was larger than when either of these conditions was present individually. These findings help resolve one of the controversies associated with GDM, i.e., is there any risk of adverse pregnancy outcomes conferred by GDM that is independent of that associated with obesity?[43]

Obesity is clearly inextricably linked to the development of GDM, presumably through a resulting reduction in insulin sensitivity. Efforts to reduce the predicted epidemic of type 2 (and gestational) diabetes are therefore critically dependent on the success of procedures to reduce obesity, particularly in women of childbearing age. To design and implement potentially suitable strategies, it is important to know causes of the current obesity epidemic. Obvious causes include the consumption of obesogenic diets and insufficient exercise. These are not the only potential causes, however, although their effect sizes are likely to be the largest. Table 9.2 shows other potential contributors to the obesity epidemic. The quality of the evidence for some

TABLE 9.1

Studies Comparing the Merits of Universal and Selective Screening of Pregnant Women for GDM

Author (Reference)	Country Where the Study Was Performed	Major Finding or Conclusion
Williams et al.[30]	United States	Selective screening would only miss a few women who actually had GDM, but approximately 90% of women would still need to be screened.
Wagaarachchi et al.[31]	Sri Lanka	Selective screening would have missed over 40% of women with GDM in Sri Lanka.
Baliutaviciene et al.[32]	Lithuania	There are sensitivity and specificity issues with the use of selective screening; therefore, universal screening is recommended.
Di Cianni et al.[33]	Italy	Universal screening should be used everywhere except where resources are very scarce and universal screening is not feasible.
Corcoy et al.[34]	Spain	Selective screening is reliable, but only a small proportion of women would not need screening. Adherence to the selective screening guidelines would make the screening policy unnecessarily complicated.
Cosson et al.[35]	France	Universal screening might improve pregnancy outcomes and reduce delays in diagnosis and initiation and care.
Shirazian et al.[36]	Iran	Selective screening does not miss substantial numbers of GDM cases.
McCarthy et al.[37]	Argentina	Universal screening is recommended due to the relatively high prevalence of GDM in those without risk factors.
Hiéronimus and Le Meaux[38]	None (review of other studies)	Selective screening limits false positives and concentrates medical resources. However, it might be more difficult to perform and could miss a high proportion of the GDM cases. Universal screening has higher sensitivity but leads to more therapeutic interventions whose benefit and cost/ effectiveness ratio need to be confirmed in low-risk women.
Teh et al.[39]	Australia	Current selective screening guidelines have high sensitivity but low specificity and offer little advantage over universal screening.

TABLE 9.1 (*Continued*)
Studies Comparing the Merits of Universal and Selective Screening of Pregnant Women for GDM

Author (Reference)	Country Where the Study Was Performed	Major Finding or Conclusion
Davis et al.[40]	Australia	Adoption of a universal screening strategy, in a population with a high prevalence of GDM, led to an improvement in pregnancy outcomes and is therefore recommended.
Avalos et al.[41]	Ireland	Depending on which diagnostic criteria were used, up to 20% of women diagnosed with GDM through universal screening would have been missed by using selective screening. This provides a strong argument for universal screening.

of these contributors is stronger than that of others, however,[45] and of course secular trends in the incidence of obesity in different populations have to be borne in mind.

9.3.2 Exercise and Gestational Diabetes

As outlined in Chapter 7, there is little evidence from randomised clinical trials to suggest that the development of GDM can be prevented by the initiation of an exercise program in at-risk individuals in pregnancy. This may be caused by the modest size of studies undertaken in this area so far, giving limited statistical power to detect clinically significant differences even when analysing studies by meta-analysis. However, given that consensus opinion suggests that regular light to moderate exercise may be beneficial to GDM risk (see Chapter 7), and that observational studies have suggested that exercise can reduce the incidence of GDM,[46] it is important that larger studies are performed, ideally with common protocols to reduce heterogeneity, in the hope of gaining convincing evidence of the benefits of exercise in this area. Several such trials have already been registered.[47] Once convincing evidence is available for an effect of exercise overall, protocols can be refined so recommendations can be made that balance the metabolic effects on the mother[48] with the safety of her unborn offspring and cost-effectiveness.[49]

9.3.3 Dietary Advice and Gestational Diabetes

Chapter 6 outlines how dietary advice forms frontline therapy for both the prevention and treatment of GDM. Whilst diets with low glycaemic indexes may hold the most promise for both dietary-mediated prevention and treatment of GDM,[50] a recent randomised controlled trial failed to show any effect of consumption of a low-glycaemic index diet on offspring birth weight or macrosomia prevalence, or in maternal insulin requirements or incidence of adverse pregnancy outcomes.[51] This negative finding

TABLE 9.2

Other Putative Contributors to the Obesity Epidemic Besides Unhealthy Diet and Insufficient Exercise

Putative Cause	Description
Reduction in smoking	Stopping smoking is associated with weight gain.
Microorganisms	There is a close interaction between adipose tissue and the immune system. Obesity-promoting viruses (e.g., canine distemper) and adiposity-enhancing gut flora do exist.
Epigenetics	There is evidence for maternal obesity having an intrauterine effect on the offspring through epigenetic mechanisms. Other epigenetic effects could also be happening.
Increasing maternal age	The age at which women have their babies has been increasing. Mothers of obese children. Comorbidities could confound. Possible mechanisms have been found in animals.
Greater fecundity among people with higher adiposity	Evidence exists that the BMI correlates with the number of offspring produced—there are a number of confounders, which first need more research.
Assortative mating for adiposity	Spousal resemblance does occur, but could be due to a number of factors after mate selection. Some studies have shown correlation before marriage and cohabitation. Animal studies suggest an impact on body weight can occur within one generation.
Sleep debt	The amount of sleep has reduced over the last 40 years. Sleep deprivation is associated with obesity.
Endocrine disrupting chemicals (EDCs)	Exposure to several EDCs is increasing. Some EDCs interfere with oestrogen and androgen signalling—this could be associated with body fat and weight.
Pharmaceutical iatrogenesis	Pharmaceutical use is increasing; some pharmaceuticals (e.g., antipsychotics, tricyclic antidepressants, beta-blockers) are associated with weight gain.
Reduction in variability of ambient temperatures	Temperature control use (e.g., air conditioning) has increased and could be associated with increase in obesity.
Intrauterine and intergenerational effects	A range of nonepigenetic mechanisms have been proposed that increase the risk of adiposity (and diabetes) in the offspring.

Source: Reproduced from Simmons, D., *Best Pract. Res. Clin. Obstet. Gynaecol.*, 25, 25–36, 2011. With permission of the publisher Elsevier, and Taylor & Francis Ltd., the publisher of the manuscript from which the text was originally collected (McAllister, E.J. et al., *Crit. Rev. Food Sci. Nutr.*, 49, 868–913, 2009).

may reflect the diet not being effective for the treatment of GDM, the difficulty in achieving a sufficiently large reduction in the overall glycaemic index of a diet, or a lack of statistical power associated with the sample sizes used ($n = 50$ in the low-glycaemic index group and 49 in the high-fibre moderate-glycaemic index diet group). As an example of the latter, the prevalence of offspring macrosomia was 2.1% ($n = 1$ out of 47 participants) in the low-glycaemic index pregnancies but 6.7% ($n = 3$ out of 45) in the others ($p = 0.16$). Clearly, even larger trials would be needed to see if there is any real benefit to the use of these diets in pregnancy,[4] although obviously these would just have greater statistical power to be able to detect differences with smaller effect sizes than are currently achievable. Whether such changes with small effect sizes would be clinically as well as statistically significant (at a population level) remains to be seen. Alternatively, as pointed out in the recent negative, randomised controlled trial,[51] it could already be that low-glycaemic index and high-fibre diets with moderate glycaemic indexes are already optimised for pregnancy outcomes.

Recent trials in Finland have been performed on women at risk of GDM testing the effects of intensified individual counselling related to physical activity, diet, and weight gain on GDM prevalence and prevalence of offspring being born large for their gestational age.[52] A further trial added the effect of maternal probiotic supplementation to the counselling.[53] Although the counselling had positive effects on reducing offspring birth weight and incidence of being large for gestational age, there was no apparent effect on the development of GDM, despite the women with intensivised counselling having increased their dietary fibre and polyunsaturated fatty acid intakes and decreased their saturated fatty acid and saccharose intakes.[52] Subsequent subanalyses showed that women in the intensive counselling group had beneficial effects on total intake of vegetables, fruits, and berries, the proportions of bread intake that was high in fibre, the proportions of all cheeses that were low fat, and the proportions of dietary fats that were of vegetable origin, and the intake of saturated fatty acids, polyunsaturated fatty acids, linoleic acid, and fibre.[54] Although with a smaller number of study participants, supplementing the dietary counselling with probiotics (*Lactobacillus rhamnosus* GG and *Bifidobacterium lactis* Bb12 in capsular form) decreased the incidence of GDM,[53] which did not occur with counselling alone. In the more recent paper from this group studying women from the Finnish Medical Birth Registry it was found that increased maternal iron intake in pregnancy was a risk factor for the development of GDM in high-risk women who were not anaemic at the start of pregnancy.[55] The authors suggested that a large prospective study is needed to confirm these findings, which may be particularly important since many women take iron supplements in pregnancy to counteract the perceived rather than clinically diagnosed anaemia.

Despite these results from Finland, a recent meta-analysis concluded that dietary counselling does significantly reduce the incidence of GDM, although the quality of the evidence for this was low and there was no clear benefit of this over other potentially useful interventions.[56] In a further meta-analysis of studies including pregnant women with raised glucose concentrations that were not high enough to classify the women as having GDM, dietary counselling and metabolic monitoring were found to reduce risk of offspring macrosomia or being large for gestational age without increasing the caesarean section and operative vaginal birth rates (although the studies included in the analysis were noted to be small and to have a moderate to high risk of bias).[57] Clearly, studies producing higher-quality evidence are required, but currently the balance is in favour of positive effects of dietary counselling on pregnancy outcomes (even if it is more related to effects on the offspring rather than on GDM risk). Indeed, such counselling to increase the likelihood of women with or at high risk of developing GDM consuming a standard healthy diet may prove more effective than implementing changes such as lowering the glycaemic index of a diet.

9.4 PATHOPHYSIOLOGY OF GESTATIONAL DIABETES

Like all forms of diabetes, once any preventive measures have failed, GDM arises from a combination of insulin deficiency and insulin resistance. Its aetiology is believed to result from a relative deficiency in pancreatic β-cell function, often like that for type 2 diabetes, the resulting phenotype emerging due to insulin resistance and the inability to raise insulin concentrations sufficiently to compensate for it. For type 2 diabetes this insulin resistance is broadly associated with obesity. Part of the insulin resistance of GDM in the majority of women with the condition is related to obesity. However, GDM often emerges prior to type 2 diabetes in susceptible women because of the physiological insulin resistance of pregnancy. Much of the future research into the pathophysiology of type 2 diabetes will therefore also be of benefit to GDM research. However, what will be most important in the study of the pathophysiology of GDM in this area will be research that is specific to the condition, i.e., the causes of pregnancy-related insulin resistance and pancreatic β-cell inadequacy. Once the pathophysiology is better understood, therapeutic targets should arise potentially translating basic science research in this area into new treatments.

It is currently thought that insulin resistance of pregnancy is mediated, at least in part, by pregnancy-specific placental hormones such placental lactogen and placental growth hormone. In humans the growth hormone gene cluster on the long arm of chromosome 17 contains the growth hormone (GH1) gene, which is expressed from the anterior pituitary, plus four placentally expressed genes: chorionic somatomammotropin hormone-like 1 (CSHL1), chorionic somatomammotropin hormone 1 (CSH1), placental-specific growth hormone (GH2), and chorionic somatomammotropin hormone 2 (CSH2).[58] The two chorionic somatomammotropin hormone genes encode human placental lactogen. In pregnancy the anterior pituitary provides maternal ligands for the growth hormone and prolactin receptors (growth hormone and prolactin, respectively), and the placenta provides foetal ligands (placental growth hormone and human placental lactogen, respectively). However, the relative balance of the two changes as pregnancy increases: toward term nearly all the growth hormone receptor ligands are the placental protein,[59] whereas the prolactin receptor ligands are still both prolactin and human placental lactogen.[60] It is not currently known what advantages there are by having one of these related systems regulated largely by the foetus and one by both the foetus and its mother. However, given that placental growth hormone's structure and, at least in rodent models, its actions are similar to those of its pituitary form,[61,62] placental growth hormone may signal to the mother to provide more fuel to the foetus, including increased nonesterified fatty acids by lipolysis and glucose by increased hepatic glucose output and decreased peripheral insulin sensitivities. In contrast to this GDM-promoting activity, recent evidence suggests that lactogenic activity may help protect the mother from excessive nutrient depletion and extraction by the foetus by stimulating an increase in maternal food intake (mediated via central leptin resistance) and in insulin secretion through the expansion of maternal pancreatic β-cells in pregnancy.[63,64] The somatogenic and lactogenic hormones therefore seem to act in concert to regulate maternal metabolism to try and balance the needs of the mother and the foetus. In disorders such as GDM the balance of this favours foetal growth. Advancement of knowledge in this area may therefore lead to treatment opportunities that normalise this balance. Unfortunately, this is made more difficult by the inability to gain much insight from rodent models, due to the differences between humans and rodents in somatogenic and lactogenic hormones.[60]

As well as placental-specific hormones, other hormones that are also present outside of pregnancy are thought to contribute to causing the insulin resistance of pregnancy. In particular, adipocytokines, which are secreted by adipose tissue outside of pregnancy and both adipose and placental tissue in pregnancy, appear to be important.[65,66] Tables 9.3 and 9.4 summarise the biological effects and roles of three of these, leptin, adiponectin, and resistin, in placental tissue and in the maternal and foetal components as they are known at present.

Areas thought to be involved with the pathogenesis of GDM, which are partially regulated by adipokines,[67,68] are inflammation and the resulting endothelial dysfunction. It is believed that an altered balance of adipokines resulting from obesity leads to subclinical inflammation that favours the emergence of gestational diabetes.[69] In the HAPO study associations were tested between measures of glucose tolerance in pregnancy (HbA1c plus OGTT circulating glucose and c-peptide concentrations 0, 60, and 120 min after consumption of the glucose load) and genetic variants in 31 inflammatory pathway genes.[70] A number of significant associations between variants and metabolic markers led the authors to conclude that polymorphic variation in a number of the inflammatory pathway genes tested (including adiponectin receptor 2 (ADIPOR2), interleukin 6 (IL6), interleukin 8 (IL8), leptin receptor (LEPR), resistin (RETN), and tumour necrosis factor-α (TNF)) may influence metabolic phenotypes in pregnant women. However, they also concluded that on the basis of their results, inflammatory pathways as a whole are unlikely to have a major influence on metabolic phenotypes in pregnancy. It is possible that measurement of markers of inflammatory pathway activity will instead become useful biomarkers of risk for the development of GDM in pregnancy, just as it has been hypothesised that they are for type 2 diabetes.[71,72] Indeed, consistent with this, a recent study of nearly 34,000 women attending a tertiary medical centre in Israel found future risk of GDM (as well as other obstetric complications) to be related to first trimester leucocyte count.[73]

Progress in understanding the pathophysiology of GDM is undoubtedly hampered by the lack of a good nongenetically manipulated rodent model. Current models often rely on dietary-induced obesity, which may induce mild glucose intolerance and insulin resistance in pregnancy but does not produce GDM due to the ability of the pancreatic β-cells to compensate for this by increasing insulin secretion. Alternative models do produce diabetes by using chemicals that are toxic to pancreatic β-cells, such as streptozotocin or alloxan, but often produce a model that is more like type 1 diabetes in pregnancy rather than GDM (due to the severity of the hyperlglycaemia, the relative lack of insulin resistance, and the need to administer the streptozotocin prior to conception so as not to affect foetal β-cells). Still more models use a lower dose of these chemicals to produce a milder hyperglycaemia that is closer to that observed in GDM. Dietary manipulation can also be used to induce insulin resistance in these animals. However, lower doses of streptozotocin do not reliably lead to hyperglycaemia in all animals, and second, like for the animals given the higher dose, the hyperglycaemia needs to be established prior to conception so as

TABLE 9.3
Biological Effects of Adipokines on Placental Tissue

Adipokines In Placental Unit	Leptin	Adiponectin	Resistin
Cellular expression	Syncitiotrophoblast Extravillous trophoblast Foetal vascular endothelial cells	Syncitiotrophoblast? Extravillous trophoblast?	Extravillous trophoblast Placental villi
Effects on trophoblast cells	↑ Proliferation Increase of IL1, E17b expression Progression to G2/S Inhibition of apoptosis ↑ Migration upregulation of fibronectin ↑ Invasion Increase MMP-2	↓ Proliferation, ↑ Differentiation, increase of hCG ↑ Invasion Increase of MMP-2, -9 Downregulation of TIMP-2 ↑ Immunomodulation Stimulation of CD24/ Siglec10	↑ Invasion Increase MMP-2, -9 Downregulation of TIMP-1, -2
Effects on angiogenesis	↑ ? Enhances angiogenic differentiation in human venous and porcine aortic endothelial cells Increases cytotrophoblasts' VEGF secretion Leptin receptors on endothelial cells of blood vessels of chorionic villi	? Favours angiogenic differentiation in HUVEC and in peripheral blood CD14+ monocytes Increases endothelial cells' apoptosis	↑ Stimulates HUVEC and HCAEC angiogenesis Upregulates angiogenic-related molecules: VEGF, VEGFR-1, -2, and MMP-1, -2

Source: D'Ippolito, S. et al., *Biofactors,* 38, 14–23, 2012. With permission from John Wiley & Sons.

Note: HCAEC, human coronary artery endothelial cell; HUVEC, human umbilical vein endothelial cell; MMP, matrix metalloproteinase; TIMP, tissue inhibitor of metalloproteinase; VEGF, vascular endothelial growth factor; VEGFR, vascular endothelial growth factor receptor.

to not kill foetal pancreatic β-cells (therefore more closely modelling undiagnosed type 2 diabetes in pregnancy rather than GDM).

Despite the above limitations in the usefulness of current GDM models, one area that has proved fruitful in recent years in terms of using rodents is that of pancreatic β-cell adaptations to pregnancy. The inaccessibility of human (maternal) pancreatic tissue in pregnancy, combined with the current scanning techniques not having the resolution to accurately quantify pancreatic β-cell mass,[74] has made mice and rats the principal source of progress in understanding β-cell physiology in pregnancy. As scanning techniques improve, however, assessing changes in pancreatic β-cell

TABLE 9.4

Role of Adipokines during Pregnancy in the Maternal and Foetal Compartments

Adipokines		Leptin	Adiponectin	Resistin
In the mother	Circulating levels during pregnancy	↑	↓	↑
	Metabolic effects	Fat deposits mobilisation	Insulin sensitivity modulation	Decreased insulin sensitivity
In the foetus	Umbilical levels at term	↑	↑	↑
	Functions	Marker of foetal adipose tissue stores? Cell- and tissue-specific growth factor? Favours foetal growth through increased placental lipolysis and transplacental amino acid transport	Increased foetal tissue sensitivity to insulin and IGFs Stimulates osteoblast activity	Increased fuel availability Increased hepatic glucose production Prevention of neonatal hypoglycaemia

Source: Adapted from D'Ippolito, S. et al., *Biofactors*, 38, 14–23, 2012. Used by permission from John Wiley & Sons.

Note: IGF, insulin-like growth factor.

mass in humans should help confirm whether they are the same, similar, or vastly different from the changes that occur in rodent pregnancies. Once mechanisms of any increases in human pancreatic β-cell mass associated with pregnancy are established, therapeutic targets may emerge that could be manipulated to help stimulate the increases, especially in women who are already at high risk of developing GDM, such as those that have had it in previous pregnancies.

The timing of the peak of pancreatic β-cell DNA synthesis in rodent pregnancies matches the timing of increased circulating lactogen (i.e., prolactin and placental lactogen) concentrations, suggesting that lactogenic activity is crucial in the response to pregnancy[75] (Figure 9.1). Further evidence for this comes from studies of prolactin receptor knockout mice that exhibit impaired glucose tolerance in pregnancy associated with reduced β-cell size, mass, and proliferation.[76] More recently, discovered factors involved in the increase in β-cell mass include hepatocyte growth factor and 5-hydroxytryptamine,[77] with effects mediated by transcription factors such as hepatocyte nuclear factor-4α and the forkhead box proteins M1[78] and D3,[79] and cell cycle regulators such as menin,[80] p27, and p18 (reviewed in Ernst[81] and Rieck and Kaestner[82]) (Figure 9.1). What is clear from such rodent models and other in vitro

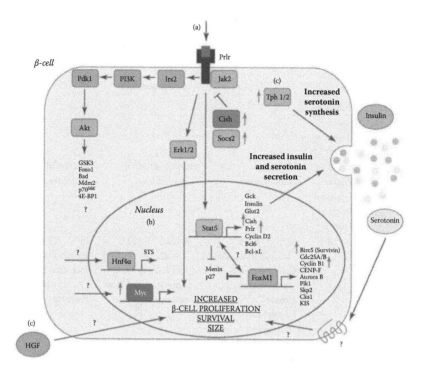

FIGURE 9.1   Summary of some of the known mechanisms responsible for pancreatic β-cell gain in rodent pregnancies. (a) Activation of prolactin receptors upon binding of lactogens (prolactin or placental lactogen) plays a pivotal role in the adaptation of the β-cell to pregnancy. Downstream signalling pathways of the prolactin receptor include signal transducer and activator of transcription 5A, phosphatidylinositol 3-kinase, and mitogen-activated protein kinase pathways, targets of which have been implicated to lead to increased β-cell proliferation, survival, and size. (b) Known transcription factors that regulate the increase in β-cell mass during pregnancy. The arrow indicates an increase in expression of islet genes during the start of the last week of the 3-week pregnancy. (c) Possible prolactin receptor-independent mechanisms leading to β-cell gain mechanisms. Abbreviations: 4E-BP1, 4E binding protein 1; Akt, protein kinase B; Aurora B, Aurora kinase B; Bad, BCL2-associated agonist of cell death; Bcl6, B-cell lymphoma 6; Bcl-xL, B-cell lymphoma—extra large; Birc5, baculoviral IAP repeat containing 5; Cdc25A/B, cell division cycle 25 A and B; CENP-F, centromere protein F; Cish, cytokine-inducible SH2-containing protein; Cks1, CDC28 protein kinase regulatory subunit 1; Erk1/2, extracellular signal-regulated kinases 1 and 2; FoxM1, forkhead box protein M1; Gck, glucokinase; Glut2, glucose transporter 2; GSK3, glycogen synthase kinase 3; HGF, hepatocyte growth factor; Hnf4α, hepatocyte nuclear factor 4α; Irs2, insulin receptor substrate 2; Jak2, janus kinase 2; KIS, kinase interacting with stathmin; Mdm2, mouse double minute 2; p70^{s6k}, 70 kDa ribosomal protein S6 kinase; Myc, myelocytomatosis viral oncogene homolog; p27, cyclin-dependent kinase inhibitor 1B; Pdk1, phosphoinositide-dependent kinase 1; PI3K, phosphatidylinositol 3-kinase; Plk1, polo-like kinase 1; PRL, prolactin, Prlr, prolactin receptor, Skp2, S-phase kinase-associated protein 2; Socs2, suppressor of cytokine signalling 2; ST5, suppression of tumourigenicity 5; STAT5, signal transducer and activator of transcriptions 5A and 5B; Tph1/2, tryptophan hydroxylase 1 and 2. (Reprinted from Rieck, S., and Kaestner, K.H., *Trends Endocrinol. Metab.*, 21, 151–158, 2009. With permission from Elsevier.)

experiments is that to compensate for the effects of pregnancy as well as increasing rates of β-cell proliferation, there also needs to be a decrease in apoptotic signalling; otherwise, diabetes can still develop.[83] This suggests that the requirements for increased proliferation and decreased apoptosis will both need to be addressed in future therapies for GDM.[82]

9.5 TREATMENT OF GESTATIONAL DIABETES

It is now clear that treatment of GDM leads to a reduction in the risk of adverse pregnancy outcomes.[84,85] Dietary and pharmacological approaches (along with exercise, at least theoretically) form the most important GDM treatments. The current pharmacological options are reviewed in Chapter 8. Whilst treatment options and chances of having a healthy pregnancy without an adverse outcome are better now than they have ever been before, they are clearly still not optimal, and the overall incidence of GDM-related complications continues to rise, fuelled by the rise in the number of women with this condition.

Perhaps the route that is most likely to achieve optimal glycaemic control for women with GDM using current treatments is closed-loop insulin therapy (which is commonly called the artificial pancreas), consisting of an insulin pump, continuous glucose monitoring, and a computerised algorithm regulating insulin release according to the circulating glucose concentrations. Whilst trials are currently underway in women with GDM, closed-loop insulin therapy has proved to be safe in pregnant women with preexisting type 1 diabetes.[86,87] Current protocols appear to be suboptimal, although no worse in terms of glucose concentrations achieved than those achieved using conventional continuous subcutaneous insulin infusion. Also, in one study use of the closed-loop insulin therapy reduced the time spent in the hypoglycaemic region.[87] Future improvements in the accuracy of recordings made by the continuous glucose monitors, in the algorithms matching circulating glucose concentrations with the insulin dose (especially in nonhomeostatic, postprandial conditions[88]) and in fault detection, along with manufacture in a more portable form,[89] have the potential to make closed-loop insulin treatment the optimal treatment for women GDM, as long as all this can be achieved in a cost-effective manner.

Alternatives to any type of insulin treatment to treat GDM will always be needed, particularly for those women presenting with a needle phobia. Promising alternatives such as metformin are already commonly used to treat GDM. In the future, we will have evidence to suggest that the apparent short-term safety of its use in pregnancy is matched by long-term safety of in utero exposure to metformin. It is hoped that as greater knowledge about the pathogenesis of GDM is gained, further therapeutic targets will emerge for its treatment, such as those that modulate insulin sensitivities or pancreatic β-cell responses to pregnancy such that more appropriate circulating insulin concentrations are reached. One possible treatment is vitamin D supplementation, although large prospective randomised clinical trials testing its potential effects on GDM incidence have not reported outcomes yet.[90] However, meta-analyses of observational studies have reported inverse relationships between maternal plasma vitamin D levels and the incidence of GDM,[91,92] possibly due to an association between reduced vitamin D levels and increased insulin resistance.[93] One study found improved glucose concentrations in women with GDM who started taking vitamin D supplements,[94] but it was not randomised. Studies producing results with higher-quality evidence are therefore required, particularly as vitamin D supplementation has other potential benefits, proven safety, and low cost.[91] Patents exist for other potential therapeutic agents, including, amongst others, glucagon-like peptide 1 and gastric inhibitory polypeptide analogues, which would theoretically improve insulin secretion in GDM, although it would clearly be a long time before any of these would be able to be used clinically.

9.6   WHAT HAPPENS AFTER GESTATIONAL DIABETES?

It is well established that GDM is associated with an increased risk of developing type 2 diabetes postpartum.[95] Indeed, whilst around 1/10 of women with GDM have a condition that more closely resembles type 1 diabetes than type 2, the remaining 90% have a condition that some believe to be the same as type 2 diabetes with the earlier onset of disease (i.e., GDM) occurring as a consequence of the insulin resistance of pregnancy. For the majority of women who go on to develop type 2 diabetes, GDM does resolve immediately postpartum (with the loss of placental hormones and reduction in circulating adipokines), but their glucose tolerance worsens with time, such that after 5 years around 13% of such women have developed type 2 diabetes.[96] It appears that the time taken to develop type 2 diabetes after having had GDM is actually dropping, possibly caused by increased prevalences of obesity. Having had GDM and knowing that they are at high risk of developing type 2 diabetes, it is these women who are given the unique opportunity to reduce their risk by lifestyle modifications, such as attempts at weight loss through alterations in dietary and exercise regimes. However, in reviewing this situation, the fact that compliance to such lifestyle alterations is poor, leading to higher than potential rates of progression to type 2 diabetes, led the authors to highlight the need for translational research in this area to develop intervention strategies.[97] As well as a reduction in the risk of progression to type 2 diabetes, such lifestyle interventions are also likely to limit the chance of GDM recurrence in subsequent pregnancies.

If type 2 diabetes does occur in a woman who has previously had GDM, it is important to detect it so that treatment may be started in order to try and prevent the onset of diabetic complications. Exactly how and when to test for the presence of diabetes is another area of controversy in the field of GDM-related regimens, however. Criteria from the American Diabetes Association (ADA) depend on what a woman's glucose tolerance is postpartum.[29] If it is designated normal, then glycaemia should be retested at least every 3 years. If the woman has either impaired fasting glycaemia or impaired glucose tolerance in the postpartum period, the ADA suggests that testing should be repeated annually. The American College of Obstetrics and Gynecology take these guidelines further by suggesting that all women who had GDM either have their fasting blood glucose measured or undergo a full 75 g oral glucose tolerance test at 6–12 weeks postpartum.[29] If these assessments are normal, then glucose tolerance should be reassessed every 3 years. However, if impaired fasting glycaemia or impaired glucose tolerance is present postpartum, then treatment with metformin should be considered due to the very high risk of subsequent progression to type 2 diabetes. Guidelines from the UK National Institute for Health and Clinical Excellence suggest measuring fasting blood glucose concentrations 6 weeks postpartum and annually thereafter.[29] Such a guideline has the advantages of not requiring women to consume rather unpleasant glucose loads and having greater analytical precision. However, they have been criticised for having lower sensitivities for detecting type 2 diabetes, due to the relatively high percentage of people who are diagnosed with type 2 diabetes on the basis of their circulating glucose concentrations 2 h after the consumption of the glucose load.[29]

The success of these different guidelines is based on cost-effectiveness (which will depend on such factors as the prevalence of GDM and type 2 diabetes within a given population, the cost of the screening program, and the cost of treating women diagnosed with type 2 diabetes relative to the savings that may be made by treating in comparison to the cost of treating diabetic complications). At present, all of them appear to be cost-effective.[29] However, in the future such guidelines are likely to be critically informed by follow-up of the HAPO mothers (see http://projectreporter.nih.gov/project_info_description.cfm?aid=8277164&icde=0 for details of the follow-up protocol) and mothers from other cohorts, assuming that this is able to continue in a sufficient number of women for a sufficient length of time. This may then lead to a more unified set of guidelines for screening women previously who had GDM for longer-term glucose intolerance. Whether or not these are acted upon would then depend on the balance of short- and long-term cost-effectiveness.

As well as risks to the mother, there appears to be increased risks to the offspring exposed to GDM in utero (reviewed in Chapter 5 and in Petry[4]). Larger and more long-term studies will confirm or refute potential links between this early exposure and increased future risk of obesity, the metabolic syndrome, and type 2 diabetes. Follow-up of HAPO offspring is again likely to prove highly instructive in this respect due to the size of the cohorts and the range of phenotypic information, including detailed measurements of maternal glucose tolerance in pregnancy that has been recorded from the cohort and its multiethnic mix. They will be most informative if they are studied longitudinally throughout their lives (in a fashion similar to that of the Framingham Study[98]), although the cost of this may be prohibitive. Obviously, information from follow-up of other cohorts of offspring of women with GDM will also provide original findings, and be valuable for confirmation and to allow meta-analyses to be performed. These studies may take many years to provide optimal information, however, due to the length of time taken to potentially develop diabetes and its sequelae, such as cardiovascular disease. In the meantime, useful insight may arise from transgenerational rodent studies, even allowing for the limitations to such models described earlier.

9.7 KEY RESEARCH QUESTIONS AND CONCLUSIONS

It is clear from the research findings outlined in this book that much progress has been made in the understanding and treatment of GDM in recent years. It is also clear that there is still much to learn, and if we are to stem the predicted massive increase in the incidence of GDM, things have to be put into practice quickly. To this end, reports have emerged from the Agency for Healthcare Research and Quality in the United States following research performed at the Johns Hopkins University Evidence-Based Practice Center, with the aim of identifying which key questions need prioritising in future research studies to improve current management of gestational diabetes.[99–101] With the help of consensus from stakeholder experts, the authors found 15 research questions that were considered of high clinical importance (Table 9.5). This list of questions was designed to inform researchers, policy makers, and funders to help direct future research projects and targeting of (limited) resources to better care for women with GDM.[100] Whilst such a series of questions can never be complete due to the limited number of stakeholders that put their own priorities on the original expanded series of questions, it is likely that some of the most effective changes in the care of women with GDM in the short to medium term will be made if answers are found to them. In the longer term, novel therapeutic targets and predictive biomarkers should emerge given more research into the pathophysiology of the condition. These and results from the other emergent and forthcoming studies outlined in this chapter (summarised in Figure 9.2) should make the future prospects for gestational diabetes rather brighter than the potential effects associated with transgenerational transmission of diabetes risk might currently lead us to believe.

TABLE 9.5

Initial Key Questions Followed by the List of Research Questions Arising From These That Were Rated as Having High Clinical Benefit or Importance[a]

Question Number	Question
I	**What are the risks and benefits of an oral diabetes agent (e.g., glyburide), compared to all types of insulin, for GDM?**
I-1	What are the effectiveness and safety of any of the second-generation sulphonylureas compared to any insulin in the treatment of gestational diabetes with regard to the following short- and long-term maternal outcomes, neonatal outcomes, and long-term offspring outcomes?[b]
I-2	What are the effectiveness and safety of metformin compared to any insulin in the treatment of gestational diabetes with regard to the following short- and long-term maternal outcomes, neonatal outcomes, and long-term offspring outcomes?[b]
I-3	What are the comparative effectiveness and safety of various insulin regimens in terms of type/duration, dosing, and frequency of administration in the treatment of gestational diabetes with regard to the following short- and long-term maternal outcomes, neonatal outcomes, and long-term offspring outcomes?[b]
I-4	What are the effectiveness and safety of other hypoglycaemic drug classes (e.g., thiazolidinediones, DPP-4 inhibitors, GLP-1 agonists, meglitinides) compared to any insulin or other hypoglycaemic drugs in the treatment of gestational diabetes with regard to the following short- and long-term maternal outcomes, neonatal outcomes, and long-term offspring outcomes?[b]
II	**What is the evidence that elective labour induction, caesarean delivery, or timing of induction is associated with benefits or harm to the mother and neonate?**
II-1	What are the effectiveness and safety of elective labour induction at 40 weeks compared to expectant management in women with gestational diabetes with regard to the following maternal and neonatal outcomes?[c]
	Populations of interest:
	• All women with gestational diabetes
	• Women with insulin-requiring (class A2) gestational diabetes
	• Obese women with gestational diabetes
	• Women with gestational diabetes with high estimated foetal weight (e.g., >4,000 or >4,500 g)
	• Women with different parities
	• Women of various races/ethnicities
II-2	What are the effectiveness and safety of elective caesarean delivery at 40 weeks compared to expectant management in women with gestational diabetes with regard to the following maternal and neonatal outcomes?[c]
	Populations of interest:
	• All women with gestational diabetes
	• Women with insulin-requiring (class A2) gestational diabetes
	• Obese women with gestational diabetes
	• Women with gestational diabetes with high estimated feotal weight (e.g., >4,000 or >4,500 g)
	• Women with different parities
	• Women of various races/ethnicities

Continued

TABLE 9.5 (*Continued*)

Initial Key Questions Followed by the List of Research Questions Arising From These That Were Rated as Having High Clinical Benefit or Importance[a]

Question Number	Question
III	**What risk factors are associated with the development of type 2 diabetes after a pregnancy with GDM?**
III-1	What is the evidence that maternal health behaviours (e.g., breastfeeding, physical activity, diet) are associated with the risk of developing type 2 diabetes or glucose intolerance/impaired fasting glucose following a pregnancy with gestational diabetes?
III-3	What is the evidence that maternal metabolic measures (e.g., fasting insulin levels, OGTT measures, HPA axis stress (subclinical hypercortisolism)) are associated with the risk of developing type 2 diabetes or glucose intolerance/impaired fasting glucose following a pregnancy with gestational diabetes?
III-4	What is the evidence that comorbid conditions (e.g., advanced maternal age, obesity, hypertension, hypercholesterolaemia) are associated with the risk of developing type 2 diabetes or glucose intolerance/impaired fasting glucose following a pregnancy with gestational diabetes?
III-7	What is the evidence that family history, gene mutations, genotypes, gene-environment interactions, epigenetic modifications, or other biomarkers are associated with the risk of developing type 2 diabetes or glucose intolerance/impaired fasting glucose among women with gestational diabetes? Are there differences in these associations by race or ethnic group?
III-8	What is the comparative effectiveness of various lifestyle interventions (e.g., diet, physical activity, smoking) for prevention of type 2 diabetes, glucose intolerance/impaired fasting glucose, and obesity in women with a history of gestational diabetes?
III-9	What is the comparative effectiveness of various educational and behavioural change strategies (e.g., patient education about diabetes risk, lactation support, diet, physical activity) for prevention of type 2 diabetes and glucose intolerance/impaired fasting glucose in women with a history of gestational diabetes?
IV	**What are the performance characteristics of diagnostic tests for type 2 diabetes in women with GDM?**
IV-1	What are the performance characteristics (sensitivity, specificity, and reproducibility) of a single fasting blood glucose test compared to the full 2 h 75 g OGTT in screening for type 2 diabetes and glucose intolerance/impaired fasting glucose following a pregnancy with gestational diabetes? Does the accuracy of the fasting blood glucose test compared to the full 2 h 75 g OGTT vary with the postpartum testing interval in screening for type 2 diabetes and glucose intolerance/impaired fasting glucose following a pregnancy with gestational diabetes?
IV-2	What are the performance characteristics (sensitivity, specificity, and reproducibility) of the HbA1c test compared to the 2 h 75 g OGTT in screening for type 2 diabetes and glucose intolerance/impaired fasting glucose following a pregnancy with gestational diabetes? Does the accuracy of the HbA1c test compared to the full 2 h 75 g OGTT vary with the postpartum testing interval in screening for type 2 diabetes and glucose intolerance/impaired fasting glucose following a pregnancy with gestational diabetes?

TABLE 9.5 (*Continued*)
Initial Key Questions Followed by the List of Research Questions Arising From These That Were Rated as Having High Clinical Benefit or Importance[a]

Question Number	Question
IV-3	What is the comparative effectiveness of strategies or interventions to improve clinician compliance with postpartum screening guidelines for type 2 diabetes and glucose intolerance/impaired fasting glucose in women with a history of gestational diabetes?

Source: Bennett, W.L. et al., *Future Research Needs for the Management of Gestational Diabetes*, Future Research Needs Paper 7 (prepared by Johns Hopkins University under Contract 290-2007-10061-I), AHRQ Publication 11-EHC005-EF, Agency for Healthcare Research and Quality, Rockville, MD, 2010. Available from www.effectivehealthcare.ahrq.gov/reports/final.cfm

Note: DDP-4, dipeptidyl peptidase 4; GLP-1, glucagon-like peptide 1; HbA1c, glycated haemoglobin; HPA, hypothalamic pituitary adrenal; OGTT, oral glucose tolerance test.

[a] Key questions are shown in bold and research questions resulting from them are shown in regular font.

[b] Outcomes for research questions I-1, I-2, I-3, and I-4:

Short-term maternal outcomes: Gestational weight gain, hypertensive disorders of pregnancy (e.g., gestational hypertension, preeclampsia), hypoglycaemia, glycaemic control (e.g., fasting blood glucose, 2 h postprandial glucose), patient-reported outcomes (e.g., patient treatment preference, quality of life), medication adherence, caesarean delivery (including primary caesarean and repeat caesarean) and indication for caesarean delivery, complications of caesarean delivery (e.g., wound infection, wound dehiscence), vaginal delivery (and specify type: spontaneous or operative), perineal lacerations, postpartum haemorrhage, shoulder dystocia, and peripartum mortality.

Long-term maternal outcomes: Postpartum weight retention, obesity, patient-reported outcomes (e.g., quality of life), development of postpartum type 2 diabetes or glucose intolerance/impaired fasting glucose, and mortality.

Neonatal outcomes: Hypoxia/anoxia, birth trauma (e.g., bone fractures, brachial plexus palsy), birth weight, hyperbilirubinaemia, hypoglycaemia, large for gestational age and macrosomia, small for gestational age, neonatal intensive care admission, respiratory distress syndrome, and perinatal mortality.

Long-term offspring outcomes: Infant and child growth, anthropometrics, and chronic diseases (e.g., obesity, type 2 diabetes).

[c] Outcomes for research questions II-1 and II-2:

Maternal outcomes: Caesarean delivery (including primary caesarean and repeat caesarean) and indication for caesarean delivery, complications of caesarean delivery (e.g., wound infection, wound dehiscence), vaginal delivery (spontaneous, operative), perineal lacerations, haemorrhage, patient-reported outcomes (e.g., patient preference, quality of life), length of hospital stay, pulmonary embolism, and mortality.

Neonatal outcomes: Hypoxia/anoxia, birth trauma (e.g., bone fractures, brachial plexus palsy), birth weight, hyperbilirubinaemia, hypoglycaemia, large for gestational age and macrosomia, small for gestational age, neonatal intensive care admission, respiratory distress syndrome, and perinatal mortality.

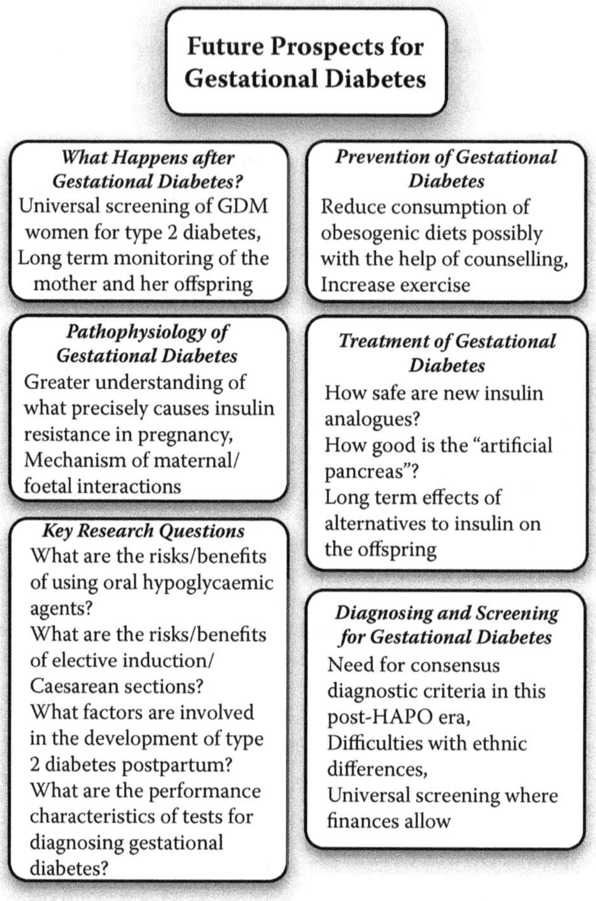

Future Prospects for Gestational Diabetes

What Happens after Gestational Diabetes?
Universal screening of GDM women for type 2 diabetes, Long term monitoring of the mother and her offspring

Prevention of Gestational Diabetes
Reduce consumption of obesogenic diets possibly with the help of counselling, Increase exercise

Pathophysiology of Gestational Diabetes
Greater understanding of what precisely causes insulin resistance in pregnancy, Mechanism of maternal/foetal interactions

Treatment of Gestational Diabetes
How safe are new insulin analogues?
How good is the "artificial pancreas"?
Long term effects of alternatives to insulin on the offspring

Key Research Questions
What are the risks/benefits of using oral hypoglycaemic agents?
What are the risks/benefits of elective induction/Caesarean sections?
What factors are involved in the development of type 2 diabetes postpartum?
What are the performance characteristics of tests for diagnosing gestational diabetes?

Diagnosing and Screening for Gestational Diabetes
Need for consensus diagnostic criteria in this post-HAPO era,
Difficulties with ethnic differences,
Universal screening where finances allow

FIGURE 9.2   Summary of some of the areas in which progress either is likely to be made in the near future or needs to be made in the field of gestational diabetes.

REFERENCES

Key references are in bold.

1. Hex, N., Bartlett, C., Wright, D., Taylor, M., and Varley, D. 2012. Estimating the current and future costs of type 1 and type 2 diabetes in the UK, including direct health costs and indirect societal and productivity costs. *Diabet Med* 29:855–62.
2. Diabetes UK news page about the Impact Diabetes Report. Available from http://www.diabetes.org.uk/About_us/News_Landing_Page/NHS-spending-on-diabetes-to-reach-169-billion-by-2035/ (accessed May 23, 2013).
3. Zhang, P., Zhang, X., Brown, J., et al. 2010. Global healthcare expenditure on diabetes for 2010 and 2030. *Diabetes Res Clin Pract* 87:293–301.
4. Petry, C.J. 2010. Gestational diabetes: risk factors and recent advances in its genetics and treatment. *Br J Nutr* 104:775–87.

5. HAPO Study Cooperative Research Group, Metzger, B.E., Lowe, L.P., Dyer, A.R., et al. 2008. Hyperglycemia and adverse pregnancy outcomes. *N Engl J Med* 358:1991–2002.
6. DCCT Research Group. 1993. The effect of intensive treatment of diabetes on the development and progression of long-term complications in insulin-dependent diabetes mellitus. The Diabetes Control and Complications Trial Research Group. *N Engl J Med* 329:977–86.
7. UKPDS Group. 1998. Intensive blood-glucose control with sulphonylureas or insulin compared with conventional treatment and risk of complications in patients with type 2 diabetes (UKPDS 33). UK Prospective Diabetes Study (UKPDS) Group. *Lancet* 352:837–53.
8. UKPDS Group. 1998. Effect of intensive blood-glucose control with metformin on complications in overweight patients with type 2 diabetes (UKPDS 34). UK Prospective Diabetes Study (UKPDS) Group. *Lancet* 352:854–65.
9. O'Sullivan, J.B. 1961. Gestational diabetes. Unsuspected, asymptomatic diabetes in pregnancy. *N Engl J Med* 264:1082–85.
10. **International Association of Diabetes and Pregnancy Study Groups Consensus Panel, Metzger, B.E., Gabbe, S.G., Persson, B., et al. 2010. International association of diabetes and pregnancy study groups recommendations on the diagnosis and classification of hyperglycemia in pregnancy. *Diabetes Care* 33:676–82.** *Modern consensus guidelines for the screening and diagnosis of gestational diabetes based on the risk of adverse pregnancy outcomes at different levels of maternal glucose tolerance using data from the multinational HAPO study.*
11. National Diabetes Data Group. 1979. Classification and diagnosis of diabetes mellitus and other categories of glucose intolerance. National Diabetes Data Group. *Diabetes* 28:1039–57.
12. [No authors listed]. 1980. WHO Expert Committee on Diabetes Mellitus: second report. *World Health Organ Tech Rep Ser* 646:1–80.
13. Long, H., and Cundy, T. 2013. Establishing consensus in the diagnosis of gestational diabetes following HAPO: where do we stand? *Curr Diab Rep* 13:43–50.
14. Langer, O., Umans, J.G., and Miodovnik, M. 2013. Perspectives on the proposed gestational diabetes mellitus diagnostic criteria. *Obstet Gynecol* 121:177–82.
15. Werner, E.F., Pettker, C.M., Zuckerwise, L., et al. 2012. Screening for gestational diabetes mellitus: are the criteria proposed by the International Association of the Diabetes and Pregnancy Study Groups cost-effective? *Diabetes Care* 35:529–35.
16. O'Sullivan, E.P., Avalos, G., O'Reilly, M., Dennedy, M.C., Gaffney, G., and Dunne, F.; Atlantic DIP collaborators. 2011. Atlantic Diabetes in Pregnancy (DIP): the prevalence and outcomes of gestational diabetes mellitus using new diagnostic criteria. *Diabetologia* 54:1670–75.
17. **International Association of Diabetes and Pregnancy Study Groups (IADPSG) Consensus Panel Writing Group and the Hyperglycemia and Adverse Pregnancy Outcome (HAPO) Study Steering Committee. 2012. The diagnosis of gestational diabetes mellitus: new paradigms or status quo? *J Matern Fetal Neonatal Med* 25:2564–69.** *Further details on the process undertaken by the IADPSG and the justification of their recommendations for the screening and diagnosis of gestational diabetes.*
18. Wendland, E.M., Torloni, M.R., Falavigna, M., et al. 2012. Gestational diabetes and pregnancy outcomes—a systematic review of the World Health Organization (WHO) and the International Association of Diabetes in Pregnancy Study Groups (IADPSG) diagnostic criteria. *BMC Pregnancy Childbirth* 12:23.
19. Jenum, A.K., Mørkrid, K., Sletner, L., et al. 2012. Impact of ethnicity on gestational diabetes identified with the WHO and the modified International Association of Diabetes and Pregnancy Study Groups criteria: a population-based cohort study. *Eur J Endocrinol* 166:317–24.

20. **Hedderson, M., Ehrlich, S., Sridhar, S., Darbinian, J., Moore, S., and Assiamira, F. 2012. Racial/ethnic disparities in the prevalence of gestational diabetes by BMI. *Diabetes Care* 35:1492–98.** *A study highlighting ethnic differences in the increased risk for gestational diabetes by maternal BMI.*

21. Doyle, M.A., Khan, S., Al-Mohanadi, D., and Keely, E. 2012. International survey on gestational diabetes. *J Matern Fetal Neonatal Med* 25:2035–38.

22. Rajput, R., Yadav, Y., Rajput, M., and Nanda, S. 2012. Utility of HbA(1c) for diagnosis of gestational diabetes mellitus. *Diabetes Res Clin Pract* 98:104–7.

23. O'Shea, P., O'Connor, C., Owens, L., Carmody, L., Avalos, G., Nestor, L., Lydon, K., and Dunne, F.P. 2012. Trimester-specific reference intervals for IFCC standardised haemoglobin A(1c): new criterion to diagnose gestational diabetes mellitus (GDM)? *Ir Med J* 105(5 Suppl):29–31.

24. Balaji, V., Balaji, M., Anjalakshi, C., Cynthia, A., Arthi, T. and Seshiah, V. 2011. Inadequacy of fasting plasma glucose to diagnose gestational diabetes mellitus in Asian Indian women. *Diabetes Res Clin Pract* 94:e21–23.

25. Consensus Development Panel. 2013. National Institutes of Health Consensus Development conference statement on gestational diabetes. Available from http://prevention.nih.gov/cdp/conferences/2013/gdm/files/GDM-FINAL-Statement.pdf (accessed May 23, 2013).

26. Bodmer-Roy, S., Morin, L., Cousineau, J., and Rey, E. 2012. Pregnancy outcomes in women with and without gestational diabetes mellitus according to the International Association of the Diabetes and Pregnancy Study Groups criteria. *Obstet Gynecol* 120:746–52.

27. Institute for Quality and Efficiency in Health Care: Executive Summaries. 2005. Screening for gestational diabetes: Executive summary of final report S07-01. Version 1.1. Cologne, Germany: Institute for Quality and Efficiency in Health Care (IQWiG). Available from http://www.ncbi.nlm.nih.gov/books/NBK84140/ (accessed August 25, 2009.)

28. Hammoud, N.M., de Valk, H.W., Biesma, D.H., and Visser, G.H. 2013. Gestational diabetes mellitus diagnosed by screening or symptoms: does it matter? *J Matern Fetal Neonatal Med* 26:103–5.

29. Simmons, D., McElduff, A., McIntyre, H.D., and Elrishi, M. 2010. Gestational diabetes mellitus: NICE for the U.S.? A comparison of the American Diabetes Association and the American College of Obstetricians and Gynecologists guidelines with the U.K. National Institute for Health and Clinical Excellence guidelines. *Diabetes Care* 33:34–37.

30. Williams, C.B., Iqbal, S., Zawacki, C.M., Yu, D., Brown, M.B., and Herman, W.H. 1999. Effect of selective screening for gestational diabetes. *Diabetes Care* 22:418–21.

31. Wagaarachchi, P.T., Fernando, L., Premachadra, P., and Fernando, D.J. 2001. Screening based on risk factors for gestational diabetes in an Asian population. *J Obstet Gynaecol* 21:32–34.

32. Baliutaviciene, D., Petrenko, V., and Zalinkevicius, R. 2002. Selective or universal diagnostic testing for gestational diabetes mellitus. *Int J Gynaecol Obstet* 78:207–11.

33. Di Cianni, G., Volpe, L., Casadidio, I., et al. 2002. Universal screening and intensive metabolic management of gestational diabetes: cost-effectiveness in Italy. *Acta Diabetol* 39:69–73.

34. Corcoy, R., García-Patterson, A., Pau, E., Pascual, E., Altirriba, O., Adelantado, J.M., and de Leiva, A. 2004. Is selective screening for gestational diabetes mellitus worthwhile everywhere? *Acta Diabetol* 41:154–57.

35. Cosson, E., Benchimol, M., Carbillon, L., et al. 2006. Universal rather than selective screening for gestational diabetes mellitus may improve fetal outcomes. *Diabetes Metab* 32:140–46.

36. Shirazian N., Emdadi, R., Mahboubi, M., et al. 2009. Screening for gestational diabetes: usefulness of clinical risk factors. *Arch Gynecol Obstet* 280:933–37.
37. McCarthy, A.D., Curciarello, R., Castiglione, N., et al. 2010. Universal versus selective screening for the detection, control and prognosis of gestational diabetes mellitus in Argentina. *Acta Diabetol* 47:97–103.
38. Hiéronimus, S., and Le Meaux, J.P. 2010. Relevance of gestational diabetes mellitus screening and comparison of selective with universal strategies. *Diabetes Metab* 36:575–86.
39. Teh, W.T., Teede, H.J., Paul, E., Harrison, C.L., Wallace, E.M., and Allan, C. 2011. Risk factors for gestational diabetes mellitus: implications for the application of screening guidelines. *Aust N Z J Obstet Gynaecol* 51:26–30.
40. Davis, B., McLean, A., Sinha, A.K., and Falhammar, H. 2013. A threefold increase in gestational diabetes over two years: review of screening practices and pregnancy outcomes in indigenous women of Cape York, Australia. *Aust N Z J Obstet Gynaecol* 53:363–68.
41. Avalos, G.E., Owens, L.A., and Dunne, F.; Atlantic DIP Collaborators. 2013. Applying current screening tools for gestational diabetes mellitus to a European population—is it time for change? *Diabetes Care*, doi: 10.2337/dc12-2669.
42. Catalano, P.M., McIntyre, H.D., Cruickshank, J.K., et al. 2012. The Hyperglycemia and Adverse Pregnancy Outcome study: associations of GDM and obesity with pregnancy outcomes. *Diabetes Care* 35:780–86.
43. Nolan, C.J. 2011. Controversies in gestational diabetes. *Best Pract Res Clin Obstet Gynaecol* 25:37–49.
44. Simmons, D. 2011. Diabetes and obesity in pregnancy. *Best Pract Res Clin Obstet Gynaecol* 25:25–36.
45. McAllister, E.J., Dhurandhar, N.V., Keith, S.W., et al. 2009. Ten putative contributors to the obesity epidemic. *Crit Rev Food Sci Nutr* 49:868–913.
46. Tobias, D.K., Zhang, C., van Dam, R.M., Bowers, K., and Hu, F.B. 2011. Physical activity before and during pregnancy and risk of gestational diabetes mellitus: a meta-analysis. *Diabetes Care* 34:223–29.
47. Han, S., Middleton, P., and Crowther, C.A. 2012. Exercise for pregnant women for preventing gestational diabetes mellitus. *Cochrane Database Syst Rev* 7:CD009021.
48. Ruchat, S.M., Davenport, M.H., Giroux, I., et al. 2012. Effect of exercise intensity and duration on capillary glucose responses in pregnant women at low and high risk for gestational diabetes. *Diabetes Metab Res Rev* 28:669–78.
49. Oostdam, N., Bosmans, J., Wouters, M.G., Eekhoff, E.M., van Mechelen, W., and van Poppel, M.N. 2012. Cost-effectiveness of an exercise program during pregnancy to prevent gestational diabetes: results of an economic evaluation alongside a randomised controlled trial. *BMC Pregnancy Childbirth* 12:64.
50. Louie, J.C., Brand-Miller, J.C., and Moses, R.G. 2013. Carbohydrates, glycemic index, and pregnancy outcomes in gestational diabetes. *Curr Diab Rep* 13:6–11.
51. Louie, J.C., Markovic, T.P., Perera, N., Foote, D., Petocz, P., Ross, G.P., and Brand-Miller, J.C. 2011. A randomized controlled trial investigating the effects of a low-glycemic index diet on pregnancy outcomes in gestational diabetes mellitus. *Diabetes Care* 34:2341–46.
52. Luoto, R., Kinnunen, T.I., Aittasalo, M., et al. 2011. Primary prevention of gestational diabetes mellitus and large-for-gestational-age newborns by lifestyle counseling: a cluster-randomized controlled trial. *PLoS Med* 8:e1001036.
53. Luoto, R., Laitinen, K., Nermes, M., and Isolauri, E. 2010. Impact of maternal probiotic-supplemented dietary counselling on pregnancy outcome and prenatal and postnatal growth: a double-blind, placebo-controlled study. *Br J Nutr* 103:1792–99.

54. Kinnunen, T.I., Puhkala, J., Raitanen, J., Ahonen, S., Aittasalo, M., Virtanen, S.M., and Luoto, R. 2012. Effects of dietary counselling on food habits and dietary intake of Finnish pregnant women at increased risk for gestational diabetes—a secondary analysis of a cluster-randomized controlled trial. *Matern Child Nutr*, doi: 10.1111/j.1740-8709.2012.00426.x.
55. Helin, A., Kinnunen, T.I., Raitanen, J., Ahonen, S., Virtanen, S.M., and Luoto, R. 2012. Iron intake, haemoglobin and risk of gestational diabetes: a prospective cohort study. *BMJ Open* 2 pii:e001730.
56. Oostdam, N., van Poppel, M.N., Wouters, M.G., and van Mechelen, W. 2011. Interventions for preventing gestational diabetes mellitus: a systematic review and meta-analysis. *J Womens Health (Larchmt)* 20:1551–63.
57. Han, S., Crowther, C.A., and Middleton, P. 2012. Interventions for pregnant women with hyperglycaemia not meeting gestational diabetes and type 2 diabetes diagnostic criteria. *Cochrane Database Syst Rev* 1:CD009037.
58. Chen, E.Y., Liao, Y.C., Smith, D.H., Barrera-Saldaña, H.A., Gelinas, R.E., and Seeburg, P.H. 1989. The human growth hormone locus: nucleotide sequence, biology, and evolution. *Genomics* 4:479–97.
59. Baumann, G.P. 2009. Growth hormone isoforms. *Growth Horm IGF Res* 19:333–40.
60. Haig, D. 2008. Placental growth hormone-related proteins and prolactin-related proteins. *Placenta* 29(Suppl A):S36–41.
61. Goodman, H.M., Tai, L.R., Ray, J., Cooke, N.E., and Liebhaber, S.A. 1991. Human growth hormone variant produces insulin-like and lipolytic responses in rat adipose tissue. *Endocrinology* 129:1779–83.
62. Barbour, L.A., Shao, J., Qiao, L., et al. 2002. Human placental growth hormone causes severe insulin resistance in transgenic mice. *Am J Obstet Gynecol* 186:512–17.
63. Ramos-Román, M.A. 2011. Prolactin and lactation as modifiers of diabetes risk in gestational diabetes. *Horm Metab Res* 43:593–600.
64. Newbern, D., and Freemark, M. 2011. Placental hormones and the control of maternal metabolism and fetal growth. *Curr Opin Endocrinol Diabetes Obes* 18:409–16.
65. Valsamakis, G., Kumar, S., Creatsas, G., and Mastorakos, G. 2010. The effects of adipose tissue and adipocytokines in human pregnancy. *Ann N Y Acad Sci* 1205:76–81.
66. D'Ippolito, S., Tersigni, C., Scambia, G., and Di Simone, N. 2012. Adipokines, an adipose tissue and placental product with biological functions during pregnancy. *Biofactors* 38:14–23.
67. Fantuzzi, G. 2005. Adipose tissue, adipokines, and inflammation. *J Allergy Clin Immunol* 115:911–19.
68. Ouchi, N., Parker, J.L., Lugus, J.J., and Walsh, K. 2011. Adipokines in inflammation and metabolic disease. *Nat Rev Immunol* 11:85–97.
69. Volpe, L., Di Cianni, G., Lencioni, C., Cuccuru, I., Benzi, L., and Del Prato, S. 2007. Gestational diabetes, inflammation, and late vascular disease. *J Endocrinol Invest* 30:873–79.
70. Urbanek, M., Hayes, M.G., Lee, H., et al. 2012. The role of inflammatory pathway genetic variation on maternal metabolic phenotypes during pregnancy. *PLoS One* 7:e32958.
71. Visser, M., Bouter, L.M., McQuillan, G.M., Wener, M.H., and Harris, T.B. 1999. Elevated C-reactive protein levels in overweight and obese adults. *JAMA* 282:2131–35.
72. Pradhan, A.D., Manson, J.E., Rifai, N., Buring, J.E., and Ridker, P.M. 2001. C-reactive protein, interleukin 6, and risk of developing type 2 diabetes mellitus. *JAMA* 286:327–34.
73. Tzur, T., Weintraub, A.Y., Sergienko, R., and Sheiner, E. 2013. Can leukocyte count during the first trimester of pregnancy predict later gestational complications? *Arch Gynecol Obstet* 287:421–27.

74. Arifin, D.R., and Bulte, J.W. 2011. Imaging of pancreatic islet cells. *Diabetes Metab Res Rev* 27:761–66.

75. Parsons, J.A., Brelje, T.C., and Sorenson, R.L. 1992. Adaptation of islets of Langerhans to pregnancy: increased islet cell proliferation and insulin secretion correlates with the onset of placental lactogen secretion. *Endocrinology* 130:1459–66.

76. Huang, C., Snider, F., and Cross, J.C. 2009. Prolactin receptor is required for normal glucose homeostasis and modulation of beta-cell mass during pregnancy. *Endocrinology* 150:1618–26.

77. Kim, H., Toyofuku, Y., Lynn, F.C., et al. 2010. Serotonin regulates pancreatic beta cell mass during pregnancy. *Nat Med* 16:804–8.

78. Zhang, H., Zhang, J., Pope, C.F., et al. 2010. Gestational diabetes mellitus resulting from impaired beta-cell compensation in the absence of FoxM1, a novel downstream effector of placental lactogen. *Diabetes* 59:143–52.

79. Plank, J.L., Frist, A.Y., LeGrone, A.W., Magnuson, M.A., and Labosky, P.A. 2011. Loss of Foxd3 results in decreased β-cell proliferation and glucose intolerance during pregnancy. *Endocrinology* 152:4589–600.

80. **Karnik, S.K., Chen, H., McLean, G.W., et al. 2007. Menin controls growth of pancreatic beta-cells in pregnant mice and promotes gestational diabetes mellitus. *Science* 318:806–9.** *A key early study investigating the mechanism of pancreatic β-cell proliferation during pregnancy.*

81. Ernst, S., Demirci, C., Valle, S., Velazquez-Garcia, S., and Garcia-Ocaña, A. 2011. Mechanisms in the adaptation of maternal β-cells during pregnancy. *Diabetes Manag (Lond)* 1:239–48.

82. Rieck, S., and Kaestner, K.H. 2010. Expansion of beta-cell mass in response to pregnancy. *Trends Endocrinol Metab* 21:151–158.

83. Laybutt, D.R., Weir, G.C., Kaneto, H., et al. 2002. Overexpression of c-Myc in beta-cells of transgenic mice causes proliferation and apoptosis, downregulation of insulin gene expression, and diabetes. *Diabetes* 51:1793–1804.

84. Crowther, C.A., Hiller, J.E., Moss, J.R., McPhee, A.J., Jeffries, W.S., and Robinson, J.S.; Australian Carbohydrate Intolerance Study in Pregnant Women (ACHOIS) Trial Group. 2005. Effect of treatment of gestational diabetes mellitus on pregnancy outcomes. *N Engl J Med* 352:2477–86.

85. Landon, M.B., Spong, C.Y., Thom, E., et al.; Eunice Kennedy Shriver National Institute of Child Health and Human Development Maternal-Fetal Medicine Units Network. 2009. A multicenter, randomized trial of treatment for mild gestational diabetes. *N Engl J Med* 361:1339–48.

86. Murphy, H.R., Elleri, D., Allen, J.M., et al. 2011. Closed-loop insulin delivery during pregnancy complicated by type 1 diabetes. *Diabetes Care* 34:406–11.

87. **Murphy, H.R., Kumareswaran, K., Elleri, D., et al. 2011. Safety and efficacy of 24-h closed-loop insulin delivery in well-controlled pregnant women with type 1 diabetes: a randomized crossover case series. *Diabetes Care* 34:2527–29.** *A study showing that the artificial pancreas was safe to use in women with type 1 diabetes in pregnancy and was as efficacious as conventional continuous subcutaneous insulin infusion with a reduced amount of time spent with hypoglycaemic glucose concentrations.*

88. Hovorka, R. 2011. Closed-loop insulin delivery: from bench to clinical practice. *Nat Rev Endocrinol* 7:385–95.

89. Clarke, W.L., and Renard, E. 2012. Clinical requirements for closed-loop control systems. *J Diabetes Sci Technol* 6:444–52.

90. De-Regil, L.M., Palacios, C., Ansary, A., Kulier, R., and Peña-Rosas, J.P. 2012. Vitamin D supplementation for women during pregnancy. *Cochrane Database Syst Rev* 2:CD008873.

91. Poel, Y.H., Hummel, P., Lips, P., Stam, F., van der Ploeg, T., and Simsek, S. 2012. Vitamin D and gestational diabetes: a systematic review and meta-analysis. *Eur J Intern Med* 23:465–69.

92. Senti, J., Thiele, D.K., and Anderson, C.M. 2012. Maternal vitamin D status as a critical determinant in gestational diabetes. *J Obstet Gynecol Neonatal Nurs* 41:328–38.

93. Walsh, J.M., McGowan, C.A., Kilbane, M., McKenna, M.J., and McAuliffe, F.M. 2013. The relationship between maternal and fetal vitamin D, insulin resistance, and fetal growth. *Reprod Sci* 20:536–41.

94. Rudnicki, P.M., and Mølsted-Pedersen, L. 1997. Effect of 1,25-dihydroxycholecalciferol on glucose metabolism in gestational diabetes mellitus. *Diabetologia* 40:40–44.

95. Ferrara, A., and Ehrlich, S.F. 2011. Strategies for diabetes prevention before and after pregnancy in women with GDM. *Curr Diabetes Rev* 7:75–83.

96. Feig, D.S., Zinman, B., Wang, X., and Hux, J.E. 2008. Risk of development of diabetes mellitus after diagnosis of gestational diabetes. *CMAJ* 179:229–34.

97. England, L.J., Dietz, P.M., Njoroge, T., et al. 2009. Preventing type 2 diabetes: public health implications for women with a history of gestational diabetes mellitus. *Am J Obstet Gynecol* 200:365.e1–8.

98. Bhargava, A. 2003. A longitudinal analysis of the risk factors for diabetes and coronary heart disease in the Framingham Offspring Study. *Popul Health Metr* 1:3.

99. Nicholson, W.K., Wilson, L.M., Witkop, C.T., et al. 2008. Therapeutic management, delivery, and postpartum risk assessment and screening in gestational diabetes. *Evid Rep Technol Assess (Full Rep)* 162:1–96.

100. **Bennett, W.L., Nicholson, W.K., Saldanha, I.J., Wilson, L.M., Mckoy, N.A., and Robinson, K.A. 2010. *Future Research Needs for the Management of Gestational Diabetes*. Future Research Needs Paper 7 (prepared by Johns Hopkins University under Contract 290-2007-10061-I), AHRQ Publication 11-EHC005-EF. Rockville, MD: Agency for Healthcare Research and Quality. Available from www.effective-healthcare.ahrq.gov/reports/final.cfm.** *A survey of key priorities for clinical research in gestational diabetes.*

101. Bennett, W.L., Robinson, K.A., Saldanha, I.J., Wilson, L.M., and Nicholson, W.K. 2012. High priority research needs for gestational diabetes mellitus. *J Womens Health (Larchmt)* 21:925–32.

Index

Milton Keynes UK
Ingram Content Group UK Ltd.
UKHW040103071024
449327UK00019B/770